Critical Care Nursing
DeMYSTiFieD

Critical Care Nursing
DeMYSTiFieD

Cynthia L. Terry, CNE, MSN, CCRN, RN

Associate Professor/Certified Nurse Educator
Lehigh Carbon Community College
Schnecksville, Pennsylvania

Aurora L. Weaver, MSN, MEd, BS, RN, CNE

Retired Nurse Educator
Lehigh Valley, Pennsylvania

 Medical

New York   Chicago   San Francisco   Lisbon   London   Madrid   Mexico City   Milan
New Delhi   San Juan   Seoul   Singapore   Sydney   Toronto

The McGraw·Hill Companies

Critical Care Nursing/Demystified

1 2 3 4 5 6 7 8 9 0   DOC/DOC   15 14 13 12 11

ISBN 978-0-07-160638-7
MHID 0-07-160638-6

This book was set in Berling by Glyph International.
The editors were Joseph Morita and Brian Kearns.
The production supervisor was Sherri Souffrance.
Project management was provided by Manisha Singh at Glyph International.
The designer was Mary McKeon; the cover illustration is by Lance Lekander.
RR Donnelley was printer and binder.

This book is printed on acid-free paper.

Library of Congress Cataloging-in-Publication Data

Terry, Cynthia Lee.
    Critical care nursing demystified / Cynthia L. Terry, Aurora L.
Weaver.
    p. ; cm.
Includes index.
ISBN-13: 978-0-07-160638-7 (pbk. : alk. paper)
ISBN-10: 0-07-160638-6 (pbk. : alk. paper)
1. Intensive care nursing.   I. Weaver, Aurora L.   II. Title.
[DNLM: 1. Critical Care—methods.   2. Critical Illness—nursing.   3. Nursing Care—methods.
WY 154]
  RT120.I5T47   2011
  610.73′6—dc22
                          2011008120

This book is dedicated to my students in all of my classes and clinicals. Through their lenses I have looked at the world in a vastly different way. It is the thing about teaching that I love the most but also the most challenging.

Also to Brenna Colleen and Padriac Glennmoore Terry, my daughter and son, "you are the wind beneath my wings" and the reason I look forward to each day.

—Cindy Terry

To my son and daughter, Ryan and Rhonda-Beth Weaver, my mainstays throughout the creation of this book. I dedicate these efforts to them, for he is my left arm and she is my right. I cannot function without either one of them. Love Forever, Mommy.

Thank you also to my co-author Cindy Terry for her continued belief and support of my active contributions to professional nursing.

—Aurora Weaver

Faculty Reviewers

Sharon Jarrow, MSN, RN
Instructor,
Nursing Program
Lehigh Carbon Community College
Schnecksville, Pennsylvania

Theresa K. Cebulski-Field, RN, MSN
Instructor
Nursing Program
Lehigh Carbon Community College
Schnecksville, Pennsylvania

Contents

Preface

Entering the world of critical care nursing is an interesting, exciting time for nurses who are making this decision. It is a journey that can produce anxiety and tension. Fear not and become demystified!

This book has been developed to lessen one's stress level easing the transition into critical care nursing. The authors believe that this transition should be smooth, seamless, comfortable, and less of a mystery to those who pursue this nursing specialty.

Critical Care Nursing Demystified serves as a guide to professional nurses who are considering a switch from their current field of nursing to that of critical care. It is also a helpful reference source to student nurses who are entering their upper level education courses and to those nurse educators seeking to clarify, simplify, and reduce the torment of presenting complicated and difficult critical care concepts.

This book is designed to be user-friendly featuring organized chapters that focus on:

lesson objectives and key terms that the nurse will use

brief overviews of basic anatomy and physiology of target organ systems

vignettes of actual nursing situations which substantiate true life-learning experiences encountered in the workplace

detailed health assessments using the body systems approach

diagnostic studies utilized to confirm an illness

common critical procedures performed

current medications used in the treatment of the critical care patient

implementation of the nursing process to identify and solve problems concerning patients

Accompanying questions and answers cap the end of each chapter and the end of the book using the NCLEX style. They include review questions that challenge the nurse to increase and strengthen critical thinking abilities.

To all nurses everywhere who aspire to greater nursing knowledge, we commend your dedication and devotion to patient care and hope that you will prevail. Although it is not designed to replace a comprehensive text on critical care, it is hoped that this book will provide sufficient insight and encouragement as you embrace the newest and advanced trends in critical care nursing. Your passion for learning and professional growth will be rewarding and evident as you realize the success and efforts of your achievements. Enjoy and demystify now!

chapter **1**

The Critical Care Nurse

LEARNING OBJECTIVES

At the end of this chapter, the student will be able to:

1 Describe the goals of choosing a career in nursing.

2 Describe the education behind a career chosen in critical care.

3 Explain the synergy model and how it can impact positive outcomes for critical care patients.

4 Discuss the regulatory issues that impact the critical care nurse and environment.

5 Explore future challenges to the critical care nurse.

KEY TERMS

AACN – American Association of Critical-Care Nurses

AJN – American Journal of Nursing

ANA – American Nurses Association

CCRN – Critical Care Registered Nurse

CCU – coronary care unit

CEU – continuing educational unit

Closed units

Competencies of critical care

HIPAA – Health Insurance Portability and Accountability Act

HRSA – Health Resources and Services Administration

ICU – intensive care unit

IHI – Institute for Health Care Improvement

Intensivist

IOM – Institute of Medicine

JCAHO – Joint Commission on Accreditation of Healthcare Organizations

Magnet Institution

NCLEX – National Council of Licensing Examinations

NLN – National League for Nursing

SCCM – Society of Critical Care Medicine

Sentinel events

Synergy model

Introduction

❶ Choosing a career in nursing should be a life's pathway—a desire to heal, protect, and serve others. Caring for patients competently is a calling that is not meant for everyone. It is hard work with numerous challenges, as well as rewards. It takes a very strong, smart individual to work in nursing and requires frequently working from the heart as well as the mind. Critical care nursing requires a nurse to have additional skills. The critical care nurse needs to

- Be well versed in advanced pathophysiology
- Be adept and calm while treating patients in environments that require quick decision-making skills under life-threatening conditions
- Stay abreast of changing advanced technology to preserve organ function
- Coordinate the care with multiple influencing factors
- Provide leadership in the management of care and
- Coordinate the multiple disciplinary team

A life in nursing, although comfortable, will not make you a millionaire, but it will provide steady, worthwhile, satisfying employment for those with the moral strength, smarts, stamina, and savvy. Working as a critical care nurse requires more training and hard work in order to be and stay competent within the field.

Education and Experience

❷ Nurses are the heartbeat of a smooth-running operation in any health care setting. Nurses are obligated to know just about everything regarding health care: the status of their patients, family information, legalities of care, physician interventions, nutrition, counseling, teaching, mentoring new health care workers and even staffing protocols of professional as well as nonprofessional personnel. We are the last link in the line of safe care of patients, families, and communities.

Nurses could be referred to as the "guardians of humanity" and the "sentinels of society," with good reason. There are few excuses for making mistakes and jeopardizing the lives of those entrusted to our care. As nurses, we must do it right the first time and every time! The consequences of performance below the standard of care can be disastrous.

Therefore, it is important to realize that the critical care nurse's accumulated knowledge extends beyond one's basic level of nursing education. Whether a graduate of a bachelors of science in nursing (B.S.N), associate's degree, or diploma program, a novice nurse is still an entry-level nurse. Due to the need to master and coordinate many cognitive and psychomotor skills, it is ideal that a nurse gains experiences prior to entering the critical care environment. Most employers require experience in medical-surgical nursing as a stepping-stone into critical care. It is very tough to accept a first job comfortably upon graduation in the critical care areas. And a very strong, supportive, prolonged preceptorship is needed to take new graduates into this type of environment without them experiencing much trauma in the socialization process.

Most acute care hospitals offer a 6- to 12-week critical care course and a lengthy orientation period for those nurses who want to increase their knowledge base and work in critical care areas of the hospital. Critical care areas are usually defined as intensive care, postoperative recovery, burn, emergency care, and telemetry units. Nurses need to have a sound knowledge and mastery of medical-surgical skills like intravenous therapy, medication administration, fluid and electrolyte monitoring, etc., prior to entering critical care training. Length of time in the medical-surgical areas will vary according to institutional policies.

NURSING ALERT

Critical care nursing is highly technical and is generally considered beyond the level of a new graduate. Often, experience in medical-surgical nursing is required prior to entering the critical care environment.

Standards, Organizations, and Certification: Promoting Excellence

Standards

Nurses must be patient advocates, know the law, and practice their profession ethically, according to established standards of care. Such expectations require that nurses have professional knowledge at their level of practice and be proficient in technological skills. Nursing Standards of Care are guidelines within the profession that ensure acceptable quality of care to our patients. They also announce to the public what nurses can do. Law, health care institutions, and professional organizations develop standards. An example of such standards is the Nurse Practice Act, which defines the boundaries of nursing practice according to individual states.

Critical care nurses also have standards of care, and these standards provide a framework for the quality of care delivered by the nurse as well as a guide for how care is to be delivered. The Standards of Care for Acute and Critical Nursing are based on the Nursing Standards and the nursing process. They can be found on the American Association of Critical-Care Nurses' (AACN) web site under Clinical Practice. Table 1–1 summarizes those standards.

TABLE 1–1	AACN Standards of Care for Acute and Critical Care Nursing	
	Standard	**Description**
I	Assessment	The nurse caring for acute and critically ill patients collects relevant patient health data.
II	Diagnosis	The nurse caring for acute and critically ill patients analyzes assessment data in determining diagnoses.
III	Outcome identification	The nurse caring for acute and critically ill patients develops plans of care that identify individualized, expected outcomes for patients.
IV	Planning	The nurse caring for acute and critically ill patients develops plans of care that prescribe interventions to attain expected outcomes.
V	Implementation	The nurse caring for acute and critically ill patients implements interventions identified in the plans of care.
VI	Evaluation	The nurse caring for acute and critically ill patients evaluates patients' progress toward attaining expected outcomes.

From AACN web site at http://www.aacn.org/WD/Practice/Content/standards.for.acute. and.ccnursing.practice.pcms?menu=Practice.

Organizations

The critical care nurse can be part of many different organizations, from the nurse's place of employment to local, state, and nationally recognized professional organizations. One of the first places a nurse is employed is the organization the nurse chooses. There are many organizational influences that create job satisfaction for the nurse entering those places. Many studies have been done on what creates a healthy work environment, and the AACN has been a voice to promote critical care nurses staying at the bedside. The leading factors for a nurse's job satisfaction and magnet-drawing institutional attributes are listed. Magnet-drawing institutions are designated as tops in their field in Table 1–2.

The nurse needs to be mindful of these healthy work environments and will adjust better if his or her philosophy of nursing fits with the organizational philosophy. Frequently, this does not occur until the nurse is well entrenched in the position. However, the astute nurse will do homework before committing to an institution. Attending job fairs sponsored by the organization, checking if the institution has Magnet status and talking to friends that are employed there. Reviewing such research can help the nurse make a wise decision for a healthy, rewarding, growing experience. Besides institutions, the nurse is also influenced by national organizations.

TABLE 1–2 Nurses' Work Satisfaction Elements and Organizational Attributes Drawing Nurses

Nurses' Work Satisfaction Elements	Magnet-Organizational Attributes
Pay	Clear work values
Autonomy	Nurse autonomy
	Self–governance
Clear delineation of tasks/duties	Quality patient care conditions
Sound organizational policies	Organizational support and structure
Fostering of environment of formal and informal interactions	Input and control over work environment
Status and respect for professional status	Respectful, collegial nurse–physician interactions
	Productivity
	Educational opportunities

> ## NURSING ALERT
>
> *Nurses need jobs where they can thrive and grow. They should ask questions about organizations and compare these data to their own philosophies. A good place to start is with a person the nurse knows who works within the organization.*

After graduating, nurses must pass the National Council Licensing Examination (NCLEX) to become licensed as Registered Nurses to practice their profession. The National League for Nursing (NLN) accredits most bona fide nursing programs. As nurses, we should work together to promote excellence within the field, hence the development of professional organizations. The goal of professional organizations is to set standards for professional competence and to assure the public of the quality and availability of the nursing services that are provided. Laws are in place to protect the public from poorly prepared nurses and to prevent the lack of standards in preparing such nurses. These measures, when combined with state licensure laws, assure the public that nurses are competent professionals, with safe standards of practice and appropriate ethical beliefs. For example, practice guidelines for the critical care nurse are developed by the AACN.

Professional associations also serve to communicate information to their members via newsletters, emails, conferences, or journals. Such items of interest may include pending legislation and political issues affecting nursing and health care.

Associations such as the AACN provide many different beneficial services to critical care nurses. They also

- Provide continuing education courses and free, unlimited on-line continuing education credits
- Encourage involvement in local chapters and at regional and national levels
- Provide additional educational resources
- Provide awards, grants, and scholarships
- Give the nurse an opportunity for leadership outside the job environment

The AACN is not the only organization that critical care nurses can belong to. There are many organizations that can benefit from the wisdom of nurses working in the field. The Society of Critical Care Medicine (SCCM), the American Heart Association, the American Lung Association, and the Hospice and Palliative Nurses Association all have nurses as members of their boards.

Although these organizations do not all represent nurses, nurses can have a strong voice in the path health care takes by working with other nurses, health care professionals, and the lay public.

Membership in professional organizations is recommended for nurses. They provide a source of empowerment and a collective voice for nurses where their concerns can be heard and their value as professionals is recognized.

> **NURSING ALERT**
>
> *Critical Care Nursing Organizations exist to tell the public what critical care nurses do. They provide an invaluable service to nurses by providing standards, guidelines for practice, and a communication vehicle for change and education.*

Certification

Many nurses specialize in their specific areas of practice and obtain additional certification beyond licensure to demonstrate expertise in their field of practice. The CCRN, or Critical Care Registered Nurse, is one of the certifications that can be obtained through the AACN. There are many different certifications that can be obtained from the AACN. Table 1–3 lists all of the currently available ones and within the critical care they involve.

> **NURSING ALERT**
>
> *In order to provide excellence in care, a nurse should become certified in a specific area of critical care nursing.*

TABLE 1–3 Certifications Available from AACN

CCRN	Adult, Neonatal, and Pediatric Acute/Critical Care Nursing Certification
PCCN	Progressive Care Nursing Certification
CMC	Cardiac Medicine Subspecialty Certification
CSC	Cardiac Surgery Subspecialty Certification
ACNPC	Acute Care Nurse Practitioner Certification
CCNS	Adult, Neonatal, and Pediatric Acute Care Clinical Nurse Specialist Certification
CNML	Nurse Manager and Leader Certification

Communication and Health Care Team Members: Calling the Shots

To establish and maintain trust in the delivery of health care, the nurse must be a successful communicator, which requires self-confidence, self-discipline, and respect and tolerance shown toward others. Physicians demand information, co-workers are stressed, families are frightened, and patients feel helpless. Therefore, it is essential for the nurse to practice strong interpersonal dynamics, both verbally and nonverbally. To promote positive health team interactions, nurses must not be defensive and must remain nonjudgmental as to the beliefs, cultures, and lifestyles of others. Professional nurses must also be perceptive of the needs of others in the delivery of high-quality patient care. A truly effective communicator is also an interested and active listener. Active listening is a reliable tool that is useful when dealing with numerous issues surrounding patients, families, and staff members. To maintain the loyalty and cooperation of colleagues and co-workers, their concerns must also be addressed and active listening skills employed and listened to.

In addition to providing hands-on quality patient care, critical care nurses also serve as mentors, leaders, teachers, communicators, and organizers of their clinical units. The critical care nurse, in the ideal situation, works harmoniously with a multidisciplinary team that includes: other professional nurses, physicians; medical students, pharmacists, residents, student nurses, licensed practical nurses, nurse's aides, dieticians, and physical, occupational, and respiratory therapists, as well as social workers, case managers, physician assistants, unit clerks or secretaries, and even maintenance and housekeeping workers.

Such enormous juggling requires almost superhuman qualities and efforts of the professional nurse to smoothly coordinate such daunting tasks, as well as prevent communication breakdowns. The critical care nurse must also deal with uncertainty and volatile changes in the workplace, like downsizing, increased responsibility for nosocomial infections, and substitution of the registered nurses with unlicensed health care providers. The nurse needs to develop tolerance for ambiguity and an increase in understanding of the political nature of health care, and see changes as an opportunity to expand the profession.

An attitude of respect for other health team members and their contributions, regardless of their status, is crucial. The end result is a job well done. With respect comes job retention, trust, loyalty, work commitment, and increased productivity. The delivery of adequate and sufficient health care will dramatically suffer without the benefits or efforts of effective communication.

> ### NURSING ALERT
>
> *Communication skills and leadership are essential characteristics of the critical care nurse. The AACN has touted these to be essential elements for a healthy work environment.*

Defining the Critical Care Nurse

❸ So what is a critical care nurse? A critical care nurse is someone who directly administers nursing care to patients who are critically ill or injured. In order to set aside what is unique about critical care nursing, the AACN has clearly defined eight critical care competencies that encapsulate the functions of these nurses. Table 1–4 sets aside these competencies, which can be found at the AACN web site (www.aacn.org, last accessed August 4, 2010).

The AACN has also set aside the role responsibilities of the bedside nurse. These include the 10 roles listed in Table 1–5 and can be found at the AACN web site. These competencies are part of the synergy model the AACN developed in the 1990s. The synergy model is used as a guide to help with certified critical care practice. It is based upon the assumptions that (1) patient characteristics are a driving force to nurses, (2) nursing competencies are needed to attend to patient needs, (3) the patient characteristics are a driving force behind the critical care competencies, and (4) when the patient characteristics and nursing competencies are in harmony, optimal patient care and outcomes are achieved. The following patient characteristics drive the nursing competencies:

Resiliency   Participation in care

Vulnerability   Participation in decision making

Stability   Predictability

Complexity

Resource availability

AACN Standards for Critical Care

The most common role for the critical care nurse is administering care to the patient at the bedside. Some critical care areas have set job ladders in relationship to these standards from novice critical care nurse to expert using Patricia Benner's model. This opportunity allows growth, professional recognition, and remuneration for staying at the bedside.

TABLE 1–4 Eight Critical Care Competencies	
1. Clinical inquiry	Ability to question and evaluate practice in an ongoing manner, using evidence–based practice instead of tradition.
2. Clinical judgment	Use of competent data collection with a more global grasp of signs/symptoms; implementation of nursing skills with a focus on decision making and critical thinking.
3. Caring	Implementation of a compassionate, therapeutic, and supportive environment in providing care to patients when interacting with families and other health care providers.
4. Advocacy	Ability to protect and support the basic rights and beliefs of patients and families.
5. Systems thinking	Negotiating and navigating within the system of health care to provide resources that benefit the patient and family.
6. Facilitator of learning	Promote and provide opportunities for formal and informal learning for patients, families, and members of the health care team.
7. Response to diversity	Analyzing and implementing care based on dif-ferences in sociocultural, economic, gender, and cultural–spiritual aspects of patients, families, and other members of the health care team.
8. Collaboration	Capitalizing on the unique contributions made by each person in achieving positive outcomes based on collaboration with patients, families, and members of the health care team.

This model serves to help with graduate and undergraduate education as well as hospital patient evaluation systems. The AACN also uses the model for specialty certification.

Regulatory Issues That Impact the Critical Care Environment

❹ There are many areas in critical care that are impacted by regulatory issues. The areas most impacted include patient safety, closed versus open units, and confidentiality and privacy.

TABLE 1–5 AACN 10 Critical Care Nurse's Role Responsibilities

1. Support and respect for the patient's autonomy and informed decision making
2. Intervening when it is questionable about whose interest is served
3. Helping the patient to obtain the necessary care
4. Respecting the values, beliefs, and rights of the patient
5. Educating the patient/surrogate in decision making
6. Representing the patient's right to choose
7. Supporting decisions of patient/surrogate or transferring care to an equally qualified critical care nurse
8. Interceding for patients who cannot speak for themselves and who require emergency intervention
9. Monitoring and ensuring quality care
10. Acting as liaison between the patient/significant others and others on the health care team

Patient Safety

Patient safety issues have become prominent in the last decade. The Institute of Medicine (IOM) and the Joint Commission on Accreditation of Healthcare Organizations (JCAHO) have a direct impact on the quality of care in health care institutions. Reported errors are often called sentinel events and include unplanned extubations; dysfunctional ventilators; inadvertent removal of drains, lines, or catheters; medication errors; and infusion device failures.

In 2000, the IOM concluded that there should be an emphasis on error disclosure and reporting. The AACN, IHI (Institute for Health Care Improvement), and JCAHO are working to create a culture of safety and reporting in order to be proactive in preventing errors. One of the many suggestions by the IOM included limiting the hours that critical care nurses work. As a result of acuity, understaffing, and other factors, nurses frequently work long hours, which increases the incidences of near errors or errors. The IOM recommends that nurses work fewer than 60 hours per week and fewer than 12 hours in a 24-hour period.

Closed Versus Open Units

Critical care patients require an increased knowledge base in those that minister to their care. An intensivist is a physician who specializes in the care of critical care patients. When a critical care intensivist is used, the Health Resources and Services Administration (HRSA) reports a decrease in costs, an increase in quality of life, and a decrease in mortality rates.

Confidentiality and Privacy

All nurses are morally and ethically bound to maintain the confidentiality and privacy of their patients. Nowhere is this more of an acute issue than in the tight confines of critical care units. With the advent of the Health Insurance Portability and Accountability Act of 1996 (HIPAA), the confidentiality of patient medical information is paramount for health care workers. Sharing of information about the patient is on a need-to-know basis only.

Future Challenges for the Critical Care Nurse

❺ The future challenges for critical care nurses come in many forms but include economic, staffing, and educational issues.

Economic Challenges

With increased diversity, age, and mobility of the population and increased use of technology, critical care nurses face challenges that will require dedication, perseverance to allow voices to be heard, and the smarts to enact change. A multilingual population is growing (in large numbers); therefore, it will be essential that the critical care nurse becomes more culturally competent in advocating and planning care for this unique group of individuals and families.

As the world becomes flatter and more mobile, the nurse needs to be aware of the risk of infection, which can create epidemics and pandemics. With the results of the swine flu and sudden acute respiratory distress syndrome (SARS) epidemics, the critical care nurse needs to keep abreast of current affairs and be an educator to prevent as well as treat disease. Communities are canvassing the health care professions seeking opportunities to help in local, national, and worldwide efforts to contain disease.

The advances in technology have yielded amazing and startling changes in the way we live and work. Critical care nurses must meet the challenge of staying abreast of but not be swallowed by the technology, always keeping in mind that there is a patient, family, or significant other that needs the healing touch a nurse can provide.

Staffing Challenges

As the population ages there is an emergence of chronic and new illnesses. Also, the average age of nurses is now mid-40s, and many will retire in the coming decade. The worry of who will provide and coordinate care causes much discussion yet inspires action in many professional organizations. Critical care nurses find themselves frequently overworked and stressed. Added to this is the need to assist and monitor the care of nonprofessional nurse extenders. Many times nurses might find themselves experiencing moral distress due to this challenge.

Moral distress is caused by a situation where the nurse knows the right thing to do but is prevented from doing it because of institutional restraints. Institutional restraints may range from lack of perceived or actual personal authority to lack of resources to do what the nurse feels is morally right. Moral distress is widely touted as a reason why nurses leave nursing. In order to help combat the incidence of moral distress the AACN has developed the 4A's model, which is comprised of ask, affirm, assess, and act (Table 1–6). This model was developed in order to help critical care nurses handle situations and have a course of action if they become subject to moral distress.

NURSING ALERT

A nurse needs to be ever vigilant to assess for signs and take action to prevent moral distress.

TABLE 1–6 The 4A's Model of Assessing for and Preventing Moral Distress	
Ask	"Am I experiencing or showing signs of suffering?"
Affirm	"Am I taking care of myself personally and professionally?"
Assess	"Where is my distress coming from?"
Act	"Am I developing an action plan to prevent this suffering? Who can help me? Is there institutional or unit help that can be instituted?"

Educational Challenges

There are many educational challenges that will be facing the critical care nurse in the coming years. Included in these challenges are the education of new critical care nurses and the graying of nurse educators, improving collegiality among critical care nurses, and mandating continued educational credits.

Disastrous results can occur as the recently licensed nurse is unmercifully "thrown to the lions" without the benefit of sufficient guidance and experience. If not nurtured and supported, novice nurses become immediately over-whelmed by the high levels of demands and responsibilities placed upon them. They become discouraged, disenfranchised, and sometimes angry with the pro-fession and leave nursing, thus worsening today's nursing shortage. Most nurse leaders are savvy to the loss of revenue in constantly reorienting new nurses and have learned to provide an organized, systematic, healthier work environment where the education of new nurses is fostered.

It is recommended that new nurses receive adequate mentoring and work in acute care settings for several years to develop the necessary organizational, leadership, and patient care skills prior to assuming a critical care position.

The same can be said of nurse educators, whose average age is in the mid-50s and who are actively retiring. Many nurses obtain the required credentials to teach and must balance the love of teaching with the lack of salary, distress of mastering three content areas (critical care research, education, and leadership), lack of clinical placements, and increased workload. Colleges need to recognize and provide funding for those nurses interested in jobs as nurse educators. Educators need to continue to vocalize the challenges they face and network with shareholders of power to plan for the future.

Since nurse educators are viewed as experts in their specialties and as people that student nurses turn to for answers and problem solving, they must live up to those expectations. Just as an infant learns to walk, so must the new nurse.

Curriculums should be designed to teach nursing skills at a beginning and elementary level, while gradually increasing the challenges and difficulties of the learning experiences.

NURSING ALERT

New nurses as well as nurse educators need the time and guidance to mature as experts in their specialties.

NURSING ALERT

To develop and maintain autonomy as professional nurses, we must continue to be actively creative and dedicated in our roles.

Currently, most US states are mandating that professional nurses obtain 30 continuing education units (CEUs) per year to remain licensed in nursing. This mandate is a positive step toward maintaining practice updates, evidence-based nursing, and credibility in nursing. Some nurses view this as a step forward; right now, all nurses need to do to renew their license is send in a check. Further education is one of the ways we can keep current and improve practice. Mandatory continuing education has also created much angst among those nurses who are near retirement age or considering retirement. To them, this mandate for additional educational credits has created a financial burden unpaid for by employers due to the current economic downturn. As a result of these new mandates, such individuals have decided to surrender their licenses and become inactive participants in nursing. After many years of dedicated service, this loss of seasoned nurses, who perhaps still had much to offer our profession as mentors and leaders, will now contribute to the nursing shortage.

Challenges facing critical care nurses in the future are not insurmountable. If nurses put their backbones into a task, the task will be completed, often with grace, kindness, and a wish for harmony and care. It is with education, experience, standards, organizations, certifications, and effective and skillful communication that critical care nurses will always be on the cutting edge. We continue to rank highest in the most respected professions, according to the Gallup poll, and we want to maintain this high public trust.

Recalling a True Story

Many years ago, there was a girl who wanted to be a nurse. Being one of three children, financially she couldn't afford a 4-year degree; she took the shortcut, earning an LPN instead. After working at a hospital, she became interested in critical care, but at that time she felt she was limited to practice there unless she obtained her RN. It took her 5 years of hard work to obtain her baccalaureate in nursing, but the hospital helped financially. Feeling she needed more education, she was the first at the hospital to obtain a CCRN and provided leadership by instituting the critical care procedure committee. Still sensing she needed further education, she enrolled in a distant university to complete her master's degree. She is now working on a doctorate, enjoys writing and editing texts, and loves teaching critical care to her students. Life has been a satisfying journey for her. This story illustrates how education is important to the satisfying career of a nurse.

REVIEW QUESTIONS

1. A seasoned critical care nurse is explaining the use of effective communication techniques to a novice nurse. This should consist of

   A. Interrupting others when they are speaking

   B. Keeping facial expressions the same

   C. Inability to maintain eye contact

   D. Listening actively

2. A critical care nurse is taking care of a patient who is nonverbal from the new insertion of a tracheostomy. Explain the best way for the nurse to communicate with the nonverbal patient.

3. List some reasons why an elderly patient in an ICU may not want to complain about his or her pain level.

4. A critical care nurse is working from the patient's perspective when mediating between a physician who prescribes blood and a patient who is morally opposed to receiving blood products. The critical care competency that this most likely applies to is

   A. Caring

   B. Advocacy

   C. Clinical inquiry

   D. Clinical judgment

5. The landmark study that poses to all critical care nurses that there should be a culture of safety is

   A. To Err Is Human

   B. The Nurse Practice Act

   C. The Standards for Acute and Critical Care Nursing

   D. The Synergy model

6. A critical care nurse is examining the progress of a patient with a spinal cord injury toward rehabilitation after a motor vehicle crash (MVC). The nurse is looking at the outcomes determined by another nurse. The part of the Standards of Care for Critical Care Nursing this nurse is addressing is

   A. Assessment

   B. Diagnosis

   C. Implementation

   D. Evaluation

7. **A new graduate is asking a critical care nurse what the initials CMC after her name mean. CMC means the critical care nurse is certified in**
   A. Cardiac Surgery Subspecialty
   B. Cardiac Medicine Subspecialty
   C. Progressive Care Nursing
   D. Clinical Nurse Specialist

8. **There remains an increase in sentinel events in the critical care areas. Which of the following is a sentinel event?**
   A. Planned extubation
   B. Use of infusion devices
   C. Inadvertent removal of drains, lines, or catheters
   D. Preventing medication errors

9. **What is moral distress and why is it a significant issue to critical care nurses?**

10. **According to the IOM, in order to promote safety, critical care nurses should:**
    A. Work fewer than 40 hours per week
    B. Work fewer than 10 hours per day
    C. Work fewer than 60 hours per week
    D. Work fewer than 18 hours per day

ANSWERS

CORRECT ANSWERS AND RATIONALES

1. D. An effective communicator is perceptive of the needs of others and will gain their trust and respect through active listening.
2. Ask the patient "yes" or "no" questions that require the patient to nod for "yes" or move the head from side to side for "no." If the patient can write, provide the patient with paper and pencil to communicate. The nurse can also use illustrations found on communication boards to indicate the patient's concerns, such as being cold or in pain.
3. Elderly patients do not want to be viewed as problem patients or a bother to busy nurses who do not have time to listen to their complaints. Elderly individual might also believe that their discomfort is a normal part of the aging process, which they must learn to accept as a normal part of growing old.
4. B. Advocacy is the role of the critical care nurse in the nurse's ability, to speak to patients and families and to protect and support their basic rights and beliefs. In this case it is the right of a patient to refuse treatment if he or she is morally opposed to it. The nurse is caring, but caring involves compassion; the nurse's role goes beyond this in mediating between the patient and the physician.

5. A. "To Err Is Human" is a brief that was published by the IOM.

6. D. Evaluation is always done on outcomes established by another critical care nurse and is the last step in the process. All others must come prior to performing the evaluation.

7. B. CSC is Cardiac Surgery Subspecialty; PCCN is Progressive Care Nursing; CCNS is Clinical Nurse Specialist.

8. C. Sentinel events are unplanned and can result in patient injury. The following are considered sentinel events: unplanned extubations; dysfunctional ventilators; inadvertent removal of drains, lines, or catheters; medication errors; and infusion device failures.

9. Moral distress is created when the critical care nurse knows the right thing to do but institution pressure/policies prevent the nurse from doing the right thing. This can lead to burnout if it is not resolved.

10. C. The IOM recommends fewer than 12 hours in a 24-hour period and fewer than 60 hours per week.

chapter 2

Care of the Patient With Critical Respiratory Needs

LEARNING OBJECTIVES

At the end of this chapter, the student will be able to:

1. Identify skills needed to assess the respiratory system.
2. Uses diagnostic procedures to determine respiratory status.
3. Explain various oxygen delivery systems.
4. Describe nursing care of patients requiring advanced airway techniques.
5. Prioritize modes and adjuncts of mechanical ventilation (MV) from simple to complex.
6. Identify medications commonly used to care for a patient with complex respiratory needs.
7. Develop the plan of care for the individual with a chest tube.
8. Given a case study, analyze care required in complex respiratory conditions.

KEY WORDS

ABGs – arterial blood gases
AC – assist-controlled ventilation
ALI – acute lung injury
ARDS – adult respiratory distress syndrome
ARF – acute respiratory failure
Aspiration
Atelectasis
BiPAP – bilevel positive airway pressure
BVM – bag-valve mask (manual resuscitator)
COPD – chronic obstructive pulmonary disease
CPAP – continuous positive airway pressure
CV – controlled ventilation
ETT – Endotracheal tube
FiO_2 – fraction of inspired oxygen

Lung compliance
LWP – Lateral wall pressure
Minimal leak technique
Mucus plug
MV – mechanical ventilation
PEEP – positive end-expiratory pressure
Pleural effusion
Pneumothorax
PPV – Positive pressure ventilation
Pressure support
RT – respiratory therapy
SaO_2 – pulse oximetry
SIMV – synchronized intermittent mandatory ventilation
Surfactant
Tension pneumothorax
V_T – tidal volume
Work of breathing

Anatomy and Physiology

In order to assist the patient with complex respiratory issues, an understanding of the intricacies of normal breathing and lung compliance patterns is required. The work of breathing is defined as the amount of force needed to overcome the elastic and resistive properties of the lungs. Lung compliance refers to the degree of elasticity or expandability of the lungs and thorax. Any condition that impedes lung contraction and expansion causes a decrease in compliance. Increased pressure within the thoracic cavity can interfere with lung expansion. Examples of certain conditions include emphysema, asthma, pleural effusion, hemothorax, pneumothorax, empyema, pulmonary edema, pulmonary emboli, or any other space-occupying lesions within the thoracic cavity.

Such obstructive diseases create a decrease in normal airflow because of diffuse airway narrowing. During normal, quiet ventilation only 2% to 3% of the total energy expended by the body is required by the pulmonary system. When pathology occurs from disease, the work of breathing can increase significantly above normal due to decreased lung compliance

---

KEY POINT *Normal ventilation depends on the following factors:*

1. Flexibility of the rib cage
2. Elasticity of the lungs
3. Normal action of the muscles of ventilation
4. Normal airway proficiency, which relies on:
   a. Ventilation: movement of gases into and out of the lungs
   b. Perfusion: the flow of blood through body parts
   c. Diffusion: the flow of gases across the alveolar capillary membranes from areas of higher to lower concentrations

---

Try to remember those grueling days of your anatomy and physiology classes, and how you promptly forgot everything that you memorized after completing those courses. Give yourself much credit, because you probably remember more than you realize. However, a brief review of the anatomy and physiology of the respiratory system can only strengthen your current knowledge base. To begin with, the respiratory system promotes gas exchange between the internal and external environments by inhaling and moving oxygen from the air into the blood and removing carbon dioxide or exhaling it from the blood into the external environment. The process of ventilation includes inspiration and expiration, which allows movement of air into and out of the lungs. Respiration allows for the gas exchange of oxygen delivery to the entire body and the removal of excess carbon dioxide buildup from the body.

The respiratory system also regulates the acid-base balance, metabolizes certain compounds, and filters out inhaled and unnecessary materials from the external environment. Structures of the respiratory system are described in the following text.

The thorax is a rigid yet flexible bony structure that protects major organs within the thoracic cavity. The thorax must be flexible to allow for the inhalation and inflation, as well as the exhalation and deflation, of the lungs. The bony structure of the thorax is composed of 12 vertebrae, 12 pairs of ribs, and the sternum. Ribs are attached posteriorly to vertebrae and anteriorly to the sternum. The 11th and 12th ribs are the exceptions and are known as "floating ribs" because anteriorly they are NOT attached to any other structures (see Figure 2–1).

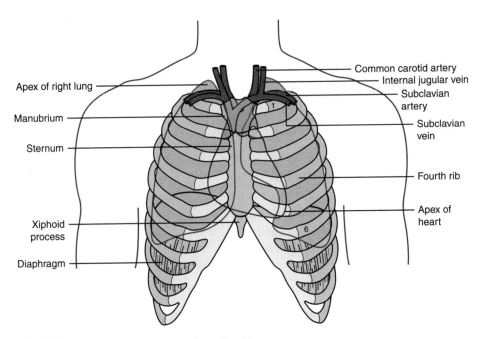

Apex of right lung

Manubrium

Sternum

Xiphoid
process

Diaphragm

Common carotid artery
Internal jugular vein
Subclavian
artery

Subclavian
vein

Fourth rib

Apex of
heart

FIGURE 2–1 • Thoracic anatomy. 1 = 1st rib, 6 = 6th rib

Contained within the thoracic cage are two air-filled, spongy lungs. The lungs are positioned one to the left and one to the right of the mediastinum. They are attached to the mediastinum by the pulmonary ligament. The right lung contains three lobes and the left lung has two lobes, due to the space limitation imposed by the heart.

The space between the two lungs is known as the mediastinum. It contains the heart, blood vessels, lymph nodes, the thymus gland, nerve fibers, and the esophagus.

Two layered pleural membranes surround the lungs and line the thoracic wall. The parietal pleura is the membrane that lines the thoracic wall, and the visceral pleura forms a protective sac that surrounds and overlays each lung. A thin, serous lubricating fluid is found in the spaces between these pleural layers. It allows these layers to slide together without friction, thus facilitating effortless lung movement during inspiration and expiration.

Similar to air in balloons, lungs remain inflated via negative pressure. Should negative pressure be lost from the intrapleural spaces due to exposure to increased atmospheric pressure, a lung collapse or **pneumothorax** will occur. An abnormal accumulation of fluid known as **pleural effusion** can also occur between pleural spaces as a result of infection, inflammation, or heart failure.

The lungs expand and contract in the following ways:

1. The downward and upward movement of the diaphragm lengthens and shortens the chest area during inhalation and exhalation. The diaphragm is a thin, dome-shaped muscle that is stimulated by the phrenic nerves. When the diaphragm contracts during inspiration, abdominal contents are forced downward and the chest expands upward to inflate the lungs. During expiration, which is primarily a passive process during normal breathing, the diaphragm relaxes, the chest wall descends, and abdominal contents return to their normal position.

2. Lung expansion and contraction also relies on the elevation and depression of the ribs, which increases and decreases the diameter of the chest cavity during breathing.

How It All Occurs

Gas exchange in the lungs is known as external respiration. Gas exchange in the body cells and tissues is known as internal respiration. The conducting or upper airways consist of the nasopharynx, the oropharynx, the trachea, bronchi, and bronchioles. Their job is to warm, humidify, and filter inhaled environmental air and channel it along the airways for further action. These structures down to the respiratory bronchioles do not participate in actual gas exchange. This is called the anatomic dead space and contains a volume of about 150 cc. of air.

The upper airway completes the job of warming, filtering, and humidifying environmental air. External respiration takes place through the respiratory bronchioles and the alveoli. The alveoli are the gas exchange units of the lungs. The adult lungs contain several million alveoli. Gas exchange takes place through the Type 1 alveolar cells, which are flat, squamous epithelial cells comprising 90% of the total alveolar surface area. Type 2 alveolar cells secrete surfactant—a very important lipoprotein that promotes alveolar inflation during inspiration and prevents the collapse of the smaller airways during expiration.

Lungs have a dual blood supply. The first supply system is the bronchial circulation, which does not participate in gas exchange but distributes blood to the airways. Pulmonary circulation, the second supply system, contributes to gas exchange by mixing with oxygenated blood that flows from the right side of the heart to the lungs. Less-oxygenated blood leaves the right ventricle of the heart and enters the pulmonary arteries. Blood passes from the pulmonary arteries through the pulmonary capillary beds in the lungs, becomes oxygenated, flows back to the main pulmonary veins, and finally flows into the left atrium of the heart. Oxygenated blood is distributed throughout the body to create internal respiration through the process of diffusion. Internal respiration can only happen through the process of diffusion, which requires an adequate number of red blood cells to transport and release oxygen to the body cells and tissues and to absorb carbon dioxide.

Ventilation is regulated by components of complex brain activity and depends on the rhythmic operation of brainstem centers and intact pathways to the respiratory muscles. Such components are identified as follows:

1. **Control of ventilation** – Several areas that work together to provide coordinated ventilation are located within the central nervous system. The medulla and pons of the brainstem regulate and stimulate automatic breathing. The cerebral cortex promotes voluntary ventilation and overrides automatic ventilation. Spinal cord neurons process information from the brain, and peripheral receptors send information to the muscles of ventilation. Efferent nerve fibers carry impulses from the controller to the effectors, while afferent nerve fibers carry impulses from sensors back to the controller.

2. **Effectors** – These are muscles of ventilation working in a coordinated and symmetrical manner. Scalene and sternocleidomastoid are the muscles of inspiration. The diaphragm, abdominal accessory, and intercostals are the muscles of expiration.

3. **Sensors** – These are chemoreceptors that respond to chemical changes in blood composition and hydrogen ion concentration. Known as central chemoreceptor sensors, they are located near the ventral surface of the medulla and are in close contact with cerebral spinal fluid. These sensors are sensitive to changes in CO_2 content and will increase respirations to blow off CO_2.

   Peripheral chemoreceptors – These are located above and below the aortic arch and at the bifurcation of the common carotid arteries. They are sensitive to changes in oxygen content in arterial blood and are thought to be the only receptors that increase ventilation in response to PaO_2 arterial hypoxemia of less than 60 mm Hg.

   Irritant sensors – These lie between airway epithelial cells and stimulate bronchoconstriction and hyperpnea in response to inhaled irritants. Stretch receptors in the airway are stimulated by changes in lung volume and will prevent inhalation of irritants and protect the lungs from overinflation, known as the Hering-Breuer reflex.

   Juxta capillary receptors or J receptors – These are found in the alveolar walls near the capillaries. Rapid, shallow breathing results from stimulation of engorged pulmonary capillaries and an increase in interstitial fluid volume of the alveolar wall.

Assessment Skills for the High-Risk Respiratory Patient

❶ When patients are critically ill with a disease that alters the functions of normal ventilation, assessment of the efficiency or inefficiency of respiration is crucial and mandatory. All nurses must possess strong assessment skills (see Tables 2–1 and 2–2).

TABLE 2–1 Physical Assessment	
History and interview	Determine the patient's chief complaint. Example: hemoptysis or bloody sputum, dyspnea, or chest pain.
	Discover elements relating to the patient's present problem such as intensity, duration of symptoms, and precipitating factors.
	Observe for clues to current health and emotional status during the interview. Example: tearful, angry, or evasive with responses.
	Question social and family history such as occupational conditions, diet, medications, recreational drug use, alcohol or tobacco use, and previous medical/surgical history.
Inspection	Observe the patient's general state of health and respiratory distress pattern.
	Inadequate nutrition and physical appearance (such as muscular atrophy, kyphosis, barrel chest) should also be noted.
	Inspect the patient from both the front and the back observing for any breathing difficulties or the obvious use of accessory muscles.
	Observe breath sounds, which should be smooth and regular with 12–20 breaths per minute.
	Factors that may reflect breathing difficulties include:
	a. Orthopnea or leaning forward to breathe.
	b. Asymmetry with lung expansion from a collapsed lung, fluid, or solid mass.
	c. Lip pursing along with an increased expiratory effort. This is often associated with chronic obstructive lung disease.
	d. Nasal flaring or air hunger from increased work of breathing due to extensively compromised alveoli.
	e. Inspect for signs of cyanosis in highly vascular areas such as the lips, nail beds, tip of the ear, and underside of the tongue.
	f. Examine the fingers for signs of "clubbing." This is often associated with chronic fibrotic lung disease, cystic fibrosis, and congenital heart disease with cyanosis.

TABLE 2–1 Physical Assessment (Continued)

Palpation	The examiner evaluates the symmetry of the chest wall by simultaneously placing the palmar surface of each hand on either side of the chest wall.
	The chest wall should feel stable and show no signs of unusual movement with respirations, no tenderness, and no masses.
	The skin surface should feel warm and smooth and have elastic turgor.
	Tactile or vocal fremitus is the vibration of the chest wall produced during vocalization and should be bilaterally equal. The nurse should simultaneously palpate both sides of the chest wall while the patient says "one, two, three" or "how now brown cow" or "9, 9, 9."
	Crepitus or subcutaneous emphysema causes a crackling under the fingers when touching the chest or neck.
	Check that the trachea is above the sternal notch; it can be deviated to the right or left in a tension pneumothorax.
Percussion	This process of assessment creates sound waves that help to distinguish whether the underlying respiratory structures are solid, fluid filled, or air filled. There are two types of percussion: direct, using the fist, and indirect, using the hand and fingers. Indirect percussion is the preferred technique for evaluating the chest wall. However, direct percussion using the fist may be required to evaluate heavily muscled or obese patients.
	Lung sounds during percussion should sound resonant. Hyperresonance indicates inflammation from emphysema, pneumothorax, or asthma.
	Dullness or flatness over the lung fields suggests atelectasis, pleural effusion, or lung consolidation.
Auscultation	Unexpected lung sounds heard on auscultation are considered to be abnormal or adventitious. Breath sounds can be diminished or absent if fluid or pus has accumulated in the pleural space, which in turn has decreased airflow to the lungs (see Table 2-2).

KEY POINT

The diaphragm of the stethoscope should be used to assess lung sounds as it makes better contact with the chest wall and covers a larger surface area. The patient, if possible, should sit upright during lung assessment and breathe slowly and deeply through the mouth to avoid hyperventilation and exhaustion. Auscultate and compare all lung fields on either side of the chest wall proceeding from left to right and right to left.

TABLE 2–2 Terms Used To Describe Adventitious Lung Sounds

Term	Description	Cause
Crackles (rales)	Popping noises heart during expiration or inspiration in the lung periphery Can be high, medium, or low pitched Do not clear with coughing	Fluid trapped in the smaller, dependent airways Pneumonia, bronchitis, heart failure, COPD, asthma
Gurgles (rhonchi)	Gurgling, louder sounds heard over larger lung tubes like the bronchi Sometimes can be felt through the chest	Sputum lodged in the larger airways Asthma, aspiration, pneumonia
Wheezes	High–pitched musical sounds Can be "squeaky" in nature Heard during expiration but in more severe cases can be heard in both expiration and inspiration	Narrowing of the larger airways or bronchial obstruction Asthma Bronchoconstriction COPD
Pleural friction rub	Low pitched Coarse and grating like leather rubbing together Heard during inspiration and expiration	Inflammation or irritation in the pleural spaces Pneumonia Pleural effusion
Stridor	Continuous audible crowing sound	Partial airways obstruction or trachea or larynx

NURSING ALERT

1. *In a dark-skinned person with central cyanosis, the facial skin may be pale gray. As such, the buccal mucosa is the most reliable area to examine for cyanosis in a dark-skinned person.*

2. *"Clubbing" is not seen with other chronic lung disorders such as asthma and emphysema.*

> **NURSING ALERT**
>
> 1. Decreased or absent fremitus is caused by excess air in the lungs and suggestive of emphysema, pleural thickening or effusion, pulmonary edema, or bronchial obstruction. Increased fremitus suggests lung consolidation caused by pneumonia, lung compression, tumor, or fibrosis.
> 2. Palpation that produces audible crackling or crepitus indicates subcutaneous emphysema in which fine beads of air are trapped under the skin. It is caused by fractured ribs that pierce the lungs and allow air to leak into the subcutaneous tissues or by air leaking from the lung into sutures from chest tube insertion sites.

> **NURSING ALERT**
>
> Increasing stridor or rapidly decreasing stridor with worsening signs of respiratory distress can indicate that a complete airways occlusion is imminent. The nurse should attempt to identify and relieve the obstruction. If unsuccessful, a rapid response should be initiated so help can be obtained right away.

Collaborative Diagnostic Tools

❷ Diagnostic procedures are performed to assess and detect the presence and severity of disease in the pulmonary system. Chest x-rays, sputum cultures, and arterial blood gases usually do not require a separate special consent form. The more invasive diagnostic tests like lung scans, bronchoscopy, and thoracentesis require that the performing practitioner explain the risks, benefits, and complications to the patient, and a consent for the procedure is usually required. Vital signs before and after such procedures as well as a thorough pulmonary assessment should be performed.

The following are common diagnostic procedures.

1. **Chest x-ray**

   This is an essential noninvasive diagnostic tool for evaluating respiratory disorders, infiltration, and abnormal lung shadows, as well as identifying foreign bodies. Chest x-rays in critical care settings are also used to check and monitor the effectiveness and placement of tubes and lines such as an endotracheal tubes, chest tubes, and pulmonary artery lines.

   Normal lung fields appear black because they are air-filled spaces. Thin, wispy white streaks are seen as vascular markings. Blood vessels can also appear gray. However, grayness in the lung fields usually suggests pleural effusion. Light white areas indicate fluid, blood, or exudate.

How to Do It–Basics of Chest X-Ray Interpretation

1. The dark material on a chest x-ray will be air and the light structures/substances will be fluid, exudate, blood, or something denser than air.

2. The diaphragm and the costophrenic angles should be sharp and easy to see. This will indicate that the lung is fully expanded and the pleural spaces are intact.

3. Look at the mediastinal area. This contains the heart. It should be a normal size and not enlarged.

4. Look at the abdominal area. If you are facing the x-ray you should see the liver below the diaphragm on the left and the stomach on the right.

2. **Sputum culture and sensitivity**

Sputum examination is microbiologic in nature and is necessary in evaluating patients with respiratory disorders. A C&S, or culture and sensitivity, is routinely performed on sputum specimens to diagnose infections and determine whether the strain is resistant to antibiotics. AFB (Acid Fast Bacillus) is a Gram stain that is done to diagnose tuberculosis.

A specimen collection trap is used to obtain sputum specimens. Whenever possible a sputum culture should be obtained in the morning, before starting antibiotics and after the patient receives oral care.

3. **Lung scan –VQ scan – ventilation perfusion scan**

Using injected radionuclide contrast material, lung scans are performed to evaluate either perfusion or ventilation, or to assess for pulmonary emboli. No specific preparation or aftercare is needed. The perfusion portion of the test consists of administering an intravenous (IV) radioactive isotope. Pulmonary structures are outlined in a photograph. For the ventilation portion of the test, the patient inhales a radioactive gas. Then another photograph is taken of the alveoli that uptakes the alveoli. A normal VQ scan shows radioactive uptake of structures. A lack of perfusion or airflow is demonstrated by diminished or absent radioactivity.

4. **Bronchoscopy**

This has numerous uses in diagnosing and treating pulmonary disorders such as direct inspection of the airways, obtaining biopsies, removing foreign objects and mucus plugs, collecting secretions for cytologic and bacteriologic culture, and to implant radioactive gold seeds for treating tumors.

Pre care – This can be done on an outpatient basis. The patient must sign a consent and remain NPO 12 hours prior to the examination. Explain the following steps to the patient: Nasal and oral pharynx are locally anesthetized. A flexible fiber-optic scope coated with lidocaine is inserted into the patient's airways. Local or general anesthesia can be used.

Post care – The patient should remain NPO until the return of a gag reflex. Monitor for recovery from sedatives and for signs of laryngeal edema.

Complications – Can include hemorrhage and pneumothorax.

5. **Lung biopsy**
Indications for lung biopsies include suspected malignancies, unexplained diffuse lung disease, and unidentified infectious processes. Tissue specimens are collected and sent to the laboratory for microbiologic, histologic, cytologic, and immunologic studies.

Pre care – Establish that consent has been signed and the patient remained NPO prior to the procedure.

Post care – A chest x-ray is done after the procedure to assess for pneumothorax. A verification of breath sounds in all lung fields and assessment for signs of hypoxia must be completed. An open lung biopsy requires assessment of the patient's postoperative recovery status: vital signs, pain, difficulty breathing, and signs of bleeding.

Complications – These include hemorrhage, hypoxia, and pneumothorax.

6. **Thoracentesis**
Pleural fluid is removed through the chest wall to determine either pleural effusion or suspected malignancies. Fluid is usually sent to the laboratory.

Pre care – Establish that a consent has been signed and explain the procedure to the patient. Position the patient with legs dangling over the side of the bed and arms and chest resting on the overbed table. Instruct the patient not to talk or cough. Local anesthesia is given. A large-bore needle is inserted through the chest wall through the plural space.

Post care – Have patient remain on the affected side after the procedure to seal the insertion site. Observe for leakage of fluid from the site. Assess for complications.

Complications – These include hemorrhage and pneumothorax.

Analyzing Arterial Blood Gas Levels

7. **Arterial blood gases (ABGs)**

   Blood gas analysis is an essential test used to diagnose and monitor individuals with respiratory disorders. Arterial blood is used because it provides more direct information about ventilatory function. Blood gas analysis determines the pH, bicarbonate levels, and partial pressures of oxygen and carbon dioxide. Indications for obtaining an arterial blood gas sample include signs of acidosis or alkalosis, cyanosis, hyperventilation, hypoventilation, or respiratory distress.

   a. **pO_2 or pO_2** – A measure of the partial pressure of oxygen dissolved in arterial blood plasma. "p" is partial pressure and "a" is arterial. Normal value is 80 to 100 mm Hg breathing room air at sea level.

   > **NURSING ALERT**
   >
   > *Values differ with the very young and the elderly. However, at any age, a pO_2 lower than 50 mm Hg represents a life-threatening situation that requires prompt action such as supplemental O_2 and/or mechanical ventilation.*

   b. **pH** – The hydrogen ion (H^+) concentration of plasma. Normal value is 7.35 to 7.45 ($\Downarrow$7.35 is acidosis; $\Uparrow$ 7.45 is alkalosis). The blood pH depends on the ratio of bicarbonate to dissolved CO_2. The ratio of 20:1 will provide a pH of 7.4.

   c. **pCO_2** – The measure of partial pressure of CO_2 dissolved in arterial blood plasma. Normal value is 35 to 45 mm Hg. This value reflects the effectiveness of ventilation in relation to the metabolic rate or an indication of whether the patient can ventilate well enough to rid the body of the CO_2 produced as a result of metabolism. A value $\Uparrow$50 mm Hg indicates ventilatory failure. A value $\Downarrow$35 mm Hg defines respiratory alkalosis created by alveolar hyperventilation.

   d. **HCO_3** – The bicarbonate level indicates the acid-base component of kidney function. Bicarbonate levels will increase or decrease in plasma levels according to renal mechanisms. Normal value is 22 to 26 mEq/L ($\Downarrow$22 mEq/L is metabolic acidosis as a result of renal failure, diarrhea, ketoacidosis, and/or lactic acidosis; $\Uparrow$26 mEq/L is metabolic alkalosis as a result of fluid loss from the upper gastrointestinal (GI) tract and medications. Examples include vomiting, nasogastric suctioning, diuretic therapy, severe hypokalemia, steroid therapy, and/or alkali administration).

Conditions That Abnormal Arterial Blood Gases Show Us

Respiratory acidosis – pH less than 7.35, pCO_2 greater than 45 mm Hg.

Causes – Central nervous system (CNS) depression of high spinal cord injury, head trauma, anesthesia, and oversedation. Further examples include pneumothorax, hyperventilation, bronchial obstruction, atelectasis, pulmonary infections, heart failure, pulmonary edema, pulmonary embolus, exacerbation of myasthenia gravis, and multiple sclerosis.

Signs and symptoms – Dyspnea, restlessness, headache, tachycardia, confusion, lethargy, drowsiness, dysrhythmias, respiratory distress, and decreased responsiveness.

Respiratory alkalosis – pH greater than 7.45, pCO_2 less than 35 mm Hg.

Causes – Fear, anxiety, pain, fever, hyperventilation, thyrotoxicosis, CNS lesions, salicylates, pregnancy, gram-negative septicemia.

Signs and symptoms – Confusion, lightheadedness, impaired concentration, paresthesias, tetany spasms in arms and legs, palpitations, dysrhythmias, dry mouth, blurred vision, and diaphoresis.

Metabolic acidosis – pH less than 7.35, HCO_3 less than 22 mEq/L.

Causes – *Increased acids* from renal failure, ketoacidosis, anaerobic metabolism, starvation, and salicylate intoxication. *Loss of base* from diarrhea and intestinal fistulas.

Signs and symptoms – Headache confusion, restlessness, lethargy, weakness, stupor, coma, Kussmaul's respirations, nausea, vomiting, dysrhythmias, warm flushed skin, increased respiratory rate, and depth.

Metabolic alkalosis – pH greater than 7.45, bicarbonate greater than 26 mEq/L.

Causes – Base gain—excessive use of bicarbonates, dialysis, lactate administration, and excessive ingestion of antacids. Loss of acids—vomiting, nasogastric suctioning, hypokalemia, hypochloremia, diuretics, and increased levels of aldosterone.

Signs and symptoms – Tetany, muscle twitching, cramps, dizziness, lethargy, weakness, disorientation, convulsions, coma, nausea, vomiting, and depressed rate and depth of respirations.

Compensation for Abnormalities of Acidemia or Alkalemia

The body attempts to compensate for abnormalities associated with acidemia or alkalemia. The respiratory or renal systems will attempt to compensate if the buffer systems cannot maintain a normal pH. If the problem is respiratory in nature, then the kidneys will work to correct it. If the problem is renal in origin, the lungs will attempt to correct it. To determine levels of compensation, examine pH, carbon dioxide (pCO_2), and bicarbonate (HCO_3).

Uncompensated, Partially Compensated, or Combined ABG Problems

There are two types of compensation to look for in an ABG. If compensation occurs, it is full or partial. If there is no compensation, the ABG is called uncompensated. If there are both respiratory and metabolic primary problems, the ABG is known as mixed or combined (see Table 2–3).

> **Uncompensated** – Here the pH is abnormal; it will be either an acidosis or an alkalosis. The pH will always point to the primary problems (acidosis/alkalosis). The nurse then needs to look at the pCO_2 or HCO_3. In an uncompensated problem, there will be a respiratory acidosis or alkalosis *or* a metabolic acidosis or alkalosis, but the value that would correct for this, the opposite organ value, will not change as there is no compensation for the problem.
>
> **Example:** Uncompensated respiratory acidosis

$$pH = 7.33, pCO_2 = 55, HCO_3 = 24$$

Reason: The pH indicates an acidosis, which is caused by the pulmonary system as the pCO_2 is elevated. The kidney would compensate, but since the HCO_3 is normal, compensation has not occurred.

Example: Uncompensated metabolic alkalosis

$$pH = 7.52, pCO_2 = 40, HCO_3 = 30$$

Reason: The pH will always tell you where the primary problem is. In this case, a pH greater than 7.45 shows an alkalosis and the HCO_3 indicates it is metabolic. There is no compensation when the pCO_2 is normal.

TABLE 2–3 ABG Interpretation Chart				Compensation	
	pH	pCO_2	HCO_3	pCO_2	HCO_3
Respiratory acidosis	↑	↓			↓
Respiratory alkalosis	↓	↑			↑
Metabolic acidosis	↑		↑	↑	
Metabolic alkalosis	↓		↓	↓	

Partially compensated – In this instance, all values are abnormal. The compensating organ system attempts to drive the pH to a more normal level but is not completely successful.

Example: Partially compensated respiratory acidosis

$$pH = 7.33, pCO_2 = 55, HCO_3 = 32$$

Reason: The pH indicates there is an acidotic state caused. Therefore, we have a respiratory acidosis. Partial compensation occurs when the renal absorption of HCO_3 causes the level to be elevated partially neutralizing an acidosis. It is not full compensation as the pH is abnormal.

Example: Partially compensated metabolic alkalosis

$$pH = 7.52, pCO_2 = 48, HCO_3 = 30$$

Reason: The pH indicates an alkalosis. Looking at the pCO_2 and the HCO_3 shows us that the alkalosis is caused by HCO_3 being retained (metabolic alkalosis). The increase in pCO_2 shows us that the lungs are partially compensating partially by retaining pCO_2.

Full or complete compensation – In this type of compensation, the pH remains normal. The pCO_2 and HCO_3 are abnormal. Because the pH remains normal, this indicates that one system has been able to fully compensate for the other.

Example: Fully compensated respiratory acidosis

$$pH = 7.35, pCO_2 = 55, HCO_3 = 30$$

Reason: The pH indicates a normal value; however, if 7.40 is absolutely normal, 7.35 is slightly acidotic. The nurse must then look at the pCO_2 and HCO_3 levels to tell where the acidosis is. In this case, a pCO_2 of 55 shows us the acidosis is respiratory. The HCO_3 is alkalotic, so it can not be the primary problem. However, it shows that there is a shift in kidney function to fully compensate for the patient's acidosis.

Example: Fully compensated metabolic alkalosis

$$pH = 7.45, pCO_2 = 48, HCO_3 = 30$$

Reason: The pH shows that the primary problem is an alkalosis, so the nurse must look at the value that indicates alkalosis, which is the HCO_3. This patient's primary problem is a metabolic alkalosis. Since the pH is on the high side of normal it indicates that this ABG is fully compensated by a change in the pCO_2.

Mixed or combined acidosis/alkalosis – At times both the respiratory and metabolic systems fail to maintain a normal pH. In this instance, both the lungs and kidneys combine efforts to create an acidosis or alkalosis. The following are examples of this potentially severe problem.

Example: Combined respiratory and metabolic acidosis

$$pH = 7.20, pCO_2 = 60, HCO_3 = 10$$

Reason: The pH indicates an acidosis. The patient is retaining carbon dioxide (respiratory acidosis) and excreting bicarbonate (metabolic acidosis).

Example: Combined respiratory and metabolic alkalosis

$$pH = 7.50, pCO_2 = 18, HCO_3 = 35$$

Reason: The pH indicates an alkalosis. The patient is excreting carbon dioxide (respiratory alkalosis) and retaining base (metabolic alkalosis).

NURSING ALERT

When the patient has a combined problem and it is not corrected, quick deterioration in the pH in the direction of an acidosis or alkalosis can cause the pH to drive to levels that are not compatible with life.

---

e. **SaO_2** – (Oxygen saturation breathing room air) measures the percentage of O_2 carried by hemoglobin in arterial blood. Normal value is 95% to 99%. No increase in value is possible, but a decrease can be caused by CO poisoning or hypoxemia. The hemoglobin level also needs to be evaluated along with the oxygenation status to determine how much O_2 is being delivered to the tissues. Pulse oximetry is an accurate, noninvasive way to continuously monitor peripheral oxygen saturation. A probe is attached to the patient's finger, ear, or toe and the saturation can be monitored intermittently or continuously (morphine patient-controlled analgesic pump).

f. **CaO_2** – This is a combined measure of the total amount of O_2 carried in the blood, the amount dissolved in plasma (pO_2) and the amount carried by hemoglobin (SaO_2). Normal value is 20 mL of O_2/100 mL of blood.

g. **Fraction of inspired air (FiO_2)** – The pO_2 level should increase if a patient is receiving supplemental O_2. Knowing the level to which the pO_2 should rise in someone with normal lung functioning who is receiving supplemental O_2 and comparing that with the level the pO_2 actually does rise in patients with pulmonary disease is valuable because it illustrates how well the lungs are functioning. Calculating the expected pO_2 is achieved by multiplying the FiO_2 value by 5. For example, 30% $FiO_2 \times 5 = 150$ mm Hg.

h. **Base excess and deficit** – These studies indicate the body's nonrespiratory contributions to acid-base balance within the normal ranges of –2 to +2 mEq/L. A negative base is reported as a base deficit, which correlates with metabolic acidosis. A positive base level is reported as a base excess, which correlates with metabolic alkalosis.

Use and Calculation of the Anion Gap

An anion gap is done to confirm metabolic problems in addition to ABGs. Anions are negatively charged ions such as bicarbonate (HCO_3^-), chloride (CL^-), and phosphate (PO_4^-). Positively charged ions are called cations, which include sodium (Na^+), potassium (K^+), and calcium (Ca^+). A total concentration of cations and anions in the blood and body fluids must remain chemically neutral and are measured in terms of mEq/L. An excess of unmeasured anions and cations present in the blood creates a "gap" between the total concentration of cations and anions. This is known as the anion gap. An equation is used that reflects unmeasured anions in the plasma. This, primarily in conjunction with ABGs, is used to diagnose metabolic acidosis. Na, K, CL, and HCO3 are responsible for maintaining a normal anion gap, which is generally less than 18 mEq/L. The normal range is 10 to 17 mEq/L. Elevations indicate acid accumulation, for example, excessive lactic acid. The anion gap is calculated by the following formula: $(Na + K) - (CL + HCO_3)$.

Example: Na^+ (135), K^+ (3.0), Cl (100), and HCO_3 (28)

Reason: $(135 + 3.0) - (100 + 28) = 10$ mEq/L, normal anion gap

Example: Na^+ (130), K^+ (5.0), CL (90), and HCO_3 (15)

Reason: $(130 + 5.0) - (90 + 15) = 30$, high anion gap = along with ABGs showing a metabolic acidosis this confirms it.

APPLYING IT

Michael Brown is a 29-year-old asthmatic who has delayed coming into the Emergency Care Unit (ECU). He is cyanotic with markedly diminished breath sounds. He is audibly wheezing and his inhalers are not working. After administering O_2 and getting the bed in a high Fowlers position, an ABG is performed. ABGs indicate the following: pH = 7.29, pCO_2 = 50, pO_2 = 50, HCO_3 = 24. Serum electrolytes show the following: Na^+ (145), K^+ (4.0), CL (110), and HCO_3 (24).

What acid-base disturbance do these ABGs indicate? Does this patient have a normal anion gap? What would your next nursing actions be?

✔ ANSWER

Uncompensated respiratory acidosis. The pH is below 7.35, indicating you have an acidosis. The pCO_2 is elevated, indicating the acidosis is caused by the lungs retaining CO_2. The patient has hypoxemia as the pO_2 is below 80 and it is severe. The HCO_3 level is normal, indicating no compensation is being done by the kidneys. The anion gap is normal $(145 + 4) - (110 + 24) = 15$. Prepare to intubate this patient as he or she has severe acidosis and is severely hypoxic and hypercarbic. You might also prepare BiPAP as an alternative to intubation and steroids to help decrease inflammation.

Frequently, arterial blood gases can be done at the bedside using an ISTAT machine. At other times, they need to be collected through an arterial line or an arterial puncture. Instructions for performing these procedures follow.

How To Do It–Collecting an ABG by Arterial Puncture

1. Wash hands and apply gloves according to facility policy.

2. Perform an Allen's test by occluding both the radial and ulnar arteries and then releasing the ulnar. The hand should turn flesh toned within seconds. If the hand is still white, do not use this artery as the dual blood supply to the hand might be compromised if you do a radial stick. Consider using an alternate arterial site.

3. Palpate the radial artery to assess for maximum pulsation in this area.

4. Cleanse the area according to facility policy—either with iodophor prep or alcohol, or both.

5. Using a prefilled, heparinized syringe, insert at a 45-degree angle into the radial artery making an oblique puncture, which allows the muscle fiber to seal the puncture as soon as the needle is withdrawn.

6. Obtain blood, remove the needle, and apply sterile gauze, keeping firm, continuous pressure over the site for at least 5 minutes.

7. Gently rotate the sample to mix heparin with the blood.

8. Send the iced specimen to the laboratory in a biohazard bag immediately or attach to an ISTAT machine.

9. Document the Allen's test results, the site of the sample, and any patient reactions to the procedure

How to Do It—Collecting a Sample From an Arterial Line

1. Wash hands and apply gloves.

2. Attach a syringe to the port closest to the patient.

3. Turn stopcock to pressurized IV line to the "open" position.

4. Remove and discard approximately 5 mL of blood, which equals the dead space in the arterial catheter and any extension tubing dead space.

5. Turn the stopcock to the "off" position.

6. Discard this blood along with the syringe.

7. Attach a heparinized syringe to the arterial line.

8. Turn the stopcock to the "open" position and withdraw the appropriate amount of blood.

9. Turn the stopcock to the "off" position.

10. Gently rotate the sample to mix heparin with the blood.

11. Flush the arterial line and stopcock according to facility protocol.

12. Replace the stopcock cap.

13. Send the iced specimen to the laboratory in a biohazard bag immediately or use in an ISTAT machine on the unit.

14. Document the time you do this and the patient's reaction to the procedure.

NURSING ALERT

Do not make more than two attempts at any one arterial puncture site. Advanced technology allows for the continuous monitoring of ABGs using a fiber-optic sensor placed in the artery.

Pulmonary Function Tests (PFTs)

PFTs are performed to determine the presence and severity of disease in the large and small airways (see Table 2–4). These functions are scrutinized by measuring the volume of air moving in and out of the lungs and then calculating various lung capacities. These tools are useful in monitoring the course of a patient with respiratory disease and to assess the patient's response to therapy.

TABLE 2–4 Description of Various Pulmonary Function Tests

Test	Description	Normal Value
Tidal volume (V_T)	Volume of air exhaled during normal respirations, exhaled volume.	Normal volume is 5.8 mL/kg of body weight.
Minute volume or V_E	Volume of air exchanged in one minute. Formulated by taking the V_T times the respiratory rate (RR) for one minute.	$V_T \times RR$ of patient $= V_E$
Respiratory dead space or V_D	Volume of air in lungs that is ventilated but not perfused. Used primarily in exercise testing.	Varies according to patient tolerance
Alveolar ventilation or V_A	The volume of air that participates in gas exchange in the lungs. Also used in exercise testing.	Varies according to patient tolerance
Expiratory reserve volume or ERV	The maximum amount of air exhaled after a resting expiratory level. Measured by simple spirometry.	1.0 L
Inspiratory reserve volume or IRV	The maximum amount of air inhaled after a normal inspiration.	3.0 L
Residual volume or RV	The volume of air remaining in the lungs at the end of maximum expiration.	1.5 L
Vital capacity or VC	Amount of air moved with maximum inspiratory and expiratory effort. Much coaching of the patient is needed to get an accurate measurement.	4.5 L
FEV_1	Forced expiratory volume in 1 second or the patient expelling at least 80% of his or her vital capacity in 1 second. A decrease in the FEV_1 suggests abnormal pulmonary air flow or a restriction of maximal lung expansion.	80%

TABLE 2–4   Description of Various Pulmonary Function Tests (*Continued*)

Test	Description	Normal Value
PEFR—peak expiratory flow rate	Maximum attainable flow rate at the beginning of forced expiration. Measured by a peak flow meter. This may be done by the patient using a peak expiratory flow meter.	Around 600 mL/breath and 600 L/minute. If the value obtained is 80%–100% of normal, then no treatment is needed. If the value is 50%–80% the patient needs to follow with prescribed medications. If the value is less than 50%, the patient needs to go to the ECU or call the family physician stat.
TLC or total lung capacity	Remaining volume of air contained in the lungs at the end of a maximal inspiration. It is useful in determining the difference between restrictive and obstructive pulmonary disease.	6 L
End tidal CO_2 (capnography)	Amount of CO_2 exhaled after intubation. Can be done on the ventilator or with a handheld monitor.	35–45 mm Hg

They are also helpful as screening tests in potentially hazardous industries, such as coal mining, and for exposure to asbestos or other toxic fumes or gases.

How to Do It-A PEFR (Peak Expiratory Flow Rate)

A PEFR is frequently used in the care of patients with asthma. It is used to aid in monitoring asthmatic bronchoconstriction. The nurse may use a peak expiratory flow meter in the Emergency Care Unit. The following describes how to use a peak expiratory flow meter:

1. Move marker to bottom of peak flow scale.

2. Have the patient take the deepest possible breath.

3. Have patient blow it out as hard and as fast as he or she can into the meter.

4. Repeat the process two more times.

5. Then take the highest of the three numbers to get the patient's peak flow result.

APPLYING IT—A PATIENT WITH ASTHMA

A 35-year-old male patient is admitted to the ECU with a diagnosis of acute respiratory failure due to asthma. He is allergic to pollen and pet dander. He has taken his fast-acting bronchodilator at home four times without any change in his condition. Since he has lost his job he acknowledges that he has stopped taking his anti-inflammatory medication. He is tachypneic, hypertensive, states he has "chest tightness," and is struggling to breathe.

He brings in his records from several months ago that document his peak expiratory flow rate (PEFR). He believes his normal value is around 600 mL. You perform a PEFR and find the values to be 250, 200, and 150. What do these PEFR values indicate? What would you anticipate as orders for this patient?

ANSWER

The PEFR is the highest of the three numbers that are recorded. In this case the PEFR is 250, which is less than 50% of this patient's past-recorded value of 600 mL. Anticipate the following orders: Nebulizers using a bronchodilator like epinephrine would be used first to increase the diameter of the bronchial tubes and ensure that following medications will get to the alveolar levels. Benadryl and IV corticosteroids, depending upon the severity of the attack, may also be added. Intubation with an endotracheal tube may be needed if his attack and symptoms do not improve with treatment.

Oxygen Delivery Systems

❸ Oxygen delivery systems are titrated according to the SaO_2, the ABGs, and patient response. From the simple to the most complex, oxygen delivery systems consist of the following (see Table 2–5):

TABLE 2–5 O_2 Delivery Devices and Percentages of O_2 Delivered	
Device	**O_2 Delivery Percentages**
Nasal cannula (nc)	Use at 2 L per minute gives flow rate of 28%.
Simple mask	Use at 6–12 L per minute gives 35%–50%.
Venturi's mask	Use at 15 L per minute gives 24%–50%.
Partial rebreather	Use at 6–10 L per minute gives 40%–60%.
Nonrebreather	Provides concentrations from 60% to 90%.

1. **Nasal cannula**

    These are two short, hollow prongs delivering direct oxygen into the nostrils. The prongs attach to tubing that connects to an oxygen source, a humidifier, and a flow meter. Benefits of this type of delivery system include a comfortable, convenient method of O_2 delivery in concentrations up to 44%. The equipment is less expensive, allows for patient activity/mobility, and is a practical system for long-term use. Disadvantages include the inability to deliver oxygen concentrations over 44%; it cannot be used if the patient has nasal problems; and a liter flow greater than 6 L will not increase the FiO_2 and can dry out the nasal passages.

NURSING ALERT

Monitor equipment daily. Evaluate for pressure sores over ears and cheek areas. Padding can be applied to reduce friction in these areas. A water-soluble lubricant can be used to prevent nasal irritation. Avoid kinking or twisting of the tubes, which will impede the flow of oxygen.

---

2. **Simple face mask**

    This mask fits over the nose and mouth and is held in place by an elastic around the head. The mask is attached to O_2 tubing, a humidifier, and a flow meter. Benefits include the delivery of higher O_2 concentrations as compared to the nasal cannula. The system does *not* tend to dry out the mucous membranes of the nose and mouth. Disadvantages include a confining mask may increase anxiety in some patients and can cause facial irritation if applied too tightly. It is difficult to talk and be understood and the airway must be protected in case emesis occurs. The simple face mask is contraindicated for patients with long-term CO_2 retention. CO_2 retainers breathe in response to a low O_2 level. Flooding the patient's respiratory system with oxygen will reduce the stimulus to breathe (hypoxic drive). Use at 6 to 12 L per minute or 35% to 50%.

3. **Venturi's mask**

This system delivers an exact concentration of oxygen regardless of the patient's ventilatory pattern. For each liter of oxygen that passes through a fixed orifice, a fixed proportion of room air will be maintained. The advantage of this delivery system is that precise amounts of oxygen can be mixed with room air and delivered to the patient. This can be used on low liter flow in patients with COPD. The disadvantages are the same as with the simple face mask. Use at 15 L per minute, giving 24% to 50% oxygen.

NURSING ALERT

A patient with COPD and CO_2 retention should not be placed on high-liter-flow O_2. This will destroy the patient's hypoxic drive, decreasing the stimulus to breathe and therefore the patient's respiratory efforts. This could cause hypoxemia, leading to a respiratory arrest. Precise O_2 via low-flow nasal cannula and Venturi's mask is recommended.

---

4. **Partial rebreather mask with reservoir bag**

This mask is similar to a simple face mask but has the addition of a reservoir oxygen bag. The purpose of the rebreather bag is to conserve oxygen by allowing it to be rebreathed from the reservoir bag. Benefits include oxygen delivery concentrations between 40% and 60%. The mask should be applied as the patient exhales and requires a tight face seal. Disadvantages include that it is impractical for long-term therapy and leaks around the face from the mask may decrease the FiO_2 if the mask is not tight fitting. Use at 6 to 10 L per minute, giving an oxygen concentration of 40% to 60%.

NURSING ALERT

The reservoir bag should remain full on expiration and partially deflate at peak inspiration. Monitor arterial blood gases, as oxygen toxicity could be a side effect.

---

5. **Nonrebreather mask with reservoir bag**

This mask has a one-way expiratory valve that prevents rebreathing of expired gases. This mask is effective as a short-term therapy modality and can provide oxygen concentrations from 60% to 90%. It has flaps that allow exhaled CO_2 to exit the side of the mask during exhalation.

Advanced Airway Techniques

❹ The purpose of advanced airway techniques is to permit ventilation. The most commonly used artificial airway for providing short-term airway management is endotracheal intubation. Endotracheal intubation is done by inserting an endotracheal tube (ETT) into the trachea by the oral route. It is indicated for airway maintenance, secretion control, oxygenation, and ventilation. It is useful in cases of emergency placement inserted via the orotracheal route and requires cuff inflation for placement stability within the trachea. One hundred percent oxygen can be given through ETT.

A tracheostomy tube is the preferred method of long-term airway maintenance in the patient requiring intubation for more than 21 days or in situations of upper airway obstruction or failed intubation attempts. These tubes are inserted via a tracheotomy procedure. The tracheostomy tube provides less resistance to airflow, making breathing easier. Secretion removal is also less difficult, patient comfort is greater, and ventilator weaning is more successful. A tracheostomy tube also requires cuff inflation for placement stability.

How to Do It–Endotracheal Intubation (ETT)

1. Explain the procedure to the patient and family.

2. Obtain baseline vital signs, SaO_2 and cardiac rhythm.

2. Manually ventilate the patient with a BVM as needed before intubation. Usually one breath every 3 to 5 seconds.

2. Check that suction is available and functioning correctly.

3. Check the ETT cuff for leaks prior to insertion by inflating it with the correct amount of air.

4. Position the patient on his/her back with a small rolled blanket or pillow under the shoulder blades to hyperextend the neck and open the airway. Do not do this if the patient has had a head/neck injury.

5. Administer sedatives, topical anesthetics, or short-acting neuromuscular blocking medications to block the cough reflex and promote rapid and non-traumatic intubation.

6. Assist the health care provider during intubation by suctioning as needed and assisting with cuff inflation.

7. Secure the ETT with a commercially prepared holder.

8. Assess the following:
   a. Vital signs, SaO_2, end-tidal CO_2 and cardiac rhythm (observe for hypotension)
   b. Breath sounds bilaterally; they should be of equal intensity
   c. Symmetry of chest wall movement (raise on the right side only could indicate intubation of the right mainstem bronchus and the ETT will need to be repositioned)
   d. Presence of the correct tidal volume on the ventilator

9. Call for an immediate portable chest x-ray after insertion to confirm proper tube placement

10. Insert a nasogastric tube to decompress the stomach and lessen the chance of aspiration.

11. Document:
    a. Patient response; vital signs, SaO_2, end-tidal CO_2
    b. Presence of breath sounds, symmetry of chest wall movement
    c. Location in centimeters of ETT as it exits the lips
    d. Premedications

NURSING ALERT

ETT placement at the lip line (documented in centimeters) must be documented to ensure continued proper placement. The patient on long term ventilation will eventually need a tracheostomy.

Nursing Interventions

1. Continuously explain all procedures to the patient and provide emotional support.

2. Suction as necessary following strict aseptic technique to prevent infection and aspiration.

3. Provide oral care to remove secretions and prevent ventilator associated pneumonia.

4. Elevate the head of the bed 30 degrees to prevent aspiration.

5. Monitor the tubing for kinks and blockages.

6. Auscultate lung sounds to determine airway patency.

7. Assess complications of accidental disconnection, tube obstruction, fractured teeth, bleeding, vocal cord paralysis and laryngospasm.

8. Teach the patient and family that communication will need to be done via signing or writing as the ETT goes in between the vocal cords and does not allow speech.

How to Do It–Minimal Leak Technique

The *minimal leak technique* is done to ensure that air flows into the lungs and not around an endotracheal or tracheostomy tube. This is done to determine the lateral wall pressure (LWP) against the tracheal wall. High LWP can cause tissue breakdown and lead to necrosis and scarring. The balloon port on the end of either device is attached to a manometer and a pressure is read. This pressure is usually kept around 25 cm/H_2O. If the pressure is too low, air is instilled into the port by manipulating a three-way stopcock until a tiny leak is heard during peak ventilator inhalation. If the pressure is too high, air is bled out of the stopcock until the manometer reads 25.

Once completed, the patient should have a slight leak around the ETT cuff at highest inhalation. The nurse confirms this by listening to the side of the tracheal wall and observing the chest rising. The slight leak should happen at the end of chest wall expansion.

Role of CPAP and BiPAP Prior to Mechanical Ventilation (MV)

There are actions that medical and nursing staff can take that might prevent implementing mechanical ventilation. These assistive devices are noninvasive and can be used when nonrebreathers do not maintain a satisfactory ventilatory level for the patient. The nurse may already be familiar with these devices, which are used for sleep apnea in medical-surgical patients or in home care. CPAP is continuous positive airway pressure. It is applied to the patient in a tight-fitting mask that covers the nose and mouth in the case of a person in respiratory distress. When the patient breathes spontaneously, a fan delivers pressure to the patient's airways all the time. If you imagine the alveolus as a balloon that expands on inspiration and gets smaller on expiration, CPAP give a positive pressure to alveoli, which keeps them expanded longer. This does two things. First, it increases the surface area of the alveolus, thus allowing more oxygen in and more carbon dioxide to diffuse in and out of the alveolus. Second, it prevents alveolar collapse by keeping positive pressure on those alveoli during the end of exhalation.

Some health care providers may skip CPAP and go to BiPAP. The only difference with this modality is the inspiratory pressures, which are set higher than expiratory pressures during the respiratory cycle.

> ### NURSING ALERT
>
> *CPAP and BiPAP are only stop-gap measures. The patient must be able to spontaneously breathe on CPAP and BiPAP. If the patient's condition continues to deteriorate, prepare for mechanical ventilation.*

Nursing care of the patient with CPAP or BiPAP involves assessing for complications of these devices. As with any mask, the patient can be uncomfortable and fight it as it is irritating and must be tight fitting for it to work. The nurse must be observant for pressure ulcers around the face. Sometimes patients feel that the tight masks are claustrophobic. Calm reassurance and antianxiety medications may help with adapting to CPAP or BiPAP. Patients may also vomit and aspirate with any mask, so close observation is important while on this therapy. These machines are also noisy and loud, but quieter models are now available.

What Is Mechanical Ventilation

❺ Mechanical ventilation (MV) is a term used to describe the delivery of life support to a patient using an invasive airway and a machine that gives pressurized oxygen. So MV is just a big air pump. Through an ETT or a tracheostomy, air is pumped into the patient's lungs just like a bike pump delivers air into the inner tube of a tire. MV is done until the patient can breathe spontaneously and cough on his or her own. MV can be based on positive pressure or negative pressure. Negative pressure ventilators (chest cuirass, iron lung, or chest ponchos) are rarely found in critical care, so the focus will be on positive pressure ventilation. Ventilation is delivered with limits set for pressure, time, and volume.

> ### NURSING ALERT
>
> *An artificial airway is always needed to provide positive pressure ventilatory support for a patient.*

Positive pressure ventilation (PPV) works in reverse of normal breathing. At the end of inspiration during normal ventilation, pressures in the lungs are negative. Using an invasive airway, PPV actively forces air into the lungs during inspiration, creating positive pressure at the end of expiration. During exhalation, the air is allowed to passively flow out of the lungs similar to normal breathing. Because of PPV, there are hemodynamic changes in the chest during the initiation of MV. PPV can impede blood flow back to the heart in patients who are sensitive to these pressures, dehydrated, or who are hypotensive.

> **NURSING ALERT**
>
> *A patient's blood pressure (BP) must be frequently monitored after being placed on positive pressure ventilation. Anticipate a drop in BP due to changes in chest pressures. NURSING ACTION: Isotonic fluids like normal saline and vasopressors like dopamine may be necessary to maintain a BP greater than 100 systolic.*

Assessment of the Patient Who Is at High Risk for MV

Patients at the highest risk for MV are those who cannot maintain a normal blood arterial oxygen level (pO_2) or have a high carbon dioxide level (pCO_2). As a rule of thumb, with a decrease in pO_2 toward 50 and an increase in pCO_2 greater than 50, aggressive intervention with MV is usually required. There are four broad groups of patients that are at risk for MV. These groups, the problems, and the medical diagnoses are summarized in Table 2–6.

TABLE 2–6 High Priority Patients for MV		
Problem	**Defining the Problem**	**Medical Diagnoses**
Failure to oxygenate (lower airway and gas exchange)	Air gets into the lungs but does not get into the alveolus	COPD leading to pneumonia*
		Pneumonia
		Adult respiratory distress syndrome (ARDS)
		Pulmonary embolus (PE)
		Pulmonary edema
		Shock
		Cardiac arrest

TABLE 2–6 High Priority Patients for MV (*Continued*)

Problem	Defining the Problem	Medical Diagnoses
Failure to ventilate (upper airway)	Air can not get down the tubes to the lungs due to poor neuromuscular effort or swelling of the airways	Asthma Bronchospasm after extubation Musculoskeletal diseases Spinal cord injury Edema of the upper airways such as in traumatic airways injury
Failure to protect the airway (aspiration and airway clearance)	Inability to cough effectively and clear secretions	Drug overdose Aspiration pneumonia Mucous plugging Neuromuscular blockade
General surgery	Inability to perform surgery without control of organs or paralysis of organ	Open-heart surgery Lung surgeries Abdominal surgery Head and neck surgery

*indicates the largest group requiring MV.

By far the largest group of patients who frequently require MV are those with pneumonia* from chronic obstructive pulmonary disease (COPD). Patients with COPD have long-standing decreased lung capacities that cause them to retain pCO_2. When they develop pneumonia on top of their disease, their lungs cannot keep up with the work of breathing. Decreased oxygen entering the alveolus and increase carbon dioxide retention, leading to severe oxygen deficits. The end result is cerebral hypoxia, which can lead to infarction, permanent brain damage, and death within 4 to 6 minutes.

NURSING ALERT

Always monitor the SaO_2 in high-risk patients, especially if they are symptomatic. A turn for the worse is signified by a decreasing SaO_2 while increasing the oxygen delivery, and a steady trend in elevation of other vital signs (VS) (heart rate [HR], respirations, and BP). NURSING ACTION: The nurse must act swiftly in this instance. Obtain ABGs and prepare for administration of oxygen from a (bag-valve-mask) BVM and equipment for emergency intubation.

A smaller percentage of patients require MV because they cannot get air into their lungs. These patients fail to ventilate their alveoli due to either swelling of the airways (status asthmaticus, bronchospasm) or musculoskeletal weakening diseases (multiple sclerosis, Guillain-Barré syndrome). Occasionally, damage done to the central nervous system creates conditions where the brain fails to tell the lungs to work (stroke), or paralysis of the diaphragm (cervical level 4–5 spinal cord injuries) occurs.

> **NURSING ALERT**
>
> *A patient with a head injury or spinal cord injury should be monitored carefully for respiratory depression. NURSING ACTION: Resuscitation equipment must be handy for emergent care of patients with these diagnoses.*

Another reason why MV may be performed is to protect the airway. In a patient who is unable to cough, many interventions are performed to help aid the mobilization of secretions. When normal nursing interventions fail, the patient may need intubation and MV to prevent secretions solidifying into mucus plugs. Mucus plugs act like a cork plugging a bottle. If they are large enough and lodge in the main stem bronchus, they can prevent airflow to an entire lung, leading to pneumothorax. Also, atelectasis or collapse of alveoli can occur from underinflated alveoli and thick secretions.

Patients who have aspirated or have an increased potential to do so from drug or alcoholic intoxication may need MV until they can protect their own airways. Aspiration of stomach contents can irritate delicate lung tissue and can cause chemically induced pneumonia.

When the muscles of respiration require paralysis to administer general anesthesia and surgical intervention, a temporary ETT and MV are used. Open-heart surgery, abdominal surgery, and open lung biopsies are done under general anesthesia. These surgeries require the target organs to be immobilized. Once the surgery is completed and the patient has recovered successfully, the tube is withdrawn and MV is stopped.

Ventilator Settings

Ventilator settings are ordered by the health care provider. Generally, a respiratory therapist (RT) sets up the ventilator and changes the settings. Settings are regulated according to the patient's assessment, expected outcome, and changes in ABGs. Table 2–7 contains settings and modes that can be used in the treatment of the patient. Get ready for lots of initials and terminology.

TABLE 2–7 Ventilator Setting and Modes of Ventilation	
	Description
Settings	
Tidal volume (V_T)	Amount of oxygen pumped into the lungs with one breath
Respiratory rate	The number of breaths the machine gives the patient in a minute
Fraction of inspired oxygen (FiO_2)	The concentration of oxygen delivered. Can be ordered as a percentage (%) or fraction. For example, 50% FiO_2 = 0.5
Modes	
Assist controlled (AC)	All breaths that are given to the patient have the same tidal volume even if they are spontaneously generated by the patient.
Synchronized intermittent mandatory ventilation (SIMV)	The patient can breathe spontaneously between ventilator breaths but at his or her own tidal volume. Tidal volume will vary depending upon how much and how often the patient breathes.
Positive end–expiratory pressure (PEEP)	Keeps a small positive pressure in the airway at the end of inspiration. Increases oxygenation and keeps alveoli open.
Continuous positive airway pressure (CPAP)	Used when patient is ready to be weaned off the ventilator. Physiologically like PEEP but with the patient breathing without ventilator breaths. In other words, breathing on his or her own but still hooked up to the ventilator.
Pressure support	Boost given to the patient while inhaling. Like a fan, helps aid in patient comfort and decreases the work of breathing.

Ventilator Alarms

Ventilator alarms are designed to tell the nurse when something is wrong with the system or the patient and can be scary for the nurse and the patient. The nurse is not expected to solve every problem with a ventilator alarm. However, the nurse is expected to support the patient while troubleshooting in an organized fashion from the patient to the machine. There are basically two types of alarms: high pressure and low pressure (see Table 2–8).

Low-pressure alarms sound most commonly when the ventilator disconnects from the patient. The nurse should check all circuits and reattach the tubing that was disconnected. Another reason could be an underinflated airway balloon on the ETT or tracheostomy. Measure the lateral wall pressure and instill more air using the minimal leak technique described under Advanced Airway Techniques. If the airway balloon will not hold air, prepare to remove

TABLE 2–8 Ventilator Alarms	
Causes	**Nursing Actions**
Low-pressure alarms	
Disconnection from patient	Find the location of the disconnect and reconnect the tubing to the patient
Underinflated balloon of ETT or tracheostomy	Determine the LWP by minimal leak technique and recheck the LWP. If leak continues, notify the person responsible for reintubating the patient and gather supplies to assist with the procedure.
High-pressure alarms	
Tubing is kinked or caught somewhere	Release the kink. Usually this is a situation where the patient is lying on the tubing or it is accidentally caught in the bedside rail.
Patient is biting on the ETT	Insert a bite block (oral airway) so the patient can not bite on the ETT; patient may need sedation.
Patient needs suctioning	Auscultate the lung fields; suction the patient and then reassess the lung fields. If it is an emergency, suction first! Auscultation then can be done after clearing the airway.
Patient is anxious and fighting or "bucking" the ETT and ventilator	Use therapeutic communications to help relax the patient. Ask yes/no questions, which give the patient a sense of control. Sedatives and paralytics might be needed as a last resort.
Change in lung compliance	Perform a physical assessment. If the lungs fill with fluid (heart failure, pulmonary edema), the patient may need a chest x-ray (CXR), diuretic, and cardiac medications to improve cardiac functioning. If the patient has a pneumothorax, it is best to ventilate with a BVM until help arrives.

and reinsert another invasive airway. This should be done by a respiratory therapist or trained health care provider.

A high alarm can sound when too much pressure is needed to pump air into the lungs. Check all ventilator tubing; sometimes the tubing is kinked or caught in something like the bedside rails. The patient maybe biting on the airway, in which case a bite block or sedation may be tried. The peak airway pressure gauge should be checked. When there is nothing that can be found wrong with the tubing, the problem may be in the patient.

A high alarm usually trips because the patient needs suctioning, is fighting the ventilator, or there has been a change in the patient's lung status. Mucus in the airways impedes the delivery of gas to the patient. In other words, if you are using a pump on a bicycle tire and there is fluid in the tire, it will require more force to inflate the tire. The MV will deliver more force to give the patient the desired tidal volume, but when a preset pressure limit is reached, it will trip an alarm requiring the nurse to assess the patient. If the patient is fighting the ETT or bucking against the delivery of gas, it will trip the high alarm. Calming patients by talking to them, and keeping them informed of their progress and that someone will come to their aid goes a long way in reassuring them. Sometimes a sedative or, in extreme cases, a neuromuscular blocking agent may be needed to calm the patient.

Perhaps the patient's lung **compliance** has changed. Compliance is the degree or ease of expansion of the lungs. When the lungs are fluid filled or blocked with thick sputum, the compliance or distensibility of the lungs is harder. This requires more pressure from the ventilator to overcome resistance to pumping air into the lungs. This will trip the high-pressure alarm. Most of the time, an increase in pressure can be caused by mucus and the patient will need to be suctioned. A thorough pulmonary assessment is imperative if this continues; the patient could be developing a pneumothorax, heart failure, or pneumonia. It also may require notification of the health care provider to order a chest x-ray and ABGs to assist with confirming assessment findings.

NURSING ALERT

If the ventilator alarms keep sounding and you can not determine the cause support the patient with a BVM. NURSING ACTION: A BVM with oxygen connection is kept at the bedside at all times. Attach the bag to the patient's airway, turn the oxygen up as far as it will go, and ventilate the patient with one breath every 5 seconds. Then calmly call for help! You are not expected to know everything about a ventilator, but you are expected to support the patient. NEVER IGNORE ALARMS!

APPLYING IT

You have been assigned Jose Mendez, a 35-year-old patient who was in a motor vehicle accident. You hear his ventilator alarming. Proceeding to his bedside, you note alarms going off on the ventilator. What should be your FIRST nursing action?

ANSWER

Observe the patient to see if he is attached to the ventilator; look at the tubing to see if it is kinked. Then auscultate his lung sounds to see if they have changed from the morning assessment. If you can not find the problem quickly, remove the manual resuscitation bag, turn the oxygen up high, and give the patient one breath every 5 seconds, then call for help.

Nursing Care Planning for the MV Patient

Nursing Diagnoses	Expected Outcomes
Ineffective airway clearance, risk for	The airway will remain open and clear
Aspiration, risk for	The patient will have a clear chest x-ray
	The patient will have baseline ABGs
	The patient will have normal breath sounds
Ventilation, impaired spontaneous	The patient's respiratory status will be within five spontaneous breaths of baseline
Gas exchange, impaired	Arterial blood gases will return to baseline
Cardiac output decreased	The vital signs will be within normal limits
	The urine output will be >30 mL/hr
Infection, risk for	The patient will have a clear chest x-ray
	The patient will have normal sputum cultures

Nursing Interventions and Rationales for the Patient During MV

1. Ongoing respiratory assessments: inspection, palpation, percussion, and auscultation. Assess the ventilator settings at the beginning of the shift and ensure they are as prescribed. Assess tubing for fluid buildup and drain, as well as humidification and temperature.

   Observe for s/s of respiratory distress. Assess serial blood gases. Monitor the color, amount, and thickness of secretions. Assess for aspiration.

   Monitor for tracheal deviation (tension pneumothorax) and subcutaneous emphysema *to prevent complications*.

   Check for placement of ETT tube by verifying mark at the end of the tube is as per intubation record *to prevent sliding down or out of proper alignment above the carina*.

   Check for minimal leak technique by auscultating a small leak at the side of the trachea during the height of inspiration *to prevent tracheal necrosis balloon from overinflation and ensure correct tidal volumes (Vt)*.

   Ensure that the ETT is taped securely *to prevent accidental extubation*.

   Ensure that the patient is not biting down on the ETT *to prevent kinking and increasing pressure to give ventilator breaths*.

2. Perform frequent suctioning with closed suctioning or individual suction kits. Perform continuous subglottic aspiration of secretions *to prevent infection and aspiration*.

3. Turn *to prevent skin breakdown, pneumonia*.

4. Reposition *to prevent contractures, pneumonia, etc.*
5. Oral care and watching for skin breakdown around the airway *to prevent ventilator-associated pneumonia (VAP).*
6. Keep a BVM at the bedside at all times to *use to support the patient in the event of electrical or MV malfunction.*
7. Keep the stomach decompressed by inserting a nasogastric *tube to prevent aspiration.*
8. Monitor the urinary intake and total output *for signs of dehydration or fluid overload.*
9. Initiate nutritional support when ready with tube feedings or hyperalimentation *to prevent negative nitrogen balance and malnutrition.*
10. Get the patient out of bed as soon as possible *to prevent hazards of immobility.*
11. Administer antiulcer medications *to prevent stress ulcers.*
12. Explain all procedures to the patient and *family to prevent undue stress.*
13. Develop a method of communication *so the patient has a voice in his or her care.*
14. Let the patient control what he or she can *to provide a decreased sense of powerlessness.*

Ongoing Assessments for Complications of MV

Aspiration Pneumonia

Aspiration pneumonia occurs when a patient inhales his or her secretions or tube feedings. It occurs with such frequency that when a patient is intubated and placed on a ventilator, a nasogastric tube is inserted to keep the stomach decompressed. This is prophylactic for the prevention of vomiting and aspiration. The gastric tube is then connected to suction. A chest x-ray confirming ETT placement will also confirm the gastric tube location.

Aspiration pneumonia is also possible if the patient is receiving tube feedings as nutritional supplementation during MV. There are many controversies in preventing aspiration pneumonia. A chest x-ray is a must to confirm the placement of a feeding tube, but a chest x-ray cannot be done once every shift to confirm placement. All sources are in agreement that aspiration of tube feedings should be done at frequent intervals throughout the day; every 4 hours is usually the minimum and whenever needed. According to guidelines, aspiration of tube feedings should be done at frequent intervals throughout the day: usually every 4 hours and whenever needed. According to guidelines, aspiration of tube feedings should be done at frequent intervals throughout the day: usually every 4 hours and whenever needed. However, when to hold the tube feedings varies from institution to institution. Consult your institutional guidelines. If the aspirate exceeds guidelines hold the feedings until it returns to baseline. Insufflating the gastric port with air and listening over the stomach is no longer an acceptable practice to determine gastric placement.

Ventilator-Associated Pneumonia (VAP)

Once the airways are violated with a device that goes into the lower airway, pneumonia is a possible consequence. There is a wealth of research in the nursing literature on VAP. Frequent hand washing is a must in preventing infection. Much research is focused on oral secretions contaminating the lung fields. Good oral hygiene several times a shift is important to prevent VAP. All suctioning must be done maintaining a sterile system. Most health care facilities use in-line suction devices in an effort to decrease suction catheter contamination. Trauma to the airways by a hard suction catheter can be decreased by the use of soft, more pliable red rubber catheters, but these can not be used in an in-line suction device. To prevent secretion pooling above ETT or tracheotomies, some tubes now come with a subglottic suction port to allow suctioning above the balloons of the tubes. Lavaging with normal saline solution is no longer an acceptable practice and has been shown to increase the chance of infection. Also, keeping the head of the bed in an elevated position of 30 degrees or higher helps decrease the chance of aspiration.

Airway Trauma From Pressure

Forcing air into the lungs can have dire effects. When PPV is instituted, the increased pressure to the lungs can rupture the alveoli. This is called a pneumothorax. Patients more prone to this are those who already have very fragile lungs; those with COPD are most prone. Also, patients on positive end-expiratory pressure (PEEP) are more prone to pneumothorax as there is always higher pressure in the lungs at expiration. The fragility of the lungs, just like a balloon if overstretched, can cause them to pop. When this occurs, the nurse will see less chest wall movement on the affected side, hear diminished breath sounds, and the high-pressure alarm will sound on the ventilator. If the nurse suspects a pneumothorax she or he should take the patient off the ventilator and use a BVM to support breathing and call the MD stat. She/he will order a chest x-ray. Manually ventilating a patient will decrease the chance of developing a tension pneumothorax.

A tension pneumothorax is caused when unrelieved pressure builds up in the chest. The pressure pushes the heart, great vessels, and trachea away from the affected side. Because these structures are compressed, the patient will lose his or her breathing and circulatory ability and a cardiac/respiratory arrest can occur quickly. The pressure that builds up would be similar to someone placing an elephant on the fragile mediastinum. The signs and symptoms of this complication depend on how fast it develops. Things to look for in a potentially lethal tension pneumothorax include a deviated trachea away from the affected side; distended jugular veins; cool, clammy skin; a profound drop in BP and tachycardia; cyanosis; and sharp pleuritic chest pain.

> ### NURSING ALERT
>
> *If a nurse allows a patient to remain on MV and a pneumothorax results, the unrelieved pressure accumulation can cause a tension pneumothorax, which is a life-threatening condition. If pneumothorax is suspected, the patient should be manually ventilated with a BVM until a chest x-ray can rule out this condition.*

The treatment for a tension pneumothorax and a pneumothorax greater than 30% involves confirmation by chest x-ray and decompression of that side of the chest with a chest tube. The oxygen level on the ventilator should be increased before the procedure and analgesics should be administered.

Controlled Ventilation (CV) Compromise and Shock

MV upsets the hemodynamics in the chest and therefore potentially the body. Because there is more positive pressure during inhalation, blood flow to the right side of the heart (preload) can be decreased. Therefore, one of the most important assessments a nurse can do right after institution of MV is monitor the blood pressure and central venous pressure if there is a central venous catheter in place. A drop in BP and a tachycardia along with a concurrent drop in urinary output indicate circulatory compromise. If this occurs, the nurse must notify the health care provider. Initiation of fluids and a vasopressor (like Levophed) can be anticipated. If the patient is dehydrated, a drop in BP can be even more profound. Initiation of fluids prior to vasopressor therapy will make the medication more effective.

> ### NURSING ALERT
>
> *The nurse must monitor the pulse and heart rate in a patient in whom MV has been started. A drop in BP and an increase in heart rate can indicate decreased cardiac output. A fluid challenge will help bring the patient's blood pressure back to baseline and prevent hypovolemic shock. If fluids do not bring up the blood pressure, administration of pressors may be initiated.*

Stress Ulcers

Being placed on MV is a very stressful event for the patient. The stress response involves producing epinephrine, which causes increased stomach acid production.

Patients can develop stress ulcers unless placed on prophylactic medications to prevent ulcers.

Ventilator Dyssynchrony

The experience of being intubated and placed on a mechanical ventilator with loss of respiratory control causes many patients to fight these uncomfortable conditions. Catecholamines are liberated when patients struggle, which causes the vital signs to elevate, increasing the work of breathing and therefore metabolism and oxygen demand. To decrease the energy expenditure and decrease metabolism, patients may need antianxiety medications like benzodiapezenes (Versed or Ativan). Diprivan (Propofol), a short-acting IV drip general anesthetic agent, can also be used to help with rapid sedation. If the results of this do not decrease the work of breathing, the patient may be chemically paralyzed with neuromuscular blockers.

NURSING ALERT

Neuromuscular blockers do not cross the blood-brain barrier, so although patients may look at peace and restful, they can feel pain and discomfort. Therefore, a strong pain medication like morphine sulfate should be administered to aid in comfort and alleviate distress.

APPLYING IT

The MV patient you are caring for suddenly appears to be in distress. You note the heart rate increasing alarmingly and the blood pressure falling dangerously low. You see neck veins distending, and breath sounds on the right side are markedly diminished from your last assessment. The trachea is deviated to the left. What do you think is happening? What would be your FIRST nursing action?

ANSWER

When there is unrelieved pressure that develops from a pneumothorax, the mediastinum is freely moveable. Pressure builds up on the affected side and pushes the trachea away from it. Because the heart and great vessels are kinked, no blood flow can enter the heart. This is the cause of the decreased breath sounds, elevated neck veins, and shock (HR up and BP down) this patient is experiencing. These are classic signs of a tension pneumothorax and you must act quickly. Take this patient off the ventilator and support him with the bag-valve mask (BVM); call a Code Blue. He needs emergency decompression of this pressure and a chest tube will probably be inserted.

Inadequate Nutrition

Patients receiving MV cannot eat because of the ETT or tracheostomy. Due to increased caloric needs to support their work of breathing, they need to have supplemental nutrition. In the short term this is usually done by feedings introduced through a nasogastric tube or small-bore feeding tube. Every effort must be made to insure safe feedings by limiting the volume initially and slowly increasing the volume and rate as well as checking for residual feedings to prevent gastric overfilling. If the patient is severely malnourished, hyperalimentation via intravenous lines may be started.

Nursing Interventions for the Weaning Patient

Once the patient can start breathing on his or her own and the reason for MV has been resolved, the health care team may decide to wean the patient. Weaning is not always done as in the case of a patient recovering from surgery. If the patient is breathing spontaneously, awake, and able to follow commands and vital signs are normal, the patient is extubated without a weaning period. Weaning is an organized trial that follows a pattern where the patient is allowed to breathe spontaneously for longer and longer periods of time until the patient is able to breathe on his or her own and is taken off MV.

To safely wean a patient, baseline vital signs and hemodynamics should be recorded, if available. Baseline PFTs like a vital capacity and tidal volumes need to be taken. Then the patient is either placed on synchronized intermittent mandatory ventilation (SIMV) with pressure support, CPAP, or a trial on a T piece. Weaning done using the first two methods is safer as the patient is still attached to the ventilator and alarms can warn the nurse of impending respiratory failure. Weaning the patient on a T piece involves disconnecting the patient from the ventilator and attaching the patient to an oxygen delivery system via a short T-shaped connector. Either way, the patient is monitored continuously and if respiratory fatigue occurs, the patient is placed back on MV. Every effort to physically and psychologically support the patient during this time is critical.

Commonly Used Respiratory Medications in Critical Care for the Patient on MV

❻ There are many medications that can be used in the care of the patient on MV. The following will detail those most frequently used for control and comfort of the patient. These medications include morphine, fentanyl, Diprivan, benzodiazepines, and paralytics.

Morphine Sulfate

Morphine sulfate is a strong opioid that has been the gold standard for pain medication control. In the critical care environment, it is used for its rapid action of depressing the patient's respirations and allowing the patient to breathe comfortably. This medication can be given IV or as a continuous drip. Because morphine can cause histamine release and resultant vasodilatation and hypotension, assessment of the patient's hemodynamic response to this medication, pain, and SaO_2 should be measured when using this therapy.

Fentanyl (Sublimaze)

Fentanyl is another opioid that has the advantages of being more potent, working faster, and having a shorter duration than morphine. It also does not have the hypotensive effects that morphine has and is safe to use in patients with renal dysfunction and allergies to morphine. Assessment of the patient's hemodynamic status as well as respiratory effort and pain response are needed when using this drug.

Diprivan (Propofol)

This short-acting general anesthetic agent is used when sedation is needed quickly and rapid metabolism is needed to assess neurologic status or readiness to wean. This should be administered through a large IV as it can result in uncomfortable burning or stinging at the administration site. The dose should be reduced daily to assess the patient's neurological and respiratory status. Analgesic agents must be added to this therapy as it does not affect pain perception. Because it is an excellent medium for infection, IV bottles and tubing must be changed every 12 hours after opening. Monitor the patient for hypotension and triglyceride levels when administering this infusion.

Benzodiazepines

Benzodiazepines have many uses, but in the critical care environment you will see them used to decrease ventilator and procedural anxieties. Commonly used benzodiazepines include alprazolam (Xanax), lorazepam (Ativan), midazolam (Versed), and diazepam (Valium). These drugs can be given IV in the case of patient intubation. The side effects to look for include sedation, dizziness, headache, dry mucous membranes, and blurred vision. Overdose with benzodiazepines can be managed with IV flumazenil (Romazicon).

Paralytics (Neuromuscular Blocking Agents)

Neuromuscular blocking agents (NMBAs) are frequently used in the critical care areas to block the transmission of impulses at the myoneural junction (see Table 2–9). These agents all decrease voluntary muscular activity and chest wall movement during breathing. Their most frequent use is when a patient is not breathing synchronously with the MV. The desired effect is to keep neuromuscular blockade in the 80% to 90% range to allow for fewer side effects of these medications. NMBAs may be monitored by peripheral nerve stimulators (PNSs). The nurse must be aware that although NMBAs block nerve transmission, the patient can still hear, feel, and sense what is going on about him or her. Therefore, concomitant administration of antianxiety medications as well as analgesics is imperative.

TABLE 2–9 Types of Neuromuscular Blocking and Musculoskeletal Relaxants	
Vecuronium bromide	Norcuron
Pancuronium bromide	Pavulon
Cisatracurium besylate	Nimbex
Succinylcholine chloride	Anectine

> **NURSING ALERT**
>
> *Even though a patient cannot respond and may appear to be unconscious, the patient can hear, feel, and sense what is going on around him or her. Therefore, the nurse MUST administer either analgesics AND/OR antianxiety medications on a round-the-clock basis when the patient is on an NMBA and Diprivan. All health care members must also be aware that the patient can hear and feel everything that goes on around the bedside.*

Respiratory Conditions Requiring Critical Care

Acute Respiratory Failure (ARF)

What Went Wrong?

ARF is a state where the body fails to maintain adequate gas exchange. There are two types: Type I and Type II. In Type I ARF, the patient has a low oxygen level (hypoxia) and a normal carbon dioxide level. In Type II, there is hypoxia again, but the carbon dioxide level is high (hypercarbia). Hypoxia results in less oxygenated blood traveling to the left side of the heart (shunting). This condition is a major cause of organ failure and death in the critical care areas. ARF can be caused by pulmonary and nonpulmonary conditions.

Common pulmonary conditions include

Pneumonia, lung tumors, cardiac and noncardiac pulmonary edema, chronic obstructive pulmonary disease, and airways obstructions

Nonpulmonary conditions that result in ARF include

Pneumothorax, pleural effusions, neuromuscular disorders (myasthenia gravis, poliomyelitis), periperheral and spinal problems (tetanus, trauma), and central nervous system problems (head trauma and drug overdose)

Prognosis

Mortality rates vary but most include an almost 50% mortality rate for those admitted to the intensive care unit with this diagnosis. This medical problem results in lengths of stay longer than a week in the ICU.

Hallmark Signs and Symptoms

Early

Neurologic changes: restlessness, agitation, confusion, anxiety.

Vital signs will elevate causing tachypnea, tachycardia, and hypertension.

Pulse oximetry will drop below the patient's baseline.

Shortness of breath and dyspnea at rest (most common).

Accessory and intercostal muscle use.

Abnormal breath sounds: crackles, gurgles.

Changes in sputum amount, color, and need for suctioning.

Cardiac dsyrhythmias.

Overall skin pallor.

Late

Neurological changes: lethargy, severe somnolence, coma.

Vital signs drop causing bradypnea, bradycardia, and hypotension.

Cyanosis/mottling and poor respiratory effort.

Cardiac arrest.

Interpreting Test Results

ABGs are examined closely to determine ARF. In a patient with normal baseline ABG values, ARF is diagnosed when the pO_2 is less than 60 mm Hg and the pCO_2 is greater than 45 mm Hg. In patients who are chronic pCO_2 retainers, the pH must also be included in the assessment, with values of less than 7.35 indicating ARF. End tidal CO_2 will also be high.

The chest x-ray will change from clear to white and cloudy (patchy infiltrates) if ARF is due to aspiration, heart failure, or fluid in the chest cavity.

Low hemoglobin and hematocrit values can cause hypoxemia if there is no iron on the hemoglobin molecule to combine with available oxygen.

NURSING ALERT

If a patient is anemic, he or she may never show signs of cyanosis due to the lack of hemoglobin. Hemoglobin combining with carbon dioxide gives the purple tinge to a patient with cyanosis.

Treatment

Early recognition and treatment of the underlying cause

Intubation before the patient is exhausted from breathing

Mechanical ventilation with PEEP and high FiO_2 added if severely hypoxic

Insertion of a nasogastric tube with nutritional support

Insertion of pulmonary artery catheter if fluid and cardiac status uncertain

Red blood cell transfusion if anemic

Medications

   Bicarbonate to correct acidosis according to the ABG values

   Neuromuscular blockade to minimize oxygen demand and allow rest

   Pain control medications if neuromuscular blockade to prevent pain from immobility

   Diuretics like furosemide to remove fluid if heart failure

   Bronchodilators/steroids to dilate airways and decrease inflammation in acute COPD

   Stomach acid blockers to prevent ulcers from stress

Nursing Diagnoses for ARF	Expected Outcomes
Impaired gas exchange	The patient will have a pO_2 that rises and a pCO_2 that drops to baseline
	The patient will have clear chest x-rays
Ineffective breathing pattern	The patient's respirations will be between 16–20 during unassisted breathing
Decreased cardiac output	The patient will have a heart rate within baseline
	The patient will have a stable cardiac rhythm

Nursing Interventions

Continuous vital sign and total body system assessments *as hypoxemia affects all organs.*

Assess daily weights as *they are the most important indicator of fluid status.*

Assess for peripheral edema *as a sign of fluid excess.*

Administer intravenous fluids to rehydrate the patient.

Insert indwelling urinary catheter with hourly intake and output to monitor cardiac/renal function.

Strict intake and output to determine if overhydration/underhydration is occurring.

Frequent position changes to prevent skin breakdown and facilitate oxygen exchange.

Oral care at least once per shift and prn to prevent ventilator-associated pneumonia.

Provide rest by pacing activities to prevent increased oxygen consumption (position changes, chest x-rays, suctioning, and bathing increase O_2 use).

Pneumonia

What Went Wrong?

Pneumonia is caused when pathogenic organisms invade the lung and produce exudate that interferes with oxygen delivery to the alveolus and carbon dioxide removal. Usually a patient's defense mechanisms prevent this from occurring, unless the patient is immunocompromised. Because hypoxemia and hypercarbia result, the patient can develop ARF. Types of pneumonia include ventilator-associated pneumonia (VAP), community acquired pneumonia (CAP), and aspiration pneumonia. VAP and aspiration are hospital-acquired pneumonias (HAPs).

Prognosis

The prevalence of HAP in critical care represents one-quarter of all nosocomial infections. One-half of all antibiotics ordered are for the treatment of HAP. This is a serious infection control issue for the critical care areas. This is also a financial issue for the patient and hospital staff, as Medicare will no longer reimburse for HAP.

Hallmark Signs and Symptoms

Elevated TPR and BP; fever

Chills and diaphoresis

Pleuritic chest pain, myalgia, and joint pain

Copious purulent sputum

Shortness of breath and dyspnea

Hemoptysis

Adventitious breath sounds: crackles (rales), gurgles (rhonchi), wheezes and friction rubs

Interpreting Test Results

There is no agreement or specific criteria for the diagnosis of pneumonia, but most resources include the following:

Positive sputum cultures

Elevated white blood cell counts

Localized chest x-ray infiltrates

Arterial blood gases may indicate respiratory acidosis if sputum obstructs oxygen and carbon dioxide exchange

NURSING ALERT

Although sputum cultures are routinely done on patients with suspected pneumonia, 50% of the time a causative agent is NOT identified. Therefore, a negative sputum does not necessarily indicate that the patient does not have pneumonia.

Treatment

HAP is a major focus in hospitals and especially critical care areas. In order to decrease occurrences, the Institute of Healthcare Improvement has recommended "bundles of care" to help improve patient outcomes. Currently there are four bundles of care in the ventilator bundle. These include

1. Positioning – keep the bed elevated at least 30 degrees, turn and reposition prn.
2. Lifting sedation – allow the patient to come out of paralyzing medications to assess the need for MV.
3. Prevention of gastric ulcers.
4. Prevention of deep vein thrombosis.

Prevention and treatment of HAP also includes:

Oxygen and mechanical ventilation (if ARF occurs)

Frequent and judicious use of hand washing and universal precautions

Antibiotics

Antipyretics to keep the patient's temperature below 101°

Hydration with fluids to reverse dehydration

(See treatment for ARF)

Bronchodilators if airway narrowing occurs

Teaching pulmonary treatments like coughing and deep breathing and incentive spirometry

Nursing Diagnoses	Expected Outcomes
Ineffective airway clearance	The patient will maintain a patient airway
	The frequency of suctioning the patient will decrease
Gas exchange impaired	The patient's ABGs will return to baseline
Hyperthermia	The patient's temperature will return to baseline
Aspiration, risk for	The patient will have clear breath sounds
	The patient's cultures (blood, sputum) will be negative

Nursing Interventions

Monitoring temperature every 2 hours and prn *to determine if infectious process is continuing*

Assessing need and effectiveness of oxygen therapy *to prevent oxygen-related problems*

Strictly enforcing standard precautions, especially the hand washing policy, *to prevent another infection from occurring*

Frequent suctioning if needed *to maintain a patent airway*

Frequent patient positioning *to prevent atelectasis and pooling of secretions*

Teaching pulmonary treatments like coughing and deep breathing and incentive spirometry *to have patient help in care and give sense of power*

(See nursing interventions for ARF)

Status Asthmaticus

What Went Wrong?

Asthma is a chronic condition of airways inflammation. The patient can have bouts of acute attacks where airway closure becomes severe. An acute attack is usually triggered by a known allergen causing an allergic reaction (extrinsic asthma) or an unknown cause usually triggered by a viral or bacterial infection (intrinsic). Attacks can also be precipitated by infection and not taking asthma control medications. Airways inflammation causes narrowing of the air passages resulting in increased work to get oxygen to the alveolar level. As the patient becomes more and more fatigued, hypercarbia and hypoxemia result, leading to a decreased blood supply to the tissues. When a patient has an acute asthmatic attack unrelieved with fast-acting medications, it is called status asthmaticus.

Prognosis

Most patients manage their asthma at home with medications. Life-threatening attacks are rare, but they require immediate medical intervention. Asthma is generally controlled on long-term asthma medications (maintenance) to control inflammation (like steroids), and patients are taught to adjust their medications according to their peak flow meter's daily values.

Hallmark Signs and Symptoms

Asymptomatic between attacks; below may indicate ARF!

Shortness of breath at rest and inability to speak in sentences or phrases

Orthopnea

Changes in the level of responsiveness like lethargy or confusion

Wheezing due to bronchoconstriction is a hallmark sign of airway closure

Absence of wheezing with no airway movement is an ominous symptom!

Bradycardia

Chest tightness

Cough

Signs of ARF

NURSING ALERT

Airways must be open for wheezing to occur. If a patient suddenly stops wheezing and still appears to be in distress, mobilize the rapid response team as the patient has a total airway obstruction. If airways swell enough, emergency endotracheal intubation maybe impossible, making an emergency tracheotomy imperative to open the airway.

Interpreting Test Results

The patient's PEFR meter will indicate a volume of less than 50% baseline.

Little to no response to short-acting bronchodilating agents ordered for the patient's plan of care.

ABGs will indicate hypoxemia with pO_2 less than 50 mm Hg and pCO_2 greater than 50 mm Hg.

SpO_2 will drop below normal levels.

Treatment

Monitor for signs and symptoms of airway obstruction *as airway closure can occur.*

Give oxygen therapy *to maintain pO_2 greater than 50 to make more O_2 available to alveoli.*

Consider early intubation if unresponsive to medications and condition worsens.

Prepare for emergency tracheostomy if patient suddenly has no airflow (silent chest).

Administer rapid-acting beta2-agonist via nebulizer to open airways.

Administer inhaled anticholinergics to relieve bronchospasm.

Administer systemic corticosteroids orally or IV to reverse airway inflammation.

Nursing Diagnoses	Expected Outcomes
Ineffective breathing pattern	The patient will have clear breath sounds
	The respiratory pattern will be within expected range for the patient

Nursing Interventions

Assess the need for advanced airway techniques.

Monitor rate, rhythm, depth, chest wall movement, and effort of respirations.

Facilitate patency of airway by positioning, suctioning, and intubation, if necessary.

Encourage hydration to help clear mucus in airways.

Monitor the effect of medication on the patient to determine when to withdraw therapy.

Teach patient relaxation techniques to decrease the work of breathing.

Teach how to cough effectively to prevent atelectasis.

Evaluate the effectiveness of rapid-acting medications.

Reassure patient during times of respiratory distress.

Acute Lung Injury (ALI)

See Chapter 6 (Care of the Traumatized Patient).

Acute Respiratory Distress Syndrome (ARDS)

What Went Wrong?

ARDS is a condition that generally comes after acute direct or indirect lung injury. Direct lung injury occurs when the lung tissue itself is affected and can include aspiration, pneumonia, fat embolism, near drowning, oxygen toxicity, pulmonary contusion, and toxic inhalation. Indirect lung injury is a result of sequelae from other insults in the body. These types of lung injury include anaphylaxis, disseminated intravascular coagulation, embolism, excessive blood transfusions, hypotension from cardiac arrest or shock/sepsis, drug overdose, long bone or pelvic fractures, and pancreatitis.

ARDS is characterized by worsening respiratory failure despite aggressive oxygen therapy. The release of inflammatory mediators allows fluid to translocate into the lungs, causing a noncardiogenic pulmonary edema. Increased fluid causes the lungs to become stiff and noncompliant, making the work of breathing more difficult for the patient. Pulmonary edema interferes with allowing carbon dioxide to be excreted (hypercarbia) and oxygen to be absorbed (hypoxemia). Increased capillary pressure can cause pulmonary hypertension leading to atelectasis and a reduction in functioning lung volumes. Ultimately this leads to blood leaving the lungs with a decrease in oxygen that is pumped by the left side of the heart to the tissues (shunting).

Prognosis

Around 150,000 cases occur each year and around half occur within the first 24 hours of hospital admission after a direct or indirect lung assault. Chronic health conditions can predispose a patient to develop ARDS like chronic lung disease and alcoholism. Inflammatory responses that are activated do not spare other organs, and multiple organ dysfunction can result from hypoxemia.

A patient who survives ARDS usually has residual lung damage that can lead to disability in activities.

Hallmark Signs and Symptoms

Changes in the level of responsiveness; restlessness and disorientation

Increasing dyspnea

Progressive lung sound changes from crackles to gurgles to bronchial breath sounds

Tachypnea and increase in accessory muscle use to breathe

Elevated central venous pressures but low to normal pulmonary capillary wedge pressures

Interpreting Test Results

Initially, respiratory alkalosis may occur as carbon dioxide has no problems diffusing.

Worsening hypoxemia despite increasing the patient's oxygenation.

Metabolic acidosis with lactic acidosis.

Chest x-rays show bilateral patchy infiltrates that have "ground glass appearance."

A hallmark is the changing of lungs from the normal black color to complete whiteout bilaterally.

PFTs decrease.

Peak inspiratory pressures rise on the ventilator, indicating decreased compliance.

Treatment

The best treatment is to initiate PEEP after mechanical ventilation.

Administration of broad-spectrum antibiotic if ARDS is due to sepsis.

Administration of corticosteroids is controversial but helpful in many cases.

Administration of Nipride to help decrease pulmonary hypertension.

Administration of continuous sedation to assist with ventilatory synchrony.

Therapeutic paralysis may be required.

Nutritional support with 35 to 45 kcal/kg per day.

Comfort and pain control.

Nursing Diagnoses	Expected Outcomes
Gas exchange impaired	The patients ABGs will return to baseline with specific watch over the pO_2
Decreased cardiac output	The patient's BP, HR, and pulmonary artery pressures will remain within normal limits after institution of PEEP therapy
Communication, verbal impaired	The patient will be assisted in making needs known by signing, writing, or other communication aids

Nursing Interventions

Assess for complications of PEEP, barotraumas, and pneumothorax to prevent complications.

Assess for signs of increasing oxygenation in SaO_2 and PaO_2 for further interventions.

Monitoring fluid management unless ARDS is due to shock.

Prone positioning using a Stryker frame; extra help or other turning devices help increase secretion removal and prevent atelectasis.

Monitor carbohydrate concentration of enteral fluids; they may increase pCO_2 retention.

Provide and monitor use of continuous sedatives and analgesics to help decrease the work of breathing.

APPLYING IT

❽ Jane Wallace is a 17-year-old high school student who was dropped off in front of her house after drinking at a weekend party. She passed out on the way to her front door and the newspaper boy found her blue and breathing shallowly in a snow bank 5 hours later. He initiated CPR after calling 911 on his cell phone.

She was successfully resuscitated in the ECU after the emergency crew initiated defibrillation and CPR at the scene. She was in ventricular fibrillation and required partial cardiopulmonary bypass to slowly warm her and convert her to a normal sinus rhythm.

You are caring for her two days post incident in the ICU. She remains on MV with an ETT on 50% oxygen with a V_T of 500 with a rate of 18, N FiO_2 of 50% on IMV. Suddenly you note pressures on the MV start to trip off the high alarm. When you suction Jane, you see that her clear secretions have changed to blood-tinged sputum from the ETT. You also note that she is in a sinus tachycardia and has an elevated BP of 150/90. A stat chest x-ray shows she has cloudy white infiltrates throughout both lung fields. ABGs are pH 7.30, pCO_2 50, pO_2 60, HCO_3 24. What do you think is happening to Jane?

✔ ANSWER

Jane was in a cardiac arrest for an undetermined period of time, which might have led to substances being released in her body to allow noncardiogenic pulmonary edema to occur. This is also based upon her worsening VS status (tachycardia, hypertension), the decreased lung compliance (signified by the alarms and hemoptysis), and whiteout appearance of her chest x-ray. Her ABGs indicate an uncompensated respiratory acidosis with severe hypoxemia. She has all the classic signs of ARDS.

Pneumothorax

What Went Wrong?

A pneumothorax is a condition where there is partial or total collapse of a lung. Conditions that cause pneumothorax include chest surgery, a buildup of tumor fluid from cancer, MV, and chest trauma. When a lung partially collapses, alveoli in the areas of collapse can not perform oxygenation; therefore, hypoxemia and hypercarbia result. The higher the percentage of pneumothorax as determined by chest x-ray, the worsening of the ventilation problems.

Prognosis

The prognosis for recovery from a pneumothorax is excellent, but catching it in time is key to the outcome. So be keenly cognizant that any patient with a pulmonary problem or on MV can develop this at any time.

Hallmark Signs and Symptoms

Elevated temperature if from empyema or malignant pleural effusion (lung fluid)

Fatigue

Cough

Pleuritic chest pain

Decreased or absence of breath sounds in the area of the pneumothorax

Dull or flat sound when percussed

Possible pleural friction rub

Interpreting Test Results

Chest x-ray (color will be blacker than black), computed tomography (CT), or ultrasound will indicate presence of fluid buildup causing a pneumothorax.

ABGs will indicate a respiratory alkalosis if the patient is in the early stages and a respiratory acidosis if the patient develops hypercarbia (later).

Treatment

Administer supplemental oxygen with a watchful eye on the SaO_2 (pulse oximetry).

Control the patient's pain.

Decompress the pneumothorax with a chest tube or temporary one-way valve or thoracentesis.

Determine the cause of the pneumothorax.

Nursing Diagnoses	Expected Outcomes
Gas exchange impaired	The patient's ABGs will return to baseline with specific watch over the pO_2
Decreased cardiac output	The patient's BP, HR, and pulmonary artery pressures will remain within normal limits after institution of PEEP therapy
Pain, acute	The patient will report a +2 level of pain after administering morphine

Nursing Interventions

Assess the patient's vital signs and SaO_2 frequently *to see if the patient is progressing or developing complications.*

Assess chest wall movement and breath sounds *as movement decreases on the affected side and breath sounds become diminished or absent.*

Assess the level of pain using a visual analogue or quantitative scale to see if therapy is effective.

Assist with thoracentesis or insertion of chest drainage tube to remove air/ fluid and reestablish negative pressure in the lungs.

Administer pain medications with an eye to the respiratory rate. Most pain medications that the patient needs, like morphine sulfate, also decrease the respiratory effort.

How to Do It—Assisting With a Thoracentesis

1. Observe for a health care provider's order and signed consent form.

2. Make sure that time is taken to verify the identity of the patient and the procedure to be performed (time out).

3. Premedicate the patient.

4. Teach the patient what will happen during the procedure.

5. Order supplies, which generally include a sterile tray with scalpel, tubing with three-way stopcock, and specimen tubes. Bring into the site analgesic and bottles into which the lung exudate will flow.

6. Prepare an over-the-bed table with a pillow for patient comfort.

7. Perform baseline vital signs and SaO_2; auscultate lung fields.

8. Monitor the sterile field during the procedure and support the patient.

9. Keep the specimen tubes in a secure area to be sent to the laboratory in a biohazard bag when the procedure is completed.

10. Keeping the physicians' field sterile, attach the tubing from the needle and three-way stopcock to the large drainage bottles if large quantities of exudate are to be removed.

11. Assist the physician with occlusive covering of the site with a sterile dressing after the procedure is completed.

12. Monitor vital signs, SaO_2, lung sounds, and insertion site for bleeding post procedure, according to hospital protocol. Palpate the site for crepitus.

13. Document the color, amount, and consistency of exudate removed and patient tolerance to the procedure.

14. Clear the area, send specimens to the laboratory, and remove drainage tubes to biohazard areas.

❼ How to Do It–Assisting With a Chest Tube Insertion

1. Observe for a health care provider's order and signed consent form.

2. Premedicate the patient.

3. Teach what will happen during the procedure.

4. Obtain supplies, which generally include chest tube insertion tray, site analgesic, chest tubes, NSS (Normal Saline Solution) (if not using a prefilled system), petroleum-impregnated gauze, chest tube clamps, and chest tube catheters.

5. Perform baseline vital signs and SaO_2; auscultate lung fields.

6. Monitor the sterile field and support the patient.

7. Set up the chest tube according to manufacturer's guidelines; this may include pouring NSS into the water seal to the "fill level" and suction control chamber to the amount of suction ordered.

8. Attach the suction control port to long tubing to wall suction. Turn the wall suction up until the suction control chamber gently bubbles.

9. Prepare the long patient tubing to attach to the chest tube catheter once the physician has the tube in place. Tape according to hospital policy.

10. Assist the physician in placing a sterile dressing over the insertion site once the tube is in place.

11. Make sure a chest x-ray is completed after the chest tube is in place.

12. Monitor the site for bleeding and crepitus after the procedure and perform vital signs as per institutional protocol.

13. Ongoing care of chest tubes includes
    a. Monitoring the insertion site for bleeding, crepitus, and infection at the beginning of the shift and prn.
    b. Observing the amount, clotting, and color of exudate in the tubing and drainage unit.
    c. Keeping the tubes unkinked and below the level of the patient.
    d. Observing the water seal chamber for fluctuation and degree of air leak if a pneumothorax is present.

e. Observing that the water seal has no bubbling if there is no pneumothorax. Bubbling in the water seal when there is no pneumothorax could indicate a leak in the system or in the patient.

f. Checking and maintaining the depth of the water if a suction control chamber is included with the unit. Some systems have dry suction where a suction control chamber is absent.

g. Keeping a petroleum gauze dressing and shodded clamps at the bedside in case of accidental disconnection and troubleshooting.

Lung Cancer/Surgery

What Went Wrong?

Lung cancer is one of the most malignant and lethal of all cancers. Cancer patients with this condition may be admitted to the intensive care unit on a ventilator due to ARF or after lung surgeries. Lung surgery is also done to remove diseased portions of a lung (wedge resection, segmental resection) or the entire lung (pneumonectomy) (see Table 2–10).

Prognosis

Prognosis is good if lung cancers are found early, but many times, since alveoli have no pain receptors, cancers can become very advanced before the patient exhibits symptoms.

TABLE 2–10 Types of Lung Surgeries

Laser surgery	A palliative measure used to shrink a tumor that is pressing on a vital structure or that is not operable.
Wedge resection	Small area near the lung surface removed using stapling devices. Generally well tolerated as it is usually a small area.
Segmental resection	One or more segments of the lungs are removed (a bronchiole and its alveoli). Remaining lung tissue expands and fills this potential space.
Lobectomy	Entire lobe of the lung is removed through a thoracotomy.
Pneumonectomy	Removal of the entire lung. Chest tube not usually present. No lung to reexpand. Empty side to fill in with exudate so tracheal shift will not occur. Balloons or implants can be used to prevent shifting.

Signs and Symptoms

Warning signals of cancer include

Hoarseness

Fever and unexplained weight loss

Fatigue

Hemoptysis

Persistent cough

Recurring pneumonias, pleural effusions, or bronchitis

Interpreting Test Results

There are many diagnostic tests that confirm the presence of lung cancer. These include

Chest x-rays

Bronchoscopy with lung biopsy

Mediastinoscopy

Thoracotomy

Treatment

Treatment for this condition includes

Radiation therapy

Chemotherapy

Surgical procedures

Nursing Diagnoses	Expected Outcomes
Gas exchange impaired	The patient's ABGs will return to baseline with specific watch over the pO_2
Pain, acute	The patient will report a +2 level of pain after administering opiates/analgesics
Infection, risk for	The patient will have a normal temperature
	The patient will have clear sputum
	The patient will have baseline chest x-ray
	The chest incision will be clean, dry, intact

Nursing Interventions

Assess vital signs *to monitor for shock, infection, or hypoxemia.*

Assess respiratory status and laboratory values *to monitor for complications.*

Assess the surgical incision site *to observe for bleeding, infection, or crepitus.*

Position the patient so the good lung is up, *so it can help with lung expansion and not be impeded by working against the weight of the patient and mattress.*

Monitor chest tube *for patency, bleeding, crepitus, and output.*

Administer chemotherapy as needed *to prevent tumor enlargement and metastasis.*

Teach the patient about radiation therapy and its potential side effects, *so the patient knows what is normal/abnormal.*

Teach the patient to cough and deep breathe *to prevent atelectasis.*

Encourage the use of incentive spirometry every hour while awake *to prevent atelectasis.*

CASE STUDY 1

❽ Melissa Black is a 39-year-old asthmatic who has delayed coming into the Emergency Care Unit (ECU). She is cyanotic with markedly diminished breath sounds. She is audibly wheezing and her inhalers are not working. After administering O_2 and getting the bed into a high Fowler's position, an ABG is performed. ABGs indicate the following: pH = 7.29, pCO_2 = 50, pO_2 = 50, HCO_3 = 24. Serum electrolytes show the following: Na^+ 145, K^+ 4.0, CL 110, and HCO_3 24.

QUESTIONS: What acid-base disturbance do these ABGs indicate? Does this patient have a normal anion gap? What would your next nursing actions be?

CASE STUDY 2

❽ Mrs. F. M. is a spry 71-year-old retired nurse who served in Vietnam. She is admitted with a diagnosis of COPD, acute respiratory distress and relates a 50-year history of smoking two packs of cigarettes per day. During the past week, Mrs. F. M. states she has had flu-like symptoms such as fever; chills; a productive cough with thick, brown purulent sputum; and chest pain when coughing. Mrs. F. M. appears anxious and irritable, taking rapid, shallow breaths while breathing through her mouth. She is also diaphoretic and has marked cyanosis around her lips. Auscultation reveals moist crackles throughout both left and right lung fields.

A chest x-ray shows lung infiltrates, and a sputum specimen contained numerous gram-positive diplococci. Baseline vital signs are T = 101°, pulse rate = 114, respiratory rate = 28, BP = 120/70. O_2 saturation is 88%. Baseline arterial blood gas values on a 50% nonrebreather mask are pH = 7.30, PCO_2 = 60 mm Hg, PaO_2 = 50 mm Hg, HCO_3 = 18 mEq/L.

QUESTIONS

1. Identify the most important things to include in your assessment.
2. Which assessment findings are of particular concern to the nurse?
3. Is the current oxygen delivery system appropriate for Mrs. FM?
4. What is a sputum culture and sensitivity test and what do Mrs. FM's results show?
5. What general information can be obtained from a chest x-ray and what do her results indicate?

CASE STUDY 3

8 Your patient is recovering from a pneumonectomy. During your second post-op check, you note that the patient's heart rate respirations and blood pressure are trending upward. His temperature is normal. He is starting to sweat slightly and his urinary output was only 15 mL/hr the last check. What might be happening? What would be your next action?

Give psychological support for a potentially lethal disease process.

REVIEW QUESTIONS

1. **A nurse is caring for a patient and hears the physician state that the patient's lung compliance has decreased. The nurse understands that decreased lung compliance indicates**

   A. Air will move more easily into the alveoli.

   B. The work of breathing will be reduced in this patient.

   C. A greater expiratory effort will be needed for this patient to exhale.

   D. A greater inspiratory effort will be needed to get air into the alveoli.

2. **The nurse is assessing a patient at risk for developing acute respiratory distress syndrome (ARDS). The nurse would assign the highest risk value for which of the following patients? The patient**

   A. Post open-heart surgery

   B. With a chest tube

   C. Who has aspirated gastric stomach contents

   D. Post motor vehicle accident (MVA)

3. **A nurse is evaluating a patient post cardiac arrest for acute respiratory distress syndrome (ARDS). The nurse would be evaluating the patient for which of the following early signs and symptoms of ARDS?**

   A. Tachypnea

   B. Hyperventilation

   C. Coma

   D. Decreased peak airway pressures

4. **An experienced nurse is explaining positive end-expiratory pressure (PEEP) to a new critical care nurse. The BEST explanation of this therapy would include**

   A. It will decrease the functional residual capacity (FRC).

   B. It will help decrease cellular oxygenation.

   C. It is used to increase alveolar surface area.

   D. It can be used very effectively to prevent the intubation of a patient with severe hypoxia

5. **To improve patient outcomes and standardize nursing during mechanical ventilation (MV), bundles of ventilator care are recommended by the Institute of Health Care Improvement. Which of the following is included in this protocol?**

   A. Using proton-pump inhibitors to decrease gastric acid secretions

   B. Suctioning the patient every 2 hours to prevent mucous pooling orally

   C. Washing hands before and after performing nursing care to prevent further introduction of pathogens

   D. Keeping the patient sedated for the first 3 days of being mechanically ventilated in the ICU

6. Your patient is ordered oxygen via a rebreather mask. The nurse providing this low-flow oxygen delivery system understands that this method of delivery
   A. Gives the highest FiO_2
   B. Delivers a precise concentration of oxygen
   C. Requires humidity during delivery
   D. Uses a reservoir without flaps on the oxygen mask

7. A 19-year-old male is admitted with a large, spontaneous pneumothorax. He is intubated with an endotracheal tube and placed on a mechanical ventilator. Which physical finding will alert the nurse to a potential problem in respiratory function before a chest x-ray confirms placement?
   A. Dullness to percussion in the third to fifth intercostal spaces, midclavicular line
   B. Decreased paradoxical motion
   C. Louder breath sounds on the right chest
   D. pH of 7.36 in arterial blood gases

8. The signs and symptoms of acute respiratory failure (ARF) can be easily over-looked. Knowing this, the nurse should be observant for which of the following that indicate the early stage of this medical emergency?
   A. Cyanosis and coma
   B. Agitation and confusion
   C. Hypotension and bradycardia
   D. Poor respiratory effort and mottling

9. A nurse is teaching a patient about status asthmaticus. Included in this teaching would be the hallmark symptom of
   A. Gurgles
   B. Pale, lifeless skin
   C. Fainting and low blood pressure
   D. Wheezes

10. A patient is admitted with a pneumothorax of the right lung from a motor ve-hicle accident. During the extrication, it was noted that the systolic blood pres-sure readings fell into the 80s. As the assigned nurse, you recognize the high risk of ARDS in the days following the accident. The diagnosis of ARDS is most readily made when
    A. The patient's pCO_2 drops below 30 mm Hg.
    B. The patient develops a metabolic acidosis.
    C. The patient's pO_2 continues to drop despite increasing the FiO_2.
    D. The patient complains of a headache and substernal chest pain.

ANSWERS

CASE STUDY 1

Uncompensated respiratory acidosis. The pH is below 7.35 indicting you have an acidosis. The pCO_2 is elevated indicating the acidosis is caused by the lungs retaining CO_2. The patient has hypoxemia as the pO_2 is below 80 and it is severe. The HCO_3 level is normal indicating no compensation is being done by the kidneys. The anion gap is normal $(145 + 4) - (110 + 24) = 14$. Prepare to intubate this patient as he has severe acidosis, is severely hypoxic, and is hypercarbic. A nurse might also prepare BiPAP as an alternative to intubation and steroids to help decrease inflammation.

CASE STUDY 2

1. As a critical care nurse, a very comprehensive assessment should be completed without exception and must include the patient's health history; occupation; comfort level; physical, emotional, and respiratory status; medication history; vital signs; and diagnostic results.
2. Since the patient has a diagnosis of COPD, acute respiratory distress, and URI (upper respiratory infection)–flu-like symptoms, the nurse should be very aware of her tachycardia, tachypnea, and rapid shallow breathing. She is febrile. She has moist crackles throughout both lung fields. She is diaphoretic and has marked circumoral cyanosis. SaO_2 is below normal levels especially since she is on a nonrebreather mask at 50%. ABG results should be analyzed (see question 3). She has a moist, productive cough with sputum that is thick and brown. Primary importance is given to maintaining a clear airway and preventing the further compromise of COPD.
3. No! Since the patient has acute respiratory distress, she requires oxygen assistance to carry the desired percentage of oxygen via hemoglobin to the tissues. Her current SaO_2 is 88% on 50% nonrebreather. This is not adequate. She is extremely hypoxic because her oxygen level is below 80%. Her ABGs indicate a combined respiratory and metabolic acidosis. Her pH is below 7.35 and her pCO_2 is above 45, which indicate a respiratory acidosis. Her HCO_3 is below 22, which shows a metabolic acidosis. Larger drops in her pH will result if she is not intubated immediately.
4. A sputum culture is a microbiologic examination of obtained sputum from the patient either through suctioning or the patient's own efforts of producing sputum from a productive cough. It is sent to the laboratory for analysis and diagnosis of infection and to determine if the strain is resistant to certain antibiotics. In this situation, the patient's sputum specimen contained numerous gram-positive diplococci, which will require antibiotic therapy.
5. Chest x-rays are noninvasive studies that are useful to identify blood, air, fluid , infiltrates, foreign bodies, and abnormal lung shadows. The chest x-ray on Mrs. F. M. shows lung infiltrates, which frequently occur if fluid is retained from pneumonia. This in conjunction with her positive sputum culture and her febrile stat could indicate she has pneumonia.

CASE STUDY 3

With the removal of an entire lung (pneumonectomy), there is a chance that the remaining lung can not handle the work of breathing. Because all vital signs are elevated, it can not be shock, as shock will trend the BP downward. This might be early respiratory failure. Do a thorough lung assessment moving through all phases: inspection, palpation, percussion, and auscultation. If protocol allows, get an ABG and a chest x-ray. Also look at the surgical site: Is there bleeding, crepitus, and are the sutures intact? Call the surgeon to let him or her know your findings.

CORRECT ANSWERS AND RATIONALES

1. D. Lung compliance is the ease of distention of the lungs during inspiration. If the patient uses more effort or work of breathing, then compliance of lung tissues have decreased.

2. C. The patient who has aspirated gastric contents might go into shock from aspirating acidic contents. There is no relationship of ARDS to chest tubes, open-heart surgery, or MVAs unless the patient's situation is complicated by shock.

3. A. Tachypnea, tachycardia, and hypertension can all be signs a patient is going into ARDS. But the cardinal sign is a decreasing pO_2 when the FiO_2 is increasing. Hypoventilation and coma are very late signs, and peak airway pressure will increase.

4. C. PEEP expands the alveolar surface area, therefore increasing pO_2 and decreasing pCO_2. PEEP increases the FRC and can only be used after the patient is intubated.

5. A. Although B to D are important in the care of the patient on MV, only A is included in the IHCI ventilator care bundle.

6. D. A rebreather has a reservoir with flaps on the side of the mask that do not open and close with breathing. It delivers less concentration than a nonrebreather, which has flaps on the mask that close during inhalation and open at exhalation. This allows the patient to breathe almost 100% FiO_2 as he or she exhales most of the carbon dioxide and inhales mostly oxygen. A Venturi's mask gives precise concentrations of oxygen. Humidity is given with masks and the highest FiO_2 without MV is delivered by a non-rebreather.

7. C. Louder breath sounds over the right chest wall indicate that the endotracheal tube may be misplaced in the right mainstem bronchus and only one lung is being mechanically ventilated.

8. B. The other signs and symptoms are late. The nurse must catch that agitation and confusion occur first!

9. D. Wheezes are musical sounds produced when the muscles between the upper airway structures constrict. Gurgles are mucus in the upper airways and usually clear with coughing. B and C are unrelated.

10. C. The classic sign of ARDS is a dropping pO_2 and rising pCO_2 in spite of increasing the oxygenation level. A metabolic acidosis might occur but it is not related to the respiratory issues the patient has. Headache and substernal chest pain are not related to ARDS.

chapter 3

Care of the Patient With Critical Cardiac and Vascular Needs

LEARNING OBJECTIVES

At the end of this chapter, the student will be able to:

1 Identify nursing assessment skills needed to assess the cardiovascular (CV) system.

2 Use diagnostic and laboratory procedures to determine CV status.

3 Explain various advanced procedural skills needed for CV assessment.

4 Describe nursing care of patients requiring hemodynamic monitoring.

5 Identify medications commonly used to care for a patient with complex CV needs.

6 Prioritize nursing care needed to safely care for patients with complex medical and surgical conditions.

7 Analyze a given case study of complex medical and surgical CV conditions.

KEY WORDS

AAA – abdominal aortic aneurysm
Angina
BNP – B-natriuretic peptide
Bruit
CABG – coronary artery bypass graft
Cardiac tamponade
Cardiomegaly
CO – cardiac output
ECG – electrocardiogram
Echocardiogram
EF – ejection fraction
Epicardial pacemaker
Gallops
HF – heart failure
Hypertensive crisis
Hypertensive urgency
IABP – intraaortic balloon pump
ICD – implantable cardiac
    defibrillator

Inotropic agent
JVD – jugular venous distention
MAP – mean arterial blood pressure
MI – myocardial infarction
Murmurs
OHS – open-heart surgery
PCI – percutaneous coronary
    intervention
Pericarditis
PMI – point of maximal impulse
PVR – peripheral vascular resistance
Remodeling
Stress test
SV – stroke volume
TEE – transesophageal echocardiogram
Thrills
Transmural infarction
Vasodilator
Vasopressor

Anatomy and Physiology of the Cardiovascular System

Structure and Function of the Cardiovascular System

The heart is the main pumping organ of the body (see Figure 3–1). About the size of a clenched human fist, the heart keeps a person alive through a system of electrical and mechanical activity. The heart is located to the left of center in the chest cavity, behind and protected by the sternum. It is surrounded by a fibrous sac known as the pericardium, pericardium which holds the heart in a fixed position and provides a physical barrier to infection. The outer membranous layer surrounding the heart is the epicardium. A very small amount of pericardial fluid is contained between these two membranes and serves as a lubricant. The next layer, or the myocardium, contains the actual pumping cells of the heart. Inner surfaces of the atria, ventricles, and heart values are known as the endocardium.

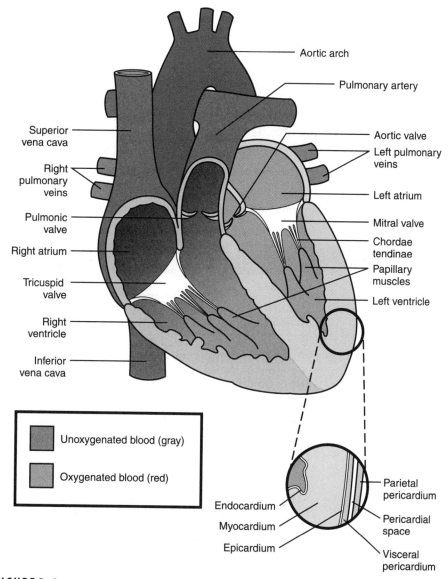

Aortic arch

Pulmonary artery

Superior
vena cava

Aortic valve

Left pulmonary
veins

Right
pulmonary
veins

Left atrium

Pulmonic
valve

Mitral valve

Right atrium

Chordae
tendinae

Tricuspid
valve

Papillary
muscles

Right
ventricle

Left ventricle

Inferior
vena cava

Unoxygenated blood (gray)

Oxygenated blood (red)

Endocardium

Parietal
pericardium

Myocardium

Pericardial
space

Epicardium

Visceral
pericardium

FIGURE 3–1 • Structure of the heart.

The heart consists of four chambers, the left and right atria and the left and right ventricles. The atria receive blood from the vena cava and pulmonary arteries and pump this blood into the ventricles. The ventricles are the main pumping forces of the heart. The right ventricle pumps blood into the pulmonary circulation. The left ventricle forcefully ejects blood into the aorta and arterial circulation.

Pulmonary circulation begins at the pulmonary artery, which receives venous blood from the right ventricle. The pulmonary artery divides into the left and right main stem branches. Oxygenated blood returns to the left side of the heart through the pulmonary veins.

Four cardiac valves exist to allow blood to flow in only one direction. The two AV (atrioventricular valves) prevent the backflow of blood into the atria during ventricular contraction. These AV valves are the tricuspid and mitral valves. The semilunar valves, or the pulmonic and aortic valves, open during systole, allowing blood to flow out of the ventricles. These valves will then close to prevent blood regurgitation back into the ventricles.

Next, consider the cardiac conduction system components in Table 3–1.

TABLE 3–1 Cardiac Conduction System Components

Components	Function	Rate
SA or sinoatrial node	Natural pacemaker of the heart, which sends off the initial electrical impulses to the atria	60–100
AV or atrioventricular node	Conducts electrical impulses initiated in the atria along to the ventricles	40–60
Bundle of His	Electrical impulses from the ventricles continue to be conducted through these firing areas. The Bundle of His divides into the right and left bundle branches several centimeters from the AV node.	Does not usually function as a pacemaker cell
Left and right bundle branches	The left bundle branch has two divisions and is thicker than the right bundle branch. The right and left bundle branches eventually divide into the Purkinje fibers.	Does not usually function as a pacemaker cell
Purkinje fibers	The Purkinje fibers have the fastest conduction rate within the entire heart muscle. They see to it that all cells depolarize.	< 40

The heart's electrical conduction system is very much like a train. Consider the train enclosed and protected within the train station, just as the heart is enclosed and protected within the structures of the chest cavity, the pericardium. As the train engine is ignited by the firing impulses of its battery, the sinoatrial (SA) node of the heart transmits its initial electrical impulses to the atria. As the train begins to move and gain speed, it is further conducted along and encouraged by electrical charges to its engine. In the heart, electrical impulses are conducted from the atria to the ventricles. The train increases its momentum with additional electrical conduction. In the heart, electrical impulses from the ventricles travel along through the Bundle of His and the Purkinje fibers to create ventricular systole and diastole. The railroad tracks diverge into many directions, as does the vascular system. The vascular system, which is composed of numerous capillaries, veins and arteries, will receive its precious cargo of oxygenated blood from the pulmonary circulation and direct it throughout the body or to the systemic circulation. The train has completed its intricate route of reaching designated circulatory destinations as has the heart.

It is crucial to remember that the heart structures are supplied with oxygenated blood through the coronary arteries. This oxygenated blood then travels to the general circulation via the coronary veins. See Figure 3–2, Nervous Conduction System.

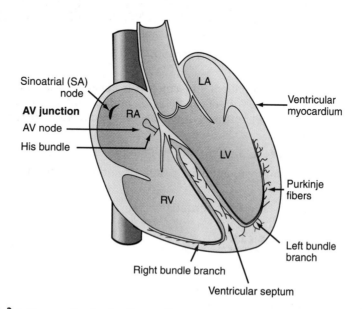

FIGURE 3–2 • Nervous Conduction System. (Reproduced, with permission, from Fauci AS et al. *Harrison's Principles of Internal Medicine*, 17th ed. McGraw-Hill, 2008.)

Assessment Skills

❶ The development of cardiac problems within the individual is very traumatic and anxiety provoking. Information pertaining to the cardiovascular system will enable the critical care nurse to provide the delivery of more thorough and comprehensive nursing care to the patient.

Again, nurse proficiency is required in the mental, emotional, and physical assessment of the individual suffering from cardiovascular issues. Strength in assessment skills and techniques will guide patient care, stabilize the patient's condition, and prevent additional cardiovascular deterioration.

History and Interview

This portion of assessment should be conducted in a nonthreatening and non-intimidating manner. The patient's presenting symptoms and complaints need to be explored using an organized framework. If the patient is experiencing active chest pain, the OPQRST organized assessment can be used so the critical care nurse is consistent and comprehensive (see Table 3–2). The OPQRST is helpful when the assessment needs to be rapid.

TABLE 3–2 OPQRST Pain Assessment	
Onset	Sudden, sometimes predictable.
Precipitating factor	Stress, exercise, or exertion.
Quality	Frequently patient's discomfort is heavy, viselike, crushing, or squeezing. Women, the elderly, and patients with diabetes may have shortness of breath, mild indigestion. May be silent.
Radiation	Poorly localized but may radiate to neck, jaw, and down arms
Severity	Discomfort to agonizing pain. Have the patient rate on a scale of 1–10.
Timing	Comes and ends abruptly. Usually responds to rest, oxygen, and nitroglycerin. Time of day when it occurs (day/night/after a heavy meal).

The nurse should ask if the pain is like any other the patient has experienced and what the patient did to relieve the pain or discomfort. Other associated symptoms such as dyspnea or shortness of breath going up and down stairs along with dizziness, extreme sweating, or diaphoresis should be noted. The nurse should also ask about the patient's diet, medication, alcohol, tobacco use, and occupational history. Determine if the patient's lifestyle is active or sedentary. A one-word response of "retired" needs further clarification by asking what the person did and what do they do now.

The patient's history, if accurately obtained, will provide substantial clues as to the onset of debilitating cardiovascular problems. If patients are emotionally distraught or in denial about recent changes in their health status, the nurse should allow them some space and quiet time to compose themselves for a few minutes prior to seeking and eliciting additional information, for example, a family history of heart disease: "My father and both brothers all died of massive heart attacks at the age of 69."

Inspection

The critical care nurse can initially garner a wealth of information by simply observing the patient's attitude, body posture, facial expressions, weight, and skin color. If the patient appears obese or overweight, this condition could suggest a cardiac risk factor. Facial expressions alone can indicate apprehension or pain, as well as lethargy, alertness, or confusion.

The skin should be assessed for color, temperature, and asymmetry. Skin color such as pallor or cyanosis is an important indicator of poor cardiac perfusion. Skin condition such as dry, scaly, cracked, shiny, tented turgor, and absence of hair growth are indicative or poor peripheral circulation. Skin temperature such as warm, cool, hot, or redness can indicate secondary complications like poor circulation and infection. Look for signs of bruising, scars, and wounds over the body. A bulge over the chest wall could signify a pacemaker or implantable cardiac defibrillator (ICD).

Systematically assess the patient for signs of edema, alterations in fluid and nutritional status, and cyanosis of the lips, conjunctiva, mucous membranes, and nail beds. Assess for "clubbing" of the nail beds, which was described in Chapter 2 as a sign of chronic hypoxia.

Body posture and position will give an indication of the effort the patient is using to breathe easier or to relieve discomfort. Respiratory rate, pattern, and effort should also be observed and recorded.

The only normal pulsation visualized on the chest wall is the apical impulse, also referred to as the PMI or point of maximal impulse. It is a quick, localized, outward movement located lateral to the left midclavicular line at the 5th intercostal space (ICS). If this pulsation is visible, describe its location, size, and character.

An abnormal pulsation that can be seen on inspection of the neck is jugular venous distention (JVD). With the patient lying supine and the head elevated 30 to 45 degrees, you should not see visible pulsation at the side of the neck. JVD is a response to increased intrathoracic pressure during the Valsalva maneuver and can temporarily be seen normally when a weightlifter bears down while lifting weights. If you see visible pulsations that occur above the jaw line, this might indicate an increase in circulating volume to the right side of the heart, which can be caused by right-sided heart failure.

NURSING ALERT

Inspect the jugular veins for pulsations and distention, which might be apparent and indicative of right-sided cardiac failure.

Inspection of the valvular areas requires that the nurse know where these valves are located. Once the nurse knows where these are, she or he can use the same areas on auscultation of these valves (see Table 3–3).

TABLE 3–3 Locations of the Heart Valves

Valve	Location
Aortic	2nd ICS (intercostal space) to right of sternum. Only region heart sounds heard to right of sternum.
Pulmonic	2nd ICS, to the left of the sternum. Right across from the aortic area.
Tricuspid	4th ICS to the left of the sternum, 4th intercostal space
Mitral	5th ICS, MCL (midclavicular line); PMI

The PMI may be seen in thin-chest-walled patients and is normal to see. All other pulsations in the chest are considered abnormal and might be due to valvular changes in the heart or heart enlargement (cardiomegaly).

Palpation

This assessment skill is best achieved by the nurse using a light sense of touch and a relaxed, unhurried approach. Palpation is used to assess pulsations in the neck, thorax, abdomen, and extremities. It is also used to assess skin turgor, capillary refill, temperature of the skin, and the presence and amount of edema (using the scale of 0 to +4). Pulse strength and volume is usually graded on a scale of 0 to +3) and includes the bilateral assessment of the following arteries: carotid, brachial, radial, ulnar, popliteal, dorsalis pedis, posterior tibial, and femoral.

NURSING ALERT

An abnormal tremor or vibration felt on palpation in the lower left abdominal area is known as a thrill and can indicate a cardiac murmur or abdominal aortic aneurysm.

NURSING ALERT

Use the pads of the fingers to assess pulse function. Never assess the carotid pulses simultaneously because doing so will obstruct oxygenated blood flow to the brain, especially if these arteries are compromised by arteriosclerosis or plaque.

Use a systematic approach when palpating areas of the patient's body. It is recommended that the nurse first locate the PMI, which represents where the apical pulse is most readily felt and is very reliable in determining the size and functioning of the left ventricle, which corresponds with the actual apex of the heart.

Applying pressure to the nail beds of the upper and lower extremities determines the status of capillary refill. Signs of pitting and nonpitting edema can be can be seen and felt not only in the feet and ankles, but also in the shins, sacrum, and abdomen.

NURSING ALERT

A patient with cardiac failure can gain as much as 10 or more pounds of excess body fluid before pitting edema becomes recognizable.

Percussion

Generally, and with good reason, this assessment technique is omitted when caring for the cardiovascular patient. If assessment is needed a chest x-ray provides the necessary data for cardiac enlargement (cardiomegaly).

Auscultation

Normal and abnormal heart sounds, bruits, and murmurs can be detected using the assessment skill of auscultation. Normal heart sounds are referred to as S1 and S2.

Normal Heart Sounds

The first heart sound, or S1, is the single sound (lub) produced when the mitral and tricuspid valves close. The second heart sound or S2 (dub) is heard loudest as the semilunar valves close (see Table 3–4).

NURSING ALERT

Both S1 and S2 are high-pitched and are heard best using the diaphragm of the stethoscope.

TABLE 3–4 The Two Normal Heart Sounds

	S1	S2
Sound	Lub	Dub
Heart cycle	Systole	Diastole
Location	Apex	Base
Closure	Mitral/tricuspid valves	Aortic/pulmonic

Abnormal Heart Sounds

Abnormal heart sounds are referred to as S3 and S4 or "gallops" when auscultated during tachycardia. They are low-pitched ventricular filling sounds that can occur during diastole and may be caused by pressure changes, valvular dysfunctions, and conduction deficits. They are referred to as gallops as they sound like the hooves of a galloping horse striking the pavement.

NURSING ALERT

S3 and S4 are best heard by placing the bell of the stethoscope over the PMI. These sounds are rhythmic and mimic a horse galloping when the patient is tachycardic.

The S3 heart sound resembles a dull, low-frequency, thudlike sound, as in ventricular galloping, for example, "lub-dub, lub-dub," or "Kentucky, Kentucky, Kentucky." A finding of S3 is normal in children and young adults and usually disappears by the mid-30s. The finding of an S3 gallop in an older adult can indicate ventricular failure.

The fourth heart sound has a hollow, low-frequency, snappy sound. It is an atrial gallop produced by atrial contractions forcing blood into a noncompliant ventricle that is resistant to filling. The sound increases in intensity during inspiration. It is heard late in diastole prior to the onset of S1 of the next cardiac cycle, and has the rhythm of the word "Tennessee," or "le-lub-dub." An S4 can be normal in an elderly person. It can also been heard in a myocardial infarction (MI) when atria contract forcefully against a distended blood-filled ventricle.

Other Heart Sounds

Murmurs Heart murmurs are prolonged extra sounds that occur during systole or diastole. They are heard loudest over the valve that is affected. They are vibrations caused by turbulent blood flow through the cardiac chambers. Murmurs are not always caused by cardiac valvular disease. Other causes include fever, anemia, exercise, or structural defects such as a patent foramen ovale. The intensity of a murmur is measured on a scale of 1 to 6. The higher the number, the louder the murmur. A grade 1 can barely be heard even with turning the patient to his or her left side. A grade 4 can usually be felt through the chest wall, and a grade 6 can be heard at the bedside without a stethoscope. Murmurs are also characterized by systolic or diastolic timing, high or low pitch, location, radiation, and quality, for example, "blowing," "harsh," or "grating."

NURSING ALERT

New, extremely loud, harsh murmurs radiating in all directions from the apex of the heart suggest an emergency situation requiring immediate intervention. Call the responsible health care provider stat.

Pericardial Friction Rubs This abnormal heart sound is described as a high-pitched back-and-forth scratching or grating sound that is equivalent to cardiac motion within the pericardial sac. It is accompanied by chest pain secondary to pericardial inflammation or effusion that can occur 1 week post cardiac surgery or post myocardial infarction. The pericardial friction rub can be auscultated at Erb's point, which is the 3rd intercostal space to the left of the sternum. When a pericardial friction rub is heard, report it to the health care provider immediately as anticoagulant therapy may need to be stopped. A pericardial friction rub can indicate bleeding in the pericardial sac that would worsen with the use of anticoagulants.

NURSING ALERT

If a pericardial friction rub is suddenly discovered by the critical care nurse, the health care provider should be notified immediately and the medication record should be scanned for the use of anticoagulants.

Other Vascular Sounds—Bruit

A bruit is an extracardiac vascular sound that is high pitched and swishing in its characteristics. It is caused by either increased blood flow through a normal vessel or blood flow through a partially occluded or torturous vessel. Assess for bruits over the carotid, renal, and femoral arteries. They can indicate stenosis of these vessels or aneurysm. Bruits can also be heard over a patent AV shunt for dialysis where turbulence of blood flow is created by anastomoses of an artery and vein.

Recounting a True Story

The critical care nurse can often have life experiences outside of work that tax his or her assessment skills. The following is one example, based on a true story.

You are attending the preceremony preparation for your daughter's wedding. The wedding is a destination wedding and all of your nearest, dearest relatives and friends are staying with you at a college inn. As you enter the car to drive your daughter to get her hair and makeup done, a call comes from your son that your father is having chest pains. Throwing the keys to your daughter, you meet your husband, mother-in-law, and father walking slowly back to the inn. You send your son for a wheelchair and start assessing your father. He is clutching his left chest, is very diaphoretic, and is reporting sudden chest pain of 5 on a 1 to 10 scale that started while walking slowly with family after breakfast. The pain has not increased in intensity with slowly walking back to the inn with his escorts. In your mind you want to call 911 and get oxygen from the hotel, but you also know your father has poorly controlled gastroesophageal reflux disease (GERD) and is not consistent in taking his medications while traveling.

Once settled back in his room, you get him to chew a baby aspirin and assess his pulse, which has been around 66 and regular since you initially assessed him. After 5 minutes of rest, he no longer has chest pain and informs you he has had episodes like this and did not take his "purple pill" this morning. He tells you not to call your daughter and does not want to spoil the wedding. He rests in the afternoon, meets you at the wedding, and dances the first dance with you. Later, you teach him about the importance of taking his pills, especially during stressful events.

Collaborative Diagnostic and Laboratory Tools

❷ There are a variety of diagnostic tools and laboratory results that can be used in the care of a patient with cardiovascular disease. First we will look at diagnostic tools.

Diagnostic Tools

Arterial Blood Gases or ABGs

Respiratory issues such as pulmonary congestion can develop in individuals with cardiovascular deficits, thereby compromising their health status. Arterial blood gas analysis may be indicated to monitor levels of blood oxygenation. Refer to Chapter 2 for procedures and interpretation of arterial blood gas results. If the patient has an intraarterial line usually placed in the radial or femoral arteries, arterial blood gas samples can be obtained from these lines using sterile techniques.

Chest X-Ray

The chest x-ray is significant in determining the following: cardiac structure and size, dilation of the main pulmonary artery, pulmonary congestion, pleural or cardiac effusion, the presence or position of pacemakers, intracardiac lines, and pulmonary artery catheters. The chest x-ray is the oldest noninvasive method used to visualize heart images. The heart, aorta, and pulmonary vessels are moderately dense structures that appear as gray areas on the x-ray film.

EKG, ECG—Electrocardiogram

A noninvasive, 12-lead EKG is recommended and is always valuable in providing cardiac diagnostic information. Electrical conduction changes that occur within the heart are recorded and monitored on rhythm strips. Diagnosis of an acute MI can be seen with an ECG. Patients who have cardiac problems like MIs will frequently have dysrhythmias. Rhythm strip analysis will be addressed in Chapter 4, "Care of the Patient with Critical Cardiac Rhythm Disturbance Needs."

Echocardiograms

This is a noninvasive study that uses ultrasonic waveforms to obtain and display images of cardiac structures, heart motion, and abnormalities such as aortic and mitral valve stenosis, mitral valve prolapse and regurgitation, aortic insufficiency, atrial septal defects, and pericardial effusions. Currently, there are three types of echocardiographic methods in use: (1) the M-mode, which is a single, vertical ultrasound beam that produces cardiac views of chamber size and wall thickness, as well as valve functioning; (2) the 2-D or 2-dimensional mode, which is a planar ultrasound beam that provides a wider view of the heart and its structures; (3) the Doppler method, which is used to demonstrate blood flow through the heart, intracardiac pressures, ejection fraction, and cardiac output.

TEE—Transesophageal Echocardiography

This study combines ultrasound with endoscopy. A transducer, or echoscope, is attached to a flexible tube similar to a gastroscope. This tube is advanced (under local anesthesia) into the esophagus where high-quality images of intracardiac structures and the thoracic aorta are produced. The interference of the chest wall, bones, and air-filled lungs is eliminated. The atrial chambers are well visualized, making it easier to detect left atrial thrombi. It is also useful in detecting suspected dissecting aortic aneurysms. TEE is a convenient way to monitor cardiac function during open-heart surgery because the transesophageal probe can be inserted and left to remain in position during surgery. TEE is particularly useful in situations where COPD, obesity, and chest wall changes due to aging create obstacles to clear image visualization.

Stress Tests

Stress tests are considered to be noninvasive and are performed to determine cardiovascular disease as well as the patient's functional ability in performing activities of daily living (ADLs). The test is also known as exercise electrocardiography, and for those individuals who can tolerate exercise, the test involves pedaling a stationary bike or walking on a treadmill while connected to an EKG machine.

Physical stress is placed on the heart and oxygen demands to the heart are increased. Any physical symptoms that develop are observed. Inadequate cardiac perfusion is also noted via a camera scanner or the EKG machine.

Some sources indicate that results of exercise testing are more effective when combined with radionuclide scanning, such as the intravenous injection of thallium. When thallium is used, it is measured for its rate of absorption by the heart muscle. Poorly perfused areas of the heart either do not absorb the thallium or do so much more slowly than the better-perfused areas of the heart.

Patients who cannot tolerate exercise may be stressed with drug-induced alternatives, which will also increase the oxygen demands and workload to the heart. Examples of pharmacological agents include adenosine, dipyridamole, or dobutamine.

Whichever stress test modalities are used, visual imaging will identify ischemic dysfunctions of the myocardium. Such results may indicate a need for further care such as a cardiac catheterization to determine the patency of the coronary arteries. Balloon angioplasty, arterial stent insertion, or even coronary artery bypass surgery might be further recommended.

Pulmonary Artery Catheter (PAC)

❹ This is a balloon-tipped invasive catheter inserted by a physician into the pulmonary capillary bed via the internal jugular, femoral, or subclavian vein (see Figure 3–3). The PAC is used to measure pulmonary venous pressure and provide data about right- and left-sided heart pressures, cardiac output, core temperature, and oxygen saturation, as well as systemic and pulmonary vascular resistance. This catheter is attached to a pressurized IV line to keep the blood from exiting the catheter. It is kept open by a slow IV drip and requires periodic flushing with a manual flush activator. The catheter has a pressure transducer

FIGURE 3–3 • Photo of PAC.

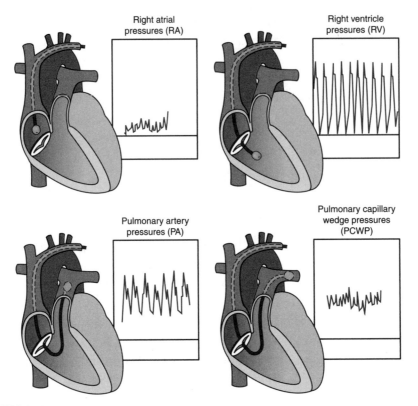

FIGURE 3–4 • Waveforms of a PAC..

near the flush activator, which converts the mechanical energy transmitted through the catheter from the heart to electrical energy that can be seen on the cardiac monitor (see Figure 3–4). This transducer can also pick up the patient's core temperature by hooking the thermistor connecter of the PAC to the cardiac monitor (see Figure 3–5).

The nurse assesses the pressures of the PAC to normal values and determines what they mean (see Table 3–5). This is usually done at the beginning of the shift and whenever the nurse deems necessary. The PAC can be attached to the monitor to read continuous PA and RA pressures. To perform a pulmonary artery wedge pressure (PAWP) and cardiac output/index (CO/CI) additional procedures need to be done.

The normal PAWP is 4 to 12 mm Hg. Increases indicate the development of pulmonary venous congestion, the occurrence of pulmonary edema, significant acute left ventricular failure, and increased resistance in the thorax. Fluid management and continuous cardiopulmonary assessment can be achieved via the assistance of a PAC or pulmonary artery catheter.

FIGURE 3–5 • Typical PAC setup..

TABLE 3–5 Pressures Obtained by Pulmonary Artery Catheter (PAC)		
Pressures	**Normal Value**	**What They Mean**
Right atrial (RA) or central venous pressure (CVP)	2–6 mm Hg	Measures preload of the right heart or amount of blood/force of blood coming into the right atrium. RA = CVP
Right ventricular (RV)	20–30/0–8 mm Hg	Pressure in the RV, only seen on insertion OR when the PAC migrates inadvertently back to RV. Only value dropping to 0 diastolically. Concurrently, life-threatening ventricular dysrhythmias can be seen if left in RV position. Catheter should never be left in this position.
Pulmonary artery pressure	20–30/8–15 mm Hg	Measures pressures within pulmonary artery. Is the pressure reading that is constant on the PAC. Not reflective of left–sided heart pressures.
Pulmonary artery wedge pressure (PAWP) or pulmonary artery occlusive pressure wedge (PAOP)	4–12 mm Hg	Measures left ventricular preload or amount/pressure of blood coming into left ventricle. Measurement involves inflation of a tiny balloon on the PCWP port of the PAC.

TABLE 3–5 Pressures Obtained by Pulmonary Artery Catheter (PAC) (*Continued*)

Pressures	Normal Value	What They Mean
Cardiac output (CO)	4–8 L/min	Volume of blood pumped out of ventricle each minute. Can be calculated via a computer after injecting the PAC with saline through the CVP port.
Cardiac index (CI)	2.5–4.2 L/min/m²	Takes into account body size and surface area. CO individualized.
Systemic vascular resistance (SVR)	770–1500 dynes/s/cm⁻⁵	Afterload. Pressure the left ventricle to work against to eject blood into the aorta.

How to Do It–Nursing Responsibilities in the Care of a Patient During Insertion of a PAC

1. Set up the pressurized line and transducing equipment according to protocols using sterile technique. The IV tubing must be kept free of air bubbles. If air enters the catheter, it can migrate into the pulmonary artery and lodge in that circulation.

2. While the patient is in a supine position, level the zeroing stopcock to the patient's phlebostatic axis (4th ICS, midaxillary line). This is the level of the atria. This is an extremely important procedure as leveling at the wrong area can change the waveforms and pressure values.

3. Attach the port to the distal end of the PAC to the monitor cable.

4. Read the values and record them as the catheter transits through the heart and finally comes to rest in the pulmonary artery.

5. Inflate the balloon through the pulmonary capillary wedge pressure (PCWP) port with less than 1 mL of air until the waveform changes from a PA to PCWP. Record your values. Let the air rebound out of the syringe, watching for the waveform to change back to PA.

6. Flush the catheter thoroughly by activating the manual flush device.

7. Place a sterile dressing on the insertion site when catheter insertion is completed: date, time, initial dressing.

NURSING ALERT

After performing the PAWP, the nurse must deflate the balloon and look for the return of the PAP waveform. If the balloon is left inflated, a pulmonary infarction could occur distal to the balloon as the circulation to that area is diminished by the balloon blocking the pulmonary artery.

NURSING ALERT

Strict sterile technique is mandated in the care and manipulation of all invasive arterial catheter insertions. Adhere to facility protocols for all tubing, catheter, flushes, dressing changes, and maintenance.

❹ How to Do It–Nursing Responsibilities in Performing a CO/CI With a Pulmonary Artery Catheter

1. Set up a cooling tower with an IV in place or use normal saline (NSS) at room temperature according to manufacturer's design. This is injectate.
2. Attach injectate to the central venous pressure (CVP) port with a screw-type adaptor. This will be injected into the CVP port 10 mL at a time.
3. Maintain the sterility of all attachments or endocarditis and sepsis can result.
4. Attach thermistor port to the cardiac monitor. This will calculate the change in temperature over the period of time that a 10-mL bolus of iced saline/NSS is injected into the CVP port.
5. Set the monitor up to measure cardiac output (CO) as per unit protocol.
6. Inject 10 mL of the iced saline or NSS into the CVP port.
7. Assess the waveform for an even upstroke and down stroke.
8. Perform CO readings three times in a patient where fluid is not a problem and twice in a patient on fluid restriction.
9. Average the two or three values.
10. Input the patient's height and weight into the monitor.
11. Read cardiac index (CI).
12. Compare the readings to previous readings. Call the primary health care provider if readings show a significant change.
13. Detach cables from the CVP port if needed as well as thermistor port.

Nursing Assessment for Complications The nurse should be observant for all possible complications when caring for a patient with a PAC.

- Pneumothorax – The introducer or catheter may accidentally pass through the vessel walls especially on insertion into the subclavian vein. Observe for diminished breath sounds in the lungs, decreased SaO_2, and chest x-ray changes.

- Infection – The PAC is an invasive procedure and the catheter passes through the heart. Look for signs of sepsis like fever and elevated white blood cells (WBCs).

- Ventricular dysrhythmias – These are caused when the catheter whips up against the endocardium creating an irritable focus. They might only be seen on insertion as the catheter coils back on itself to pass through the pulmonary artery. Notify the physician; the catheter may need to be advanced so that it does not migrate back to the right ventricle.

- Pulmonary infarction – This can be caused if the catheter is left in a "wedged position." Always watch the pattern return to a PA pattern after performing a PCWP reading. Notify the health care provider if suspected. The catheter may be pulled back and repositioned by the health care provider.

- Pulmonary artery rupture – This is one of the most serious issues and can be caused by overinflation of the balloon while performing PCWP or on insertion. Look for signs of hemorrhage and shock.

Cardiac Catheterization (CC)

A CC is a study to measure pressures in the heart and to visualize flow of blood via a dye injected into the heart chambers or coronary arteries. CC tells how the heart is functioning and whether any of the coronary arteries is blocked. An extensive medical/surgical history must be done prior to this test as well as laboratory values for coagulation (PT, PTT), bleeding (H&H), and kidney function (BUN and creatinine). Baseline coagulation studies tell if the patient will be prone to bleeding before and after the procedure. Potential hidden bleeding into the groin is monitored by the H&H and lastly, since the dye is nephrotoxic, kidney function must be screened to see if the patient can excrete the dye.

The patient's heart is accessed through a femoral puncture. If the patient has a right-heart catheterization, the femoral vein is punctured, and if it is a left-sided heart catheterization, the femoral artery is punctured. Once the pressures are obtained, dye is injected to see the function of the chambers of the heart and visualize the coronary arteries (left-sided heart catheterization only). The patient is observed at this time for rhythm disturbances, flushing, and hypotension from the dye.

Post procedure, the nurse is responsible for

- Monitoring vital signs and heart rhythm
- Assessing the patient for the presence of chest pain
- Checking the femoral site frequently for bleeding and hematoma formation
- Assessing all peripheral pulses for compromised circulation or embolus formation
- Monitoring color, movement, sensation, and temperature of extremities; paresthesias are the first signs of neurovascular compromise
- Forcing IV or oral fluids to excrete the dye injected
- Maintaining the patient on bedrest (length according to protocol) to prevent disturbance of clot formation at the insertion site
- Log rolling the patient if the patient needs to be turned or placed on a bedpan
- Providing patient education before discharge to home

Laboratory Tools: Electrolytes

❷ Serum blood levels are routinely performed to determine electrolyte concentrations that can affect cardiac function. Other organs such as the renal, liver, and pulmonary systems and glucose metabolism are examined to identify organ dysfunction. Cardiac isoenzymes determine whether death of myocardial cells have occurred. Enzyme levels are scrutinized to identify myocardial infarction. Lipid levels are important to determine coronary artery disease risk factors. A patient's hematologic status can determine anemia or infection that can be causes of cardiac disease or coagulation difficulties. Abnormal chemistry values can affect cardiac contractility and are important to evaluate.

Potassium (K+)

The normal potassium level is 3.5 to 5.5 mEq/L. An excess or deficiency of potassium will affect cardiac muscle function. Hyperkalemia is an increased potassium level that can lead to ventricular fibrillation and cardiac standstill. Hypokalemia is a decreased potassium level, which can be caused by chronic steroid therapy, diuretic therapy, and gastrointestinal fluid losses. Cardiac rhythm disturbances are noted on EKG in cases of both hypo- and hyperkalemia but are reversible with sufficient potassium drug replacement.

> **NURSING ALERT**
>
> *It is critical to keep potassium values within the normal range as potassium has a profound effect on heart rate and contractility. Always check the potassium, hold diuretics like Lasix (furosemide), and administer potassium supplements prior to giving the diuretic or dysrhythmias may occur. When administering potassium IV, infuse at a slow rate to prevent vein irritation and cardiac arrest. Only give 10 mEq in 50 mL over 1 hour.*

Calcium (Ca$^+$)

Calcium is known as the gatekeeper because it controls and maintains an adequate exchange of potassium and sodium across the cell membranes. Normal calcium levels range from 8 to 10 mg/dL. Calcium is crucial to maintain a balanced effect on cardiac contractility and excitability. Hypercalcemia is an excess of calcium. Hypocalcemia is a calcium deficit. Calcium replacement is necessary to correct the occurrence of cardiac dsyrhythmias, which develop from calcium imbalances.

Magnesium (Mg$^+$)

Magnesium is critical to normal cardiac and skeletal muscle function. The normal magnesium level ranges from 1.5 to 2.5 mEq/L. A decreased level is known as hypomagnesemia and can be caused by diuresis, chronic alcohol abuse, inadequate diet, or by TPN (total parenteral nutrition). Hypomagnesemia can easily occur in patients receiving diuretics to treat fluid overload, which is common in cases of heart failure. Intravenous magnesium sulphate replacement is required to increase Mg$^+$ levels. Hypermagnesemia is an increase in magnesium levels, which is seen less frequently then a low magnesium level or hypomagnesemia. Increased levels of magnesium may slow cardiac conduction resulting in prolonged PR intervals and a widening QRS complex. Low magnesium levels may increase cardiac irritability and aggravate cardiac dysrhythmias.

Sodium (Na$^+$)

The normal laboratory range for sodium is 135 to 145 mEq/L. This abundant cation is responsible for maintaining acid–base balance, extracellular fluid balance, and the transmission of nerve impulses. Hyponatremia refers to lower than normal levels of sodium. Hypernatremia defines higher than normal levels of sodium. Increased sodium levels leads to increased water retention and may lead to peripheral edema and exacerbate heart failure.

Laboratory Tools: Hematology

In patients with an altered cardiovascular status, the following hematologic studies are necessary.

Red Blood Cells (RBCs)

The red cell or erythrocyte count determines the number of red blood cells found in each cubic centimeter of whole blood. The primary function of RBCs is to carry hemoglobin, which provides oxygen to all cellular and tissue areas of the body. Oxygen combines chemically with the hemoglobin to perform these functions. Normal red blood cell results are as follows: males, 4.5 to 6 million and females, 4.5 to 5 million. Red blood cells are further broken down into hemoglobin or Hgb with 14 to 18 g/dL being the normal range for males and 12 to 16 g/dL being the normal female range. The hematocrit describes the volume percentage of RBCs in whole blood. The normal range for males is 40% to 54%. The normal female range is 38% to 48%.

A decrease in the serum level of total red blood cells will demonstrate a decrease in the Hgb and Hct levels. A condition such as anemia, where less oxygen is delivered to the cells and body tissues due to a reduction in the number of red blood cells, can increase cardiac workload and lead to heart failure. Increases in RBC formation, known as polycythemia, results in higher Hgb and Hct levels and can be a response to tissue hypoxia.

Erythrocyte Sedimentation Rate (ESR)

The ESR measures how quickly RBCs separate from plasma within a 1-hour period of time. With specific injuries such as endocarditis or pericarditis, or a myocardial infarction, the ESR will increase due to the faster precipitation of globulin and fibrinogen levels in the bloodstream. The ESR is a nonspecific test that can indicate a pathologic condition, but it does NOT identify the source of inflammation, infection, or tissue injury. In the adult male, a normal range would be 0 to 17 mm/hr and 1 to 25 mm/hr in the female.

> **NURSING ALERT**
>
> *Heart failure will decrease the ESR due to decreased levels of serum fibrinogen found in the bloodstream.*

White Blood Cells (WBCs)

WBCs are the absolute total number of leukocytes circulating in a cubic millimeter of blood. WBCs defend against invading organisms through the process of phagocytosis. They also provide antibodies to help fight infections and maintain immunity against diseases.

A normal white cell count is 5 to 10,000 mm³. A rise in the white cell count generally indicates the presence of disease, infection, or inflammation such as myocardial infarction (MI), rheumatic fever, and endocarditis, to name a few. Necrotic tissue is produced within the heart during an MI. The production of WBCs surrounding the pericardial sac increases the likelihood of pericarditis in an MI.

> **NURSING ALERT**
>
> *Signs and symptoms of both local and systemic infections must be explored and monitored by the nurse in instances of elevated WBCs.*

Laboratory Tools: Cholesterol Levels

The term hyperlipidemia is a broad term used to signify high plasma concentrations of cholesterol and triglycerides in the bloodstream. These are used to evaluate a patient's risk for developing atherosclerosis and coronary heart disease. Cholesterol, produced by the liver, is a lipid or fatty substance that is stored in cell membranes.

Cholesterol, HDL and LDL

Excess amounts of greater than 200 mg/dL is a precursor to the progression of atherosclerosis. About 20% of cholesterol is HDL, or high-density lipoprotein. HDL is the good or "HAPPY" cholesterol, because it removes unwanted cholesterol from body cells. LDL, or low-density lipoprotein, is the "BAD" or "LOUSY" cholesterol, because it TRANSPORTS cholesterol to the cells, where it remains waiting to cause trouble unless it is removed by the "GOOD" or "HAPPY" cholesterol. The desirable cholesterol level for adults is 130 mg/dL.

Triglycerides

Triglycerides are the most abundant group of lipids and are natural fats and oils obtained from animal fats and vegetable oils. Triglycerides are useful for energy; however, excesses are stored in the body as adipose tissue. Acceptable normal adult triglyceride levels are 40 to 150 mg/dL.

Laboratory Tools: Cardiac Enzymes (Markers)

Isoenzymes

In times of tissue damage, certain enzymes or proteins that are found in multiple organ systems are released. Specific to the heart are cardiac enzymes, which are released from damaged myocardial tissue cells and include

Creatine phophokinase (CPK), also known as CK or creatine kinase. When broken down into component parts, the result yields isoenzymes that provide diagnostic information specific to cardiac disease. CPK is composed of three isoenzymes or subunits found in varying amounts in muscle and brain tissue.

CK–BB – Indicates concentrations of creatine kinase found in the lungs, bladder, brain, and gastrointestinal tract. Results will increase after a cerebral vascular accident (CVA) or brain stroke. The normal range is 0% to 1%.

CK–MM – This isoenzyme is found within skeletal muscle and the myocardium. The normal range is 95% to 100%.

CK–MB – This isoenzyme is found exclusively within the myocardial cells. It is found in the serum as the most specific indicator or "gold standard" for diagnosing a myocardial infarction within the first 24 hours of onset and symptoms. This isoenzyme will elevate anywhere from 4 to 8 hours after an MI, peak within 15 to 24 hours, remain elevated for 48 to 72 hours, and return to normal after 3 days provided no further cardiac damage has occurred. The normal range is 0% to 6% of the total CK.

NURSING ALERT

Intramuscular injections can cause an elevated CPK–MM but not the CPK–MB. Therefore, this process should be noted on the laboratory request if the patient has been or is receiving intramuscular injections during the previous 24 to 48 hours.

Lactic Dehydrogenase (LDH)

This enzyme contributes to carbohydrate metabolism and is found in the heart, kidneys, and red blood cells. LDH is useful for the late diagnosis of an MI after the CK–MB has returned to normal. The predictive value of measuring LDH to determine if myocardial damage has occurred is 90% to 95%. Increased LDH activity begins to appear 10 to 12 hours after an MI, peaks within 48 to 72 hours, and remains elevated for as long as 14 days. The LDH is particularly necessary to assess when diagnosing MIs after the initial 24 hours of onset and the CK–MB isoenzyme peak is missed. LDH is composed of five isoenzymes, with the majority of LDH1 and LDH2 found in myocardial cells and rising after an acute MI. LDH1 and LDH2 are known as the cardiac fraction, with serum levels of LDH1 normally LESS than LDH2. With an MI, both LDH1 and LDH2 levels will rise, with the LDH1 level increasing before there is an increase in the total LDH. The LDH1 level will actually exceed or become greater than the LDH2 level. This response is known as a "FLIPPED PATTERN," or a REVERSAL of the LDH1 and LDH2 levels, confirming the diagnosis of an MI. To review, under healthy, normal circumstances, LDH2 results are generally higher than LDH1 levels. In the case of an MI, the opposite situation occurs.

LDH3 – Is found in the lungs, spleen, pancreas, thyroid, adrenal glands, and lymph nodes

LDH4 and LDH5 – Are the hepatic fractions found mostly in the liver and skeletal muscle.

Normal range of LDH percentages – LDH1, 17% to 33%; LDH2, 27% to 37%; LDH3, 18% to 25%; LDH4, 3% to 8%; and LDH5, 0% to 5%.

Troponin

Gold standard cardiac markers that have evolved to evaluate myocardial damage are the troponins. Troponins are proteins that are highly specific to cardiac muscle and will increase early and rapidly in the bloodstream as does the CK–MB after an MI. Troponins are NOT detected in healthy individuals and any muscle injury other than the heart. Troponins occur in various forms:

Troponin I – Rises in 4 to 6 hours, peaks in 14 to 18 hours, and remains elevated for 5 to 7 days. The normal range is 0 to 2 ng/mL.

Troponin T – Available for rapid cardiac damage assessment, as well as predicting the prognosis for patients with acute coronary destruction. These troponins will increase in 3 to 4 hours and remain elevated for 10 to 14 days. The normal range is 0 to 0.2 ng/mL.

> **NURSING ALERT**
>
> *Cardiac troponin remains detectable in the peripheral circulation for 8 to 12 hours after the onset of an MI and is the gold standard for early diagnosis of an MI. Many sources indicate differences in troponin testing and the interpretation of results. The above examples are only approximations and may vary according to health care facility standards and laboratory protocols.*

Myoglobin

Myoglobin is another important cardiac enzyme (marker) that can be used in the earliest detection of an MI. It is released within 30 to 60 minutes after an MI with a normal value that is gender specific. Normal values for males are less than 72 ng/mL and are less than 50 ng/mL in women. A myoglobin in combination with other markers helps in the detection of an MI but is not used solely to make a diagnosis.

B-Type Natriuretic Peptide (BNP)

BNP is a neurohormone that is secreted by the cardiac ventricles in response to ventricular stretch and overload. An excellent indicator of diagnosis and prognosis of heart failure (HF), BNP liberated in values in excess of 400 pg/mL shows significant heart failure. With the advent of this blood test, patients can be treated quickly for HF.

Advanced Procedural Skills

Intraaortic Balloon Pump (IABP)

❸ The IABP a catheter inserted into the femoral artery resting just below the subclavian artery. It used to support failing cardiac circulation. It is a temporary and mechanical circulatory assist device that inflates during diastole and deflates just prior to systole. When it inflates during diastole, the IABP forces blood backward toward the coronary arteries and forward toward the systemic circulation. When it deflates just before systole, the balloon deflation leaves a vacuum that decreases the resistance against which the heart has to work. Timing to the heart cycle and aortic BP to ensure proper inflation and looking for complications is an essential job of the critical care nurse. Special classes are designed to help nurses develop competency and confidence in managing this special lifesaving device.

The overall physiologic effect of this type of therapy is to improve the balance between myocardial oxygen supply and demand by reducing myocardial oxygen demands. The IABP can be inserted via the femoral artery and is positioned into the descending thoracic aorta. Contraindications to the IABP include aortic aneurysm, aortic valve insufficiency, bleeding tendencies, and severe peripheral vascular disease.

Left Ventricular Assist Device (LVAD)

This device is used often because left ventricular failure occurs more frequently than right ventricular failure. Blood is diverted from the left atrium to a pump outside the body that returns the blood to the aorta. The LVAD is indicated for people who demonstrate persistent cardiac failure but have the potential to regain normal heart function after the heart is given time to rest. It is used after open-heart surgery (OHS) in critical patients with severe left ventricular dysfunction not responsive to usual treatment.

Patients who have the potential to regain normal heart function, described as "pending recovery" individuals, are the first category of patients requiring an LVAD. The second category of patients requiring an LVAD are those who need circulatory support until a heart transplant can be performed. This category is termed "bridge to transplant." The LVAD is designed to support a failing heart via flow assistance. The pump diverts quantities of systemic blood flow around a failing ventricle. Ultimately, cardiac workload will be reduced and circulation maintained. Flow rates between 1 and 6 L per minute are used to maintain adequate cardiac output while decreasing ventricular workload.

Cardiovascular Medications Used in Critical Care

❺ Medications that affect the CV system may best be explained by how they affect the patient's *stroke volume (SV)*. Recall that the *cardiac output* is the amount of blood the heart pumps throughout the system in 1 minute and is calculated by taking the heart rate times of the SV. The SV is the amount of blood that is pushed out of the left ventricle with each heartbeat. SV is made up of three components: preload, contractility, and afterload. The components of SV are manipulated by cardiac medications in order to improve cardiac performance. First, we will look at medications that affect the preload of the heart.

Preload

Preload is defined as the ability of the heart's muscle fibers to stretch at the end of diastole. The components that affect this ability to stretch are determined by the amount of blood volume or pressure of that blood returning to the heart. Any medications that increase the preload will increase the stroke volume and therefore the workload of the heart, thus increasing the heart's oxygen need. The opposite occurs as well. Any medication that decreases the preload will decrease the stroke volume and ultimately decrease the workload of the heart. In diseased hearts, the critical care nurse will use more of the latter type of medications. Table 3–6 shows medications that enhance or reduce preload.

Medications like nitroglycerin and sodium nitroprusside (Nipride) are called *vasodilators* because they work to decrease the amount of wall tension in the arteries and veins, thus decreasing or reducing the preload. A decrease in pressure in the vascular circuit results in a decrease in *peripheral vascular resistance (PVR)*. The decrease in PVR results in a decrease in blood pressure.

TABLE 3–6 Preload Enhancers and Reducers

	Action	Use	Precautions
Preload Enhancers (Vasopressors)			
Dopamine	Constriction of the peripheral veins	In hypotensive crisis, heart failure and cardiac arrest	1. Must have volume replacement before therapy 2. Still practiced but being questioned 3. Monitor the site for extravasation; large-bore IVs are preferable for use
Levophed (norepinephrine)	Similar to epinephrine in action At high doses, increases vasoconstriction of alpha receptors	To elevate BP in shock states, especially in hypotension due to cardiogenic shock	1. Monitor the BP every 2–5 minutes when beginning infusion 2. Monitor MAP (keep around 80 mm Hg), VS, CVP, and urinary output 3. Use large-bore IV as severe vasoconstriction can result in smaller peripheral IVs 4. Observe for extravasation. Regitine can be injected into tissues to prevent necrosis
Preload Reducers (Vasodilators)			
Diuretics like Lasix (furosemide)	Tablets, IV push, or continuous drip	To remove excessive fluid to help the heart work with less demand	1. Monitor the patient's BP; do not give if below 90 systolic 2. Check the potassium level before giving 3. Monitor the urinary output for diuretic effects
Aldosterone inhibitors like spironolactone (Aldactone) or amiloride (Midamor)	Blocks aldosterone secretion on distal tubule, therefore increasing water excretion and decreasing sodium retention	In hypertension, heart failure, to rid the body of excess fluid Also helps decrease ventricular remodeling	1. Relatively few 2. Can cause hyperkalemia, especially if given with an ACE inhibitor or ARB 3. Contraindicated in severe renal and hepatic disease 4. Drowsiness, lethargy, or headache can occur

TABLE 3–6   Preload Enhancers and Reducers *(Continued)*

	Action	Use	Precautions
Nitroglycerin (Tridil; Nitro-Dur)	Causes both arterial and venous dilatation Selectively dilates the coronary arteries, increasing blood flow to the myocardium Decreases preload	Use for anginal episodes and prevention of angina Also used to bring the BP down acute coronary syndrome (ACS)	1. Sublingually (SL), intravenously (IV), and intranasally (IN); always take the BP before administering and 5 minutes after for a total of three SL or IN. Hold if the BP is < 110 systolic 2. May cause hypotension and headaches, which are dose related
Sodium nitroprusside (Nipride)	Profoundly and rapidly dilates the peripheral arteries by relaxing smooth muscles resulting in a drop in BP	Fast acting; only used in HTN emergencies	1. Thiocyanate and cyanide toxicity can occur. Assess for nausea, confusion, and tinnitus 2. Careful and continuous BP monitoring; arterial line might be indicated to closely monitor BP
Morphine sulfate	Dilates the venous system	The analgesic of choice for angina and ACS	1. Watch respirations as can cause depression leading to hypoxemia 2. Observe BP closely as can cause hypotension 3. Watch for oversedation, especially in elderly 4. Reversal agent is naloxone (Narcan)

The heart has to work harder to maintain this pressure. If the vessels are very small, then the pressure in the vessels is very high, which would cause more pressure in the CV system. Medications that decrease the diameter of the arteries or veins in the CV system are known as vasopressors or preload enhancers. Vasopressors are administered when the BP is too low as in a shocklike state. Commonly administered *vasopressors* in critical care include dopamine and Levophed.

Contractility

Contractility is the ability of the cardiac muscle to shorten in response to electrical stimulation. Some medications like beta-adrenergic blockers (metoprolol or Lopressor) decrease contractility by blocking the sympathetic stimulation of the heart. Medications that decrease the contraction of the heart are known as negative *inotropic agents*. Other medications do the opposite—positive inotropic agents increase contractility. Medications like digoxin and epinephrine increase the strength of contraction. A summary of these medications appears in Table 3–7.

Afterload

Afterload is the force required for the left ventricle to eject blood into the aorta. Afterload reduction is necessary to decrease the workload on a struggling left ventricle. Many drugs that are used for other purposes are afterload reducers. Table 3–8 gives some commonly used afterload reducers.

Anticoagulants

Because acute coronary artery occlusion is caused by platelets that block coronary arteries, anticoagulants are standard treatment to prevent occlusion. Anticoagulants can also be used in the prevention and occurrence of pulmonary emboli (see Table 3–9, p. 119).

Angiotension-Converting Enzyme (ACE) Inhibitors and Angiotension II Receptor Blockers (ARBs)

ACE oratory inhibitors and their alternatives, ARBs, are the mainstays in the treatment of heart failure. They have been shown to be effective in decreasing hospitalizations and in slowing the progression of heart failure, hypertension, and death (Table 3–10, p. 120).

Diuretics

Diuretics are used most in heart failure to rid the body of excessive fluid that can back up into the lungs (pulmonary edema) or the body (peripheral edema). Diuretics reduce the preload of the heart and allow the heart to work with less fluid stress. Table 3–11 (p. 121) includes a list of drugs that can be used for see heart failure.

TABLE 3–7 Drugs That Affect Contractility

	Action	Use	Precautions
Decreased Contractility (Negative Inotropic Agents)			
Beta–adrenergic blocking agents like metoprolol (Lopressor) or atenolol (Corgard) or bisoprolol (Zebeta)	Blocks the sympathetic response (fight or flight; increased HR, BP, adrenaline in the system) Reduces cardiac remodeling and reduces dysrhythmias Results in slower HR and lowered BP	ACS, acute hypertensive crisis, tachycardia Stable heart failure and reduced ejection fractions	Right ventricular heart failure from pulmonary HTN, heart block, and bradycardia
Calcium channel blockers like verapamil (Calan) or diltiazem (Cardizem)	Decreases intracellular calcium in cardiac muscle Also reduces afterload Dilates coronary arteries	Tachycardia, coronary artery spasm, angina	Do not use in bradycardias or sick sinus syndrome; do not stop abruptly. Assess for hypotension and heart failure
Increased Contractility (Positive Inotropic Agents)			
Digoxin	Decreases heart rate as well as AV conduction	Fast tachyarrhythmia	Watch for signs of digoxin toxicity, which include blurred or yellow vision Do not administer if apical HR is < 60 Do not give if patient is in heart block Observe and replace potassium level if < 4 mEq/L Hold if digoxin serum level is >1.5 Not indicated for acute decompensated heart failure

TABLE 3–7 Drugs That Affect Contractility (*Continued*)

	Action	Use	Precautions
Epinephrine	Synthetic form of adrenaline that stimulates the action of the sympathetic nervous system Causes vasoconstriction leading to increased HR	First-line drug in most advanced cardiac life support algorithms for cardiac arrest bradycardia and <BP Also given when patient is in symptomatic bradycardias and heart blocks	Continuous cardiac monitoring is needed to see HR increases Given IV push in an arrest. Infusion may be prepared via pump Assess VS frequently during initiation and infusion Destroyed in alkaline solutions like bicarbonate; so use separate line for infusion Check label as comes in varying solutions
Dobutrex (Dobutamine)	Works on B1 and B2 receptors of adrenergic system to increase contractility and reduce afterload Improves CO	In acute heart failure	Always use infusion pump for administration Assess VS frequently during initiation and during infusion Monitor SaO_2 Observe especially for hypotension and tachycardia
Milrinone (Primacor)	Phosphodiesterase inhibitor Increases contractility by blocking the breakdown of cyclic AMP Also vasodilates and reduces afterload	For acute heart failure	Always use an infusion pump Assess VS frequently during initiation and during infusion Monitor SaO_2 Observe especially for hypotension, ventricular dysrhythmias, and tachycardia

TABLE 3–8 Afterload Reducers

Drug	Action	Use	Precautions
Dobutamine (Dobutrex)	See Table 3-7		
Milrinone (Primacor)	Phosphodiesterase inhibitor Increases contractility by blocking breakdown of cyclic AMP Produces vasodilation Reduces afterload	Positive inotropic therapy in HF	1. Not actively titrated 2. Always use infusion pump 3. Assess VS, SaO_2 4. Observe for hypotension and ventricular dysrhythmias
Morphine sulfate	See Table 3-6	MI to lower the workload on the left ventricle	See Table 3-6
Nitroglycerin	See Table 3-6	Drops the BP and therefore workload of the heart	See Table 3-6

Medical CV Conditions Requiring Critical Care

Hypertensive Emergencies

What Went Wrong?

❻ Hypertensive crisis is a condition where the blood pressure (BP) soars abnormally high and does not respond to the usual treatment. Nurses are familiar with chronic hypertension (HTN) and its stages where the systolic blood pressure goes beyond 120 mm Hg. But critical care nurses need to be familiar with hypertensive emergencies.

There are two types of hypertensive emergencies: hypertensive urgency and hypertensive crisis. In hypertensive crisis, there is target organ damage. Damage to the heart, brain, blood vessels, and kidneys results from an unrelieved high BP, so health care providers must lower the BP at once to prevent further progressive damage to these structures. The patient must be admitted to the intensive care unit so that complications from HTN emergencies like stroke, acute MI, abdominal aortic aneurysm (AAA), and seizures can be prevented.

TABLE 3–9 Anticoagulants

	Drug Action	Use	Precautions
Aspirin	Stops platelets from clumping together to form a plug that blocks a coronary artery	Immediately during and for long-term management of angina and ACS	May cause GI upset. Use H2 blockers or proton pump inhibitors if GI upset/bleeding. Can be used if taking other analgesics like acetaminophen (Tylenol).
Heparin Low molecular weight heparin (LMWH) like enoxaparin (Lovenox) or dalteparin (Fragmin)	Prevents the formation and growth of blood clots LMWH may be used to treat ACS instead of heparin	In ACS	Monitoring of the aPTT is done frequently to prevent under- or overdosing of heparin LMWH do not need laboratory monitoring All heparin products require close monitoring for bleeding Monitor the platelets for reduction that can occur with heparin
Thrombolytic therapy Includes clot-busting drugs like t–PA (tissue plasminogen activator), alteplase (Activase), and reteplase (r–PA)	Busts apart clots formed during acute coronary syndromes leading to MI Decreases permanent damage done in MI and improves ventricular functioning	First–line drug used in ACS; chest pain of longer than 20 minutes not relieved by NTG and rest with ECG changes	1. Does not dissolve the plaque that lays the basis for clot formation. May need atherectomy or open heart for this. 2. Bleeding, as they are not specific for coronary arteries and can cause hemorrhage in recent trauma or hemorrhagic stroke. 3. Best given 3-6 hours post onset of symptoms. 4. Door–to–needle time should be no longer than 30 minutes. 5. Monitor lab oratory values like H&H for bleeding.

> ### NURSING ALERT
>
> *All patients placed on thrombolytic therapy should have bleeding precautions implemented like close observation of all invasive lines, minimizing venipunctures for lab draws, preventing tissue trauma, and applying pressure after any invasive procedures.*

TABLE 3–10 Angiotension-Converting Enzyme Inhibitors and Angiotension II Receptor Blockers

Drugs	Action	Use	Precautions
ACE Inhibitors			
Captopril (Capoten) Enalapril (Vasotec) Lisinopril (Prinivil; Zestril) Quinapril (Accupril)	Are part of the "Core Four" to improve patient outcomes in heart failure according to the Joint Commission's (JACHO) annual report 2007 Blocks conversion of angiotension I to angiotension II, which leads to vasodilation and decreased vascular resistance. Decreases aldosterone secretion and rids body of sodium and water. Decreases symptoms of heart failure	First–line drug used in slowing progression of heart failure	Contraindicated in allergy, angioedema, hypotension hyperkalemia, renal artery stenosis, and worsening renal disease
Angiotension II Receptor Blockers (ARBs)			
Candesartan (Atacand) Losartan (Cozaar) Valsartan (Diovan)	Blocks the attachment of angiotension II to its receptor resulting in vasodilation and decreased vascular resistance. Decreases aldosterone secretion and rids body of sodium and water. Decreases symptoms of heart failure	Can be used as an alternative in initial diagnosis of heart failure if ACE inhibitors cause intolerable side effects	Headache, dizziness, and orthostatic hypotension. Watch for angioedema and acute renal failure that are first–dose related.

In hypertensive urgency there is no organ damage so the BP can be lowered in the Emergency Department (ED) until the patient responds to treatment.

TABLE 3–11 Diuretics			
Drugs	**Action**	**Use**	**Precautions**
Loop Diuretics			
Furosemide (Lasix) Bumetanide (Bumex) Toresemide (Demadex)	Works on loop of Henle in kidney to block sodium and water reabsorption Increases urinary sodium excretion Decreases physical signs of fluid retention	To control peripheral and pulmonary edema	Monitor the potassium level prior to giving. If K^+ close to or below normal, give potassium supplements prior to giving diuretic Monitor BP; can cause hypotension, vertigo, and dizziness Monitor intake and output and daily weights
Thiazide Diuretics			
Aldosterone Inhibitors: Spironolactone (Aldactone) Eplerenone (Inspra)	Lowers the serum aldosterone, therefore reducing sodium and water retention	For moderate to severe heart failure	Can cause hyperkalemia, so monitor the K^+ level Can cause hypotension, so watch the BP

The patient maybe discharged on medications with a follow-up appointment with a clinic or primary physician to occur within 24 to 48 hours.

The most common cause of a hypertensive emergency is a previous history of chronic hypertension, although it can occur in patients without any prior history. A thorough nursing history needs to include what medications the patient is taking for HTN and when they were taken last. Other conditions that can cause HTN emergencies include kidney problems like acute glomerulonephritis and renal disease; acute aortic dissection; pheochromocytoma; ingesting tyramine-containing foods if the patient is taking tricyclic antidepressants or other sympathomimetics with a monoamine oxidase inhibitor (MAO); pregnancy conditions like eclampsia and preeclampsia; head injury; stroke; use of recreational drugs like cocaine, amphetamines, PCP, and LSD; scleroderma and other collagen vascular problems; and too-rapid withdrawal from antihypertensive medications.

Prognosis

The prognosis for HTN emergencies is good as long as the patient is treated in a timely manner. In patients over the age of 50, death from stroke or heart failure is increased with hypertensive emergencies.

Interpreting Test Results

- There may be no other test than an elevated blood pressure that shows HTN.
- EKG may show left-ventricular hypertrophy if the HTN is long standing.
- BUN and creatinine may be elevated if renal damage has occurred.

Hallmark Signs and Symptoms

First, an accurate measurement of the patient's BP in both arms must be performed and documented. A significant difference needs to be reported to the responsible health care provider. In an acute hypertensive crisis the patient may present with one or more of the following symptoms: changes in neurological status like changes in the level of responsiveness, headache, visual disturbances, nausea, and/or vomiting, chest pain, and shortness of breath.

Treatment

For hypertensive emergency, the patient's BP needs to be brought down slowly but steadily.

If the patient's BP is brought down suddenly, the abrupt lowering can cause inadequate cerebral blood flow.

Start at least one peripheral IV and begin an infusion of nitroprusside (Nipride) at 0.1 µg/kg per minute to lower the mean arterial blood pressure (MAP) at least 25% below the MAP.

The physician may also order IV labetalol (Normodyne, Trandate), nitroglycerin (Nitropaste), or a calcium channel blocker like nicardipine (Cardene) infusion; hydralazine (in eclampsia); or furosemide (Lasix).

For a hypertensive urgency, a loop diuretic and an antihypertensive medication like a beta-adrenergic blocker, calcium channel blocker, or an ACE inhibitor may be prescribed with a follow-up appointment with a clinic or primary physician to occur within 24 to 48 hours.

Nursing Diagnoses for Hypertensive Emergency	Expected Outcomes
Ineffective tissue perfusion alteration (cerebral)	The patient's mean arterial pressure (MAP) will be lowered by 25% over 2 hours
	The patient's neurological status will indicate improvement or no changes

Nursing Interventions

Monitor the patient's BP until stable; this may include intraarterial monitoring to see if therapy is effective in lowering the BP 25% within 2 hours.

Monitor for signs/symptoms of stroke (numbness/tingling in extremities, paralysis or weakness, change in ability to talk). Stroke is a major complication of acute hypertensive emergencies.

Initiate and monitor the effects of BP lowering medications to see if therapy is effective.

Assess patient's financial status, as money to buy medications is a big issue in today's economic crisis.

Teach the patient the importance of taking medications even if he or she feels well. The patient may have high BP and not feel ill.

Teach the patient ways to modify risk factors to help lower the BP and give a sense of control.

NURSING ALERT

In an acute hypertensive emergency, bringing the patient's BP down too swiftly can lead to cerebral or myocardial ischemia and hypoperfusion. Consult with the neurologist to determine the BP to stabilize the patient without causing further damage.

Angina

What Went Wrong?

Angina is a term used to describe episodic chest pain or pressure. It is a symptom of coronary artery disease or an overwhelming demand placed upon the heart where the cardiac muscle is not perfused. It is different from an MI because myocardial death does not occur in angina.

In coronary artery disease, the intimal lining (inner) of the arteries within the heart develops atherosclerotic plaques. The plaques cause an obstruction in coronary arteries, which causes a decrease in blood supply to the coronary arteries. The decrease in blood supply can occur during periods of stress, exercise, or any increase in demand upon the heart. The narrowed coronary arteries lay the foundation for the formation of a complete blockage of an artery, which can lead to an acute coronary syndrome (ACS).

The modifiable risk factors associated with angina include hypertension, high cholesterol levels, smoking, obesity, physical inactivity, metabolic syndrome, and diabetes. Nonmodifiable risk factors include heredity, aging, gender, and race. Angina can be prevented by changing as many modifiable risk factors as possible.

TABLE 3–12 Other Causes of Angina

Anemia	Lack of red blood cells within the body leads to a decrease in O_2 to the cardiac tissues. This stresses the heart, making it work hard to get available RBCs to the cells.
Hyperthyroidism	Increase in thyroid hormone causes a tachycardia, which places stress upon the heart.
Chronic lung disease	Lack of oxygenation to the blood increases the risk of tachycardia, which can lead to angina.

Angina can be classified into three stages: stable, variant, and unstable. Stable angina is predictable and does not increase in intensity or duration. Variant angina, sometimes called Prinzmetal's angina, is thought to occur with coronary artery spasm and is usually treated with calcium channel blockers. It occurs at rest. Unstable angina is unpredictable, increasing in intensity or duration, and is the beginning of ACS.

The diseases listed in Table 3–12 are known causes of angina and could lead to ACS.

Angina episodes can be caused by physical exertion; a sudden change in temperature, especially cold; stress; or eating a heavy meal.

Prognosis

Cardiovascular disease is the leading cause of mortality in the United States and the leading cause of death in men and women.

Hallmark Signs and Symptoms

It is best to use an organized pain assessment. It is important that nothing be left out in a pain assessment as angina mimics other heart and respiratory disorders. The OPQRST memory jog might be helpful to cover all your bases.

- **Onset:** sudden; sometime predictable.
- **Precipitating factor:** stress, exercise, or exertion
- **Quality:** frequently patient's discomfort is heavy, viselike, crushing, or squeezing. Women, the elderly, and patients with diabetes may have shortness of breath, mild indigestion; may not have typical chest pain or may have silent MI.
- **Radiation:** poorly localized but may radiate to neck, jaw, and down arms.
- **Severity:** discomfort to agonizing pain. Have the patient rate on a 1 to 10 scale.
- **Timing:** comes and ends abruptly. Usually responds to rest, oxygen, and nitroglycerin. Time of day when it occurs (day/night/after a heavy meal).

Other associated signs/symptoms may include

- Nausea
- Diaphoresis
- Dizziness
- Anxiety and apprehension
- Feeling of numbness or weakness in extremities

NURSING ALERT

The difference between an acute coronary event and angina is that angina is relieved with rest, oxygen, and nitroglycerin. Angina that increases in frequency, duration, or is unrelieved with nitrates, oxygen, and rest requires medical intervention.

Treatment

Rest is in order to decrease the demand upon the heart.

Oxygen to increase myocardial oxygenation.

Self-administration of nitroglycerin to dilate the veins and decrease the preload to the heart.

Aspirin to prevent platelets from adhering together and causing coronary artery thrombosis.

Metoprolol to help strengthen the heart's contractions.

NURSING ALERT

Some patients never experience pain or pressure and yet could have a coronary event. Women, the elderly, and patients with diabetes must be monitored closely as they can have atypical symptoms.

Nursing Diagnoses for Angina	Expected Outcomes
Acute pain related to coronary artery occlusion	The patient will report 0 pain on 1–10 scale after administration of nitrates and rest

Nursing Interventions

Assess the patient using organized pain assessment to ensure a complete, comprehensive assessment.

Monitor for worsening of angina intensity or duration, which can indicate unstable angina or ACS.

Have the patient rest to avoid further increase in demand on the heart and decreased oxygen need.

Administer and monitor oxygen saturation to ensure an adequate amount of oxygen to the heart muscle

Administer nitroglycerin sublingually or intranasally to help dilate coronary arteries and pool blood peripherally away from the heart.

Educate patients about nitrates to help decrease preload and O_2 demand on the heart.

Teach patients that daily acetylsalicylic acid (ASA) is needed to prevent platelets from adhering and causing a clot in the coronary arteries.

Acute Coronary Syndrome (ACS)

What Went Wrong?

ACS is an all-encompassing syndrome that includes angina, ST segment elevation myocardial infarction (MI), and acute MI. Angina was described previously in this chapter.

The plaques narrowing the coronary arteries rupture causing a progressive to complete block of blood flow to the coronary artery, which can lead to an acute MI.

The three main events that characterize ACS include ST segment elevation MI, unstable angina, and myocardial infarction. Table 3–13 summarizes the difference between these three coronary events.

TABLE 3–13 Acute Coronary Syndromes (ACSs)	
ST segment elevation myo–cardial infarction	Sometimes called a non–Q wave MI. The ST segment of the ECG in certain leads that look at the left ventricle is elevated. Cardiac enzymes are also elevated.
Unstable angina	Angina that increases in either frequency or duration. This is a clear message that an MI can occur unless intervention is swift.
MI (Q wave)	Death of myocardial tissue within three muscular coats called a transmural MI (endo–, myo–, and epicardium). This leaves a permanent "electrical scar" on a 12–lead ECG called a "Q" wave, thus the name.

An MI can also be classified according to its location by ECG. Commonly occurring MIs include those listed in Table 3–14.

TABLE 3–14 Location of MI by ECG			
Location	**Coronary Blocked**	**Lead Changes**	**Changes That Occur**
Anterior septal MI[a]	Left anterior descending (LAD)	V1–V4	ST segment elevation
			Flipped T waves
			Q waves
Inferior MI	Right coronary	II, III, and AVF	ST segment elevation
			Flipped T waves
			Q waves
Lateral MI	Circumflex or diagonal branch of LAD	V1 and V6	ST segment elevation
			Flipped T waves
			Q waves
Posterior MI (uncommon)	Distal sections of RCA and circum-flex		Reciprocal changes (reverse as in back of the heart)
			ST segment elevation
			T wave elevation
			Large R waves

[a]One–quarter of all MIs with the most severe complications and higher death rates.

Prognosis

The prognosis for ACS is very good if patients do not ignore their symptoms and seek advanced medical attention. Many medications can be administered to relieve symptoms as well as prevent the occurrence of MI. However, according to the American Heart Association, approximately one-third of patients experiencing MI will die from it.

Interpreting Test Results

- ECGs are done to look for ST segment elevation (ischemia; lack of blood supply), T wave inversion (injury; damage to myocardium), and infarction (Q waves; death to myocardium) that indicate a transmural infarction.
- Cardiac enzymes are evaluated. If elevated, they indicate damage to cardiac cells and infarction if they are above normal values.

- Chest x-rays are done to determine cardiac size and lung congestion.
- BNP (B-type natriuretic peptide) is monitored according to hospital protocol to diagnose whether the ACS is from heart failure. A BNP of greater than 400 pg/mL usually indicates significant HF. The higher this value goes, the poorer the prognosis of the patient.
- Serum electrolytes (K^+, Ca^{++}, Mg^+) are monitored to determine if treatment needs to be initiated. Alterations in serum electrolytes may increase the chance for cardiac dysrhythmias.
- An echocardiogram is done to see if there is a decrease in wall motion or malfunctioning of the heart valves.

Hallmark Signs and Symptoms

Monitor the patient using a consistent, well-defined structure for pain assessment as angina or MI can mimic noncardiovascular events such as abdominal aortic aneurysm (AAA), gastric esophageal reflux disease (GERD), pulmonary embolism (PE), cholecystitis, and pneumonia. **OPQRST** is one that is easily remembered. Classic symptoms using an organized pain assessment include

- **Onset** – When did it start? Usually sudden.
- **Precipitating factor** – What caused it? Usually stress or exertionally induced.
- **Quality** – What does the patient tell you it feels like? "Crushing, viselike, heavy." May be atypical in the elderly, in women, and/or in diabetics. They might say "stomach-ache, shortness of breath, tired feeling."
- **Radiation** – Where does it go? This can travel to the jaw, back, or arm(s).
- **Timing** – How long does it last? Longer than angina and it is not relieved with nitroglycerin (NTG) and rest. What time did it occur?

Other associated symptoms that can occur with an MI include

- Shortness of breath
- Diaphoresis
- Epigastric distress
- Nausea and vomiting
- Dysrhythmias
- Syncope (feeling like passing out)
- Feeling like something really bad is going to happen; impending doom
- Hypotension and shock

Treatment

Stop all activity.

Administer oxygen.

Give medications (ASA, anticoagulants, Lopressor, nitrates, thrombolytics).

Prepare for coronary arteriogram, angioplasty, or open-heart surgery (OHS) if needed.

Nursing Diagnoses for ACS	Expected Outcomes
Acute pain due to coronary artery blockage	The patient will have 0 pain on a 1-10 scale
Ineffective tissue perfusion, cardiac due to blockage of coronary arteries	The patient will have normal VS, CO, and peripheral pulses

Nursing Interventions

Have patient stop all activity immediately and place patient on bedrest to decrease workload and energy demand upon the heart.

Monitor the patient's vital signs (VS) at least every 15 minutes, especially if starting IV medications to identify and prevent cardiogenic shock.

Auscultate lung fields and heart sounds frequently to determine if heart failure is occurring due to MI.

Monitor the patient's telemetry because dysrhythmia disturbances often occur in ACS, and they can lead to cardiac arrest or cardiogenic shock.

Assess ECGs periodically and when chest pain reoccurs to see if the infarction has extended into other ventricular tissues.

Continue ongoing pain assessments to evaluate if therapy is effective or more advanced cardiac measures are needed like IABP, PAC, angioplasty, etc. (Refer to these sections in this chapter.)

Perform venipunctures for cardiac enzymes and possible electrolytes and check medication level as needed to see if ECG or electrolyte changes (i.e., low potassium or calcium) have occurred that can be treated.

Place the patient in a semi-Fowler's position to allow the patient to breathe easier.

Start at least one IV to allow for emergency administration of drugs. If the patient is to receive thrombolytic therapy, three separate IV lines may be needed.

Administer aspirin to help prevent platelets from sticking together.

Administer NTG sublingually and prepare for IV nitroglycerin if the patient's BP is greater than 90 mm Hg to help reduce pain and increase coronary artery perfusion.

Give supplemental oxygen to help increase myocardial oxygenation.

Administer morphine sulfate to help decrease pain and anxiety and decrease preload.

Perform a stat 12-lead ECG to see if changes indicative of an MI have occurred.

Observe for complications of MI, which can include pericarditis, cardiac tamponade, ventricular aneurysm, and cardiogenic shock.

Heart Failure (HF)

What Went Wrong?

Heart failure (HF) is a term used to describe a syndrome of cardiac conditions that affect the structure and function of the heart. In this syndrome, blood is not effectively pumped out of the heart (systolic failure) or allowed to fill it (diastolic failure). The end result is remodeling of the heart. Remodeling occurs when long-term activation of compensatory mechanisms to increase cardiac output leads to

Increased afterload

Peripheral and pulmonary edema

Chamber dilation or hypertrophy

Regardless of the cause, progressive, dysfunctional remodeling leads to progressively worsening ventricular dysfunction.

Etiologies of heart failure include those listed in Table 3–15. The most common causes of HF include ischemia of the heart and hypertension.

TABLE 3–15 Etiology of Heart Failure	
Structural abnormalities	Valvular dysfunction/heart disease; stenosis or regurgitation
	Cardiomyopathy
Functional abnormalities	Hypertension
	MI
	Unrelieved fast dysrhythmias

The risk factors of HF include hypertension, diabetes, high cholesterol levels, obesity, sleep apnea, and a family history of cardiomegaly.

A decrease in cardiac output from HF results in complex hemodynamic and neurohormonal changes. The stress on the heart from structural/functional abnormalities results in a decreased CO. This increases circulating catecholamines, chiefly epinephrine. Epinephrine increases the heart rate and the oxygen consumption, resulting in an increase in demand on the heart, which stresses the heart further.

Heart failure can happen suddenly or acutely in the instance of a patient having a fast tachy rhythm. It can also be slow and insidious in onset as with a patient having slowly rising hypertension. Compensation for heart failure includes the following mechanisms:

Compensatory Mechanisms for Heart Failure

Decrease in CO
results in
Increase in circulating catecholamines (epinephrine) Decrease in blood supply to kidneys
leads to an
Increase in HR and O_2 consumption   Stimulates renin-angiotension system
creating
Decreasing the CO   Increase sodium and water retention
leading to
Increased preload, decreased contractility, and increased afterload

Hallmark Signs and Symptoms

The American Heart Association uses a functional classification of heart failure that includes four classes. Class I includes no limitation of physical activity with no dyspnea or fatigue. Class II includes slight limitation in physical activity, but ordinary activity results in fatigue and dyspnea. Class III includes marked limitation in physical activity without symptoms and symptoms are present at rest. Any physical activity increases symptoms. Class IV includes being unable to carry on any physical activity without symptoms and if any activity is undertaken, symptoms are increased.

- Progressively worsening dyspnea and fatigue
- Tachycardia and new onset rhythm disturbances
- S3 heart sound
- Ascending crackles and worsening cough initially in left-sided HF

- Drop in the O_2 saturation levels in right-sided HF
- Hypotension
- Decreased urinary output
- Increased weight gain
- Reduction of CO elevated PAWP
- Elevated CVP if the patient has right-sided HF alone OR right AND left-sided HF

The signs and symptoms of HF can be further broken down into right- and left-sided heart failure. Left-sided HF is considered much worse as it affects oxygenation of the body and can lead to cardiogenic shock (see Table 3–16).

Prognosis

This is an insidious disease with over 5 million Americans living with HF. Thirty to sixty percent of patients are readmitted within 6 months of initial diagnosis and hospitalization.

Interpreting Test Results

ECGs are done to look for cardiac ischemia or conduction problems that could cause HF. Rhythm disturbances can include many forms of dysrhythmias

TABLE 3–16 Comparison of Right versus Left-Sided Heart Failure	
Right-Sided Heart Failure	**Left-Sided Heart Failure**
Causes	
Left–sided heart failure untreated	Left ventricular infarction
COPD	Hypertension
Tricuspid regurgitation	Aortic stenosis
Right ventricular infarction	
Signs/Symptoms (Peripheral Edema)	**Signs/Symptoms (Pulmonary Edema)**
Exercise intolerance	Exercise intolerance
Elevated JVD	Change in level of responsiveness
Tachycardia	Tachycardia
Hepatosplenomegaly	Crackles, wheezes, hemoptysis
Increased abdominal girth (ascites)	Decreased urinary output below 30 cc/2 hr
Peripheral edema (feet, ankles, legs)	S3 heart sound
Increased CVP	Increased PAWP

including atrial fibrillation or flutter, paraxoysmal atrial tachycardia, premature ventricular contractions (PVCs), ventricular tachycardia, and ventricular fibrillation.

Chest x-rays are done serially to determine if pulmonary edema has resulted or resolved.

BNP (B-type natriuretic peptide) is monitored frequently to diagnose and determine if treatment is effective. A BNP of greater than 400 pg/mL usually indicates significant HF. The higher this value is, the poorer the prognosis for the patient.

Serum electrolytes (K^+, Ca^{++}, Mg^+) are monitored to serve as a baseline for replacement therapy as these electrolytes need normalizing for effective ejection fraction.

Nursing Diagnoses for HF	Expected Outcomes
Ineffective tissue perfusion, peripheral and pulmonary	Clear lung sounds
	VS stable
	HR with normal sinus rhythm or baseline
	Pulmonary artery pressures stabilize
	Urinary output >30 cc/hr
	Resolution of peripheral edema
	Positive peripheral pulses

Interventions

Assess daily weight—the number one accurate indicator of fluid gain or loss. A weight gain of 1 kilogram = 1,000 cc of fluid retention.

Assess lung sounds. Lungs will start with bibasilar crackles that ascend if HF worsens.

Assess the results of ejection fractions and echocardiograms to help determine which therapies are most effective.

Monitor BNP levels. BNP is a significant diagnostic indicator and therapeutic tool to determine if therapy is effective.

Monitor for cardiogenic shock as indicated by a cardiac index of less than 2.0 L/min, systolic BP less than 90 mm Hg, and PAWP of above 18 mm Hg.

Administer morphine sulfate to decrease pulmonary edema and improve oxygenation.

Administer and monitor nitroglycerin to decrease preload and PAWP.

Administer and monitor nesiritide (Natrecor), a synthetic derivative of BNP that helps reduce PCWP in the short term. Monitor closely for hypotension and dysrhythmias.

Administer IV inotropics (dobutamine and milrinone) to improve effectiveness of cardiac muscle.

Insert and monitor pulmonary artery catheter to monitor pressures on right and left side of the heart. Pressures should decrease as therapy is effected.

Prepare and monitor for insertion of IABP to help reduce the afterload and improve the blood supply to the coronary arteries.

Prepare for and monitor patient post insertion of implantable cardioverter defibrillator (ICD) to help increase the heart rate when it is bradycardic and shock the heart if it fibrillates (see Chapter 4 on rhythm disturbances).

Prepare for and monitor initiation of biventricular pacing to help improve the synchronization of the heart, therefore increasing the cardiac output (see Chapter 4).

Ensure that teaching and discharge instructions include information regarding diet, weight monitoring, energy conservation techniques, and medication (ACE/ARBs, digoxin, etc.) to prevent readmission, which frequently occurs with HF.

Teach and refer for smoking cessation advice/counseling to prevent further damage to lungs/heart. For additional information on how to quit smoking check out this web site: http://www.surgeongeneral.gov/tobacco/(last accessed July 1, 2010).

> **NURSING ALERT**
>
> *Daily weights are critical to monitor in a patient with a diagnosis of heart failure. A gain of 1 kilogram = 1,000 cc of fluid retention.*

Inflammatory Disease Process (Pericarditis, Myocarditis, Endocarditis)

Inflammatory heart disease is classified into three different types of pathologies. These include pericarditis, myocarditis, and endocarditis.

What Went Wrong?

Pericarditis Pericarditis is an inflammation of the pericardium or fibrous sac that surrounds the heart. This more commonly occurs after MI but can occur after open-heart surgery (OHS) or as a result of an infection or tumor. Pericarditis becomes a severe problem when fluid builds up, placing outside pressure on the inner structures like the chambers and valves. (See cardiac tamponade in this section.)

Myocarditis Myocarditis is an infection of the myocardium. When cardiac muscle fibers are damaged, they cannot pump effectively. Like pericarditis, myocarditis is commonly seen in infections from viruses, bacteria, and fungi.

Endocarditis Infective endocarditis is an invasion of the inner lining of the heart and valves by microbes. Staphylococci and streptococci tend to invade the heart valves depositing fibrin and platelets causing stenosis of these valves. Risk factors for endocarditis include prosthetic heart valves, IV drug use, and valvular disorders. Endocarditis can lead to systemic embolization; so signs of this should be part of the nursing assessment (see Table 3–17).

The pathophysiology that all of these conditions have in common is that they affect the pumping efficiency of the heart and therefore can lead to heart failure.

Hallmark Signs and Symptoms

TABLE 3–17 Inflammatory Disease Signs/Symptoms	
Disease	**Signs/Symptoms**
Pericarditis	Pain over the heart worsening with movement or breathing deeply (pleuritic pain)
	Pericardial friction rub heard best over the lower–middle left sternal border
	Mild fever
	Signs of dyspnea if heart failure occurs
Myocarditis	Flu–like initially
	Fatigue
	Dyspnea and signs of HF if increases in severity
	May develop sudden cardiac death in severe HF
Endocarditis	Fever
	New onset heart murmurs over valves affected
	Osler nodes, which are small, painful nodes over the pads of the fingers/toes
	Conjunctival and mucous membrane petechiae
	Splinter hemorrhages (reddish–brown lines) of the fingernails
	Janeway lesions (painless, red, irregular macules) on the palms, fingers, toes, and soles of the feet
	Vague feeling of malaise

Prognosis

Prognosis is good if the patient does not go into heart failure and the symptoms are caught early.

Interpreting Test Results

In any inflammatory disease, the nurse can see

- Elevated WBCs.
- Elevated ESR.
- Positive blood cultures isolating the causing organism.
- ECG in pericarditis shows ST segment elevation with an upward concavity and PR segment depression.
- ECG in other inflammatory diseases show nonspecific ST changes.

Nursing Diagnoses for Inflammatory Heart Disease	Expected Outcomes
Decreased CO RT ineffective pumping of the heart	The patient will have normal VS
The patient will have baseline ECG
Hyperthermia RT invasion of the heart by infectious organisms	The patient will have a normal temp.

Interventions

Assess VS, especially temperature. The patient will have an elevated temperature in most inflammatory diseases and it may be present for weeks.

Assess heart sounds for S3, new or worsening murmurs, or friction rub that may indicate HF (S3), compromised valvular functioning (murmur), or pericarditis (friction rub).

Assess for systemic embolization in endocarditis, which can lead to PE and stroke.

Monitor for signs of cardiac tamponade in pericarditis as fluid accumulation can compress the heart.

Monitor laboratory values, especially BNP, for signs of worsening heart failure.

Monitor serial chest x-rays for signs of worsening heart failure.

Limit the patient's activity to prevent further stress and increased O_2 demand on the heart.

Administer and monitor the use of analgesics and anti-inflammatory drugs such as aspirin and ibuprofen in pericarditis to reduce inflammation and pain.

Administer antibiotics to help destroy causative infectious agents.

Administer medications to treat HF.

Identify and treat dysrhythmias if they occur as a result of HF.

Teach antibiotic prophylaxis before invasive procedures (endocarditis) to prevent common recurrence.

Teach patient to carry medical alert identification to communicate presence of past history of pericarditis and institution of antibiotic prophylaxis when treated.

NURSING ALERT

All patients who have had a past history of pericarditis should be treated with prophylactic antibiotics before any invasive procedure.

NURSING ALERT

Myocarditis predisposes the patient to digitalis sensitivity. Digoxin is given to patients with myocarditis to improve contractility. Nurses need to closely monitor patients for digitoxicity. Signs/symptoms include nausea, vomiting, headache, and malaise.

Cardiac Tamponade

What Went Wrong?

Cardiac tamponade occurs when fluid accumulates in the pericardial sac, preventing blood from entering the heart (preload increase) and decreasing CO so that there is a profoundly decreased cardiac output. This would be almost like someone squeezing the heart between the hands in a viselike grip. Nothing could get into the heart and nothing could get out. This is called cardiac tamponade because a tamponade means to apply pressure. This can happen suddenly due to a severe MI, rupture of a coronary artery during angioplasty, or multiple trauma as in the chest being crushed between a car seat and a steering wheel (blunt trauma). It can also occur slowly as in the build up of fluid from a pericardial tumor or radiation pericarditis.

Because the heart cannot fill properly, venous return (preload) increases dramatically, allowing very little blood to get into the heart. The increased pre-load causes blood to back up into the venous system. The heart cannot pump effectively when the atrial valves and ventricles are squeezed; therefore, contractility decreases. Since blood cannot get out, the afterload also decreases. If this process occurs slowly, the heart can compensate using neurohormonal mechanisms listed in the box on page 131. If this process occurs quickly, the following life-threatening symptoms can occur.

Hallmark Signs and Symptoms

Cardiac tamponade	Drop in BP
	Elevated right heart pressures like CVP with decreased PCWP
	Tachycardias and dysrhythmias
	Distended neck veins
	Muffled heart sounds
	Pulsus paradoxus (more than 10 mm Hg drop of systolic BP on inspiration)

NURSING ALERT

There are three classic signs (Beck's triad) of a cardiac tamponade. Hypotension, distended neck veins, and muffled heart sounds. Without prompt treatment the patient will die from a cardiac arrest, so the nurse must identify and mobilize the rapid response team ASAP.

Prognosis

If the cardiac tamponade occurs slowly, the heart can effectively propel blood forward by increasing the contractility of the myocardium. A large amount of fluid can accumulate before symptoms of HF become severe enough to be seen.

If the tamponade develops quickly, as in the case of blunt or penetrating trauma, a medical emergency can result unless pressure around the heart is relieved ASAP.

Interpreting Test Results

Echocardiogram can show fluid around the heart and compression of underlying structures.

ECG can show electrical alternans where one QRS is taller, alternating with a QRS that is shorter.

Chext x-ray (CXR) shows fluid accumulation around the pericardial sac.

Nursing Diagnoses for Cardiac Tamponade	Expected Outcomes
Decreased CO due to pressure on the myocardium from fluid around the pericardial sac	The patient will have a stable BP >100 JVD will be normal Heart sounds will be clear

Interventions

Administer 100% oxygen ASAP via nonrebreather mask to help improve myocardial oxygenation.

Establish an IV line to help with emergency medications prn.

Obtain a stat 12-lead ECG as cardiac tamponade can mimic an MI.

Obtain a chest x-ray, which will show an enlarged cardiac silhouette that occurs with a large cardiac effusion.

Prepare to administer cardiac contractility stimulators like dobutamine to improve the functioning of the myofibrils.

Prepare for an emergency thoracotomy if there are penetrating cardiac injuries.

Prepare for a pericardiocentesis (an echocardiogram-guided needle aspiration); if fluid is from a pericardial effusion it can be removed by this method.

Prepare the patient for a pericardial window, which is done by thoracotomy if fluid recurs.

How to Do It–Nursing Responsibilities in the Preparation of a Patient Having a Pericardiocentesis

1. Assess that consent form has been signed. Ensure time out is conducted.

2. Obtain a pericardiocentesis tray, which includes a cardiac needle and an alligator clip to attach the needle to an ECG machine.

3. Explain to the patient what is going to happen.

4. Make sure there is a patent IV line.

5. Administer sedation and monitor the airway for patency.

6. Take baseline VS and baseline ECG.

7. Have defibrillator and pacemaker available.

8. Obtain an ECG or echocardiogram machine. The alligator clip will be attached to the ECG machine/echocardiogram after the physician inserts the cardiac needle under the xiphoid process into the heart.

9. Watch the ECG printout for ST segment elevation. This indicates that the needle is in the myocardium and needs to be pulled out slightly.

10. Prepare test tubes for specimens, if needed. The exudate may need to be checked for cytology if a tumor is the most likely cause or if no cause is known.

11. Observe the patient closely for signs of tamponade relief, which includes an increasing BP, decreasing neck vein distention, and heart sounds increasing in intensity.

12. Assist the physician with application of a pressure dressing just below the xiphoid process.

13. Monitor the needle insertion site for bleeding. Observe, monitor for rhythm disturbances.

14. Document the procedure and the patient's tolerance.

Pulmonary Embolism (PE)

What Went Wrong?

A pulmonary embolism (PE) occurs when a clot originating in the venous circulation, usually the deep veins of the legs or the pelvis, travels to the lungs and lodges in a pulmonary artery. PE can also occur as a complication from the right side of the heart when the cardiac rhythm is atrial fibrillation or atrial flutter. The lack of complete emptying in atrial fibrillation/flutter can set up eddies within the atria that allow the formation of clots. In these rhythms, the atria do not contract uniformly, which leads to stagnation of blood flow and tendencies to clot.

The hazards of PE can be summarized by Virchow's triad. A patient at highest risk is one who has (1) venous stasis, (2) injury to blood vessels, and (3) hemoconcentrated blood. Venous stasis can be caused by immobility from bedrest and riding in the same position in a car, train, or airplane. Blood vessels can be injured through any instrumentation or surgery, especially of the pelvis and lower extremities such as total knee surgery and prostatectomy. Hypercoagulability or hemoconcentrated blood can result from pregnancy or dehydration.

With the blockage of blood flow in the lungs, the circulation in front of the clot is affected. This blockage acts like a dam where only a trickle of blood (water) gets through. The larger the clot, the more symptomatic the patient becomes. If the clot is large enough, the alveoli do not get venous flow and therefore cannot get rid of CO_2 or absorb O_2. Hypercarbia and hypoxemia result. This is a true perfusion or circulation problem but it affects oxygenation.

Also as with a dam, blood builds up behind the clot, increasing the pressure in the lungs and resulting in pulmonary hypertension.

Hallmark Signs and Symptoms

The symptoms of PE depend upon the size, location, and how much of the pulmonary circulation is blocked. In a small PE, the following symptoms can occur:

- Dyspnea is the most common symptom.
- Tachycardia.
- Atrial fibrillation/flutter may be present.
- Pleuritic chest pain that often mimics an MI.
- Shortness of breath.
- Decreased breath sounds over the affected area.

Signs of shock can occur if the PE is massive. These include

- Hypotension
- Cyanosis
- Change in the level of responsiveness
- Cold, clammy skin
- Decreased urinary output
- Hemoptysis
- Elevated CVP or RA and PA pressures (right-sided heart pressures)
- Low PCWP pressure (left-sided pressure)

Prognosis
The best thing to do is prevent PE, but once it occurs the mortality rate is high, especially if a large portion of the pulmonary circulation is blocked.

Interpreting Test Results
Because PE mimics other conditions, many studies are done to rule out those conditions.

Worsening hypoxemia and hypercapnea with respiratory acidosis.

Chest x-ray to rule out pulmonary edema or tumor.

ECG to rule out MI.

Spiral CT of the lungs.

Positive D-dimer assay, which shows presence of blood clots.

Pulmonary angiogram where dye is injected into the heart is the definitive test, but it has a high mortality rate.

Nursing Diagnoses for PE	Expected Outcomes
Tissue perfusion, ineffective (pulmonary) RT damming of blood from the right side of the heart	The patient will have stable VS
	The patient will have normal RA, PAP, and PCWP pressures
Ineffective tissue oxygenation	The patient will have normal pH, pO_2 and pCO_2 levels on room air

Interventions
Ongoing assessment of VS and SaO_2 to see if therapy returns the VS to baseline and oxygen levels rise.

Give the patient oxygen at high liter flow to help recruit functional alveoli.

Elevate the head of the bed to allow the patient to breathe easier by dropping the diaphragm using gravity.

Keep the patient on bedrest to decrease the chances that a clot can travel farther and to prevent strain on the heart.

Monitor the heart rhythm for atrial fibrillation and flutter, which can cause PE.

Prepare the patient for a spiral CAT scan, which can indicate that a clot is actually occurring.

Prepare to administer thrombolytics to dissolve the blood clot (see Table 3–9 for anticoagulants for nursing care).

Prepare the patient for a pulmonary angiogram if embolectomy is being considered.

Prepare to administer anticoagulants like heparin or low molecular weight heparin to help prevent the clot(s) from enlarging or others from occurring.

Prepare to insert a PA catheter if pressures of the heart and fluid status are in question.

Observe for heparin-induced thrombocytopenia, which is a complication of heparin therapy (a marked drop in platelets after giving heparin).

Teach the patient that he or she may need a vena caval umbrella, which can help prevent clots from going to the right side of the heart by acting like a sieve.

Teach the need for systemic anticoagulation on coumadin, usually for life, to prevent further PE.

Teach the patient to keep mobile, hydrated, and be cognizant of signs/symptoms of deep venous thrombosis (DVT)/PE so he or she can seek early help and treatment for PE.

Surgical CV Conditions Requiring Critical Care

Percutaneous Coronary Interventions (PCIs)

What Went Wrong?

❻ PCIs in the form of coronary angioplasty or cardiac stenting are generally done after a cardiac catheterization to compress the underlying plaque into the arterial wall (angioplasty) and prop the artery open by lining it with a mesh-pipe link device (stenting).

When the patient has angina and is given clot busters (thrombolytics), the clot busters open the artery dissolving the clot, but the plaque still narrows the coronary arteries. To restore unimpeded blood flow, the lumen of the artery must be widened and plaque compressed. If that is not possible, coronary artery bypass grafting (CABG) will be necessary.

Generally, the first procedure is coronary angioplasty, but this does not ensure that the artery will remain open. Since the area where the angioplasty occurs is inflamed, platelets and other sticky substances migrate to this area and can reclot what the health care workers have tried hard to keep open. Therefore, many times during an angioplasty the physician will insert a stent. The stent covers these inflamed areas, decreasing the likelihood that the vessel will reocclude.

Sometimes additional drugs will be given after PCIs to help prevent reocclusion. These drugs, II-III glycoprotein inhibitors like ReoPro and Integrilin, stop clot activation. The platelet membrane contains glycoprotein receptors that bind with fibrinogen, linking the platelets together. Glycoprotein inhibitors block this platelet-linking process, leading to less reoclussion after PCIs. Drug-emitting stents may also be placed. To prevent reocclusion after the PCIs, patients are usually prescribed aspirin and clopidogrel (Plavix) for long-term anticoagulation.

Hallmark Signs and Symptoms
Refer to the sections on angina/MI for signs and symptoms of reoclussion of the artery.

Prognosis
The prognosis is good after an angioplasty or stent, but the nurse must be observant for signs/symptoms of reocclusion of the vessel.

Interpreting Test Results
- See signs and symptoms for MI/angina.
- Baseline coagulation studies including H&H, PT, PTT, platelets.
- Baseline renal studies like BUN and creatinine can show the kidney's ability to excrete the dye injected.
- Baseline ECG and rhythm strip to monitor for postoperative complications.

Nursing Diagnoses for PCIs	Expected Outcomes
Risk for decreased CO related to reocclu-sion of the coronary artery	The patient will have 0 pain on a scale of 1-10

Interventions (Preprocedure)

Assess for consent form and time out to make sure that legally the patient knows what will occur and to identify the correct patient/procedure.

Assess baseline VS to determine normal from abnormal after the procedure.

Assess all baseline laboratories and diagnostic studies so that nurse knows what is normal for the patient.

Assess baseline peripheral pulses as clots can embolize to any organ/extremity.

Prepare the patient for angioplasty and stenting telling the patient that he or she will have to lay quiet and flat and that flushing may occur with dye insertion so the patient will know what to expect.

Ensure a patent IV; so medications maybe administered during the procedure.

Administer preprocedural sedation to decrease sympathetic stimulation and relax the patient as much as possible.

Teach the patient to report any abnormal sensations like chest pain/pressure, numbness, or tingling in extremities so the patient can self-monitor and let the nurse know what to report to him or her.

Teach the patient that he or she will be on aspirin and Plavix (clopidogrel) after the procedure to prevent reblockage of the artery.

Interventions (Post Procedure)

Assess VS and rhythm according to protocols to note early signs of complications.

Assess all peripheral pulses to make sure no clot formation has occurred.

Assess the insertion site according to protocols to monitor for hematoma and hemorrhage.

Monitor the IV and any medications that may have been added like II-III glycoprotein inhibitors.

Administer fluids as per protocol to dilute the dye injected and prevent renal failure (the dyes are nephrotoxic).

Teach the patient to lay flat and log roll if he or she needs to turn, to prevent reopening or hemorrhage at the PCI site.

Teach the patient about the importance of taking medications like ASA and Ticlid as prescribed to prevent reocclusion.

Open-Heart Surgery (OHS)

OHS is a general term for any surgery where the chest is opened and the heart is surgically corrected. Two types of OHS are common: valve replacement and coronary artery bypass grafting (CABG).

Valve Replacement

What Went Wrong?

Any valve in the heart can become stenotic (narrowed) or loose (regurgitation/insufficiency). Stenotic valves are caused by atherosclerosis and fibrosis of aging. They are also caused by vegetation collecting on them in conditions like bacterial endocarditis. Valves become loose from congenital problems like a floppy mitral value (mitral stenosis), and they can become loose when the chordae tendineae become weak or fail to close when the myocardium they are attached to become necrotic and do not function. The valves that are most prone to wear and tear are on the left side of the heart. These "keep on a ticking although they keep getting a licking" from the high-pressure state of the left heart.

Let us take stenosis first. No matter what the cause in a stenotic valve such as mitral stenosis, look at what it does to the preceding chamber, in this case the left atrium. The left atrium has to work harder to pump blood through this very tight valve. The left atrium rises to the challenge by increasing its size to meet the job it is now required to do; therefore, left atrial hypertrophy (enlarged muscle) results. Over time, this chamber becomes overworked and the muscle becomes flabby and does not eject blood as efficiently. This can lead to decreased blood flow with a damming effect. If you remember what happened in left-sided heart failure, fluid will now alarmingly build up in the lungs, causing pulmonary edema and all of the symptoms of left-sided heart failure. This is a backward problem so you will sometimes hear this referred to as backward failure.

What happens in front of this tight mitral valve is also affected. Since blood cannot get through very well, the left ventricle is stressed as well. To propel the little blood that gets through, that left ventricle also has to work harder. As it overworks due to this stress, it enlarges as well. This sets the heart up for forward failure. No matter what valve is affected, if you use the model of backward and forward flow problems, you can piece together what happens in the heart.

A valve can also be loose or cause regurgitation. Let us take the mitral valve again and piece this through. If the mitral valve is very floppy, the valve leaflets cannot maintain their shape and turn back upon themselves into the atria. Therefore the mitral valve can never really shut tight, thus allowing blood back into the previous chamber during ventricular contraction. Blood flows back into the atria instead of going forward from the ventricle into the aorta. The poor heart can never catch up as it recycles blood back and hardly forward. So again, in each chamber both atria and ventricles have to work harder to build up pressure to open the valves.

Hallmark Signs and Symptoms

- Asymptomatic at first
- Dyspnea that increases with exertion
- Fatigue
- Murmur over the valve that is affected
- Signs and symptoms of heart failure: right-sided failure if it is a right heart valve like the tricuspid and pulmonic, and left-sided failure if it is the mitral and aortic valves (see section on heart failure and Table 3–16).

Prognosis

Valvular problems are progressively disabling and affect the ADLs as signs and symptoms of HF worsen. A valve replacement is needed to help with the quality of life. Prognosis is good if this occurs.

Valves can be replaced with either porcine (pig) or mechanical valves. If the patient chooses a mechanical heart valve he or she will have to take anticoagulant medications for life, because platelets adhere to the valves possibly leading to stroke or PE.

NURSING ALERT

Patients who opt to have a mechanical heart valve will need to take coumadin for life. They will need frequent prothrombin time/international normalized ratio (PT/INR) assessments to evaluate their level of anticoagulation. They must also wear medical alerts so health care workers can take precautions to prevent bleeding.

Interpreting Test Results

- See tests for HF.
- Cardiac catheterization on the side that the valve has affected.
- Echocardiography will show either a stenotic or regurgitant valve.

Nursing Diagnoses for Valvular Dysfunction	Expected Outcomes
See section on heart failure (HF)	

Interventions

See interventions for HF and CABG.

Teach the patient wound care to monitor for early signs of mediastinal infection.

Teach the patient that he or she will need systemic anticoagulation with coumadin if the patient has a mechanical heart valve as these valves are prone to developing blood clots.

Reinforce antibiotic prophylaxis to prevent endocarditis.

Coronary Artery Bypass Grafting (CABG)

What Went Wrong?

CABG involves taking veins (saphenous) from the legs or arteries (radial, internal mammary) to bypass an obstructed coronary artery. CABG is performed when coronary angioplasty and stents do not keep an artery open or the blockage cannot be reached during angioplasty. This type of open-heart surgery may require that the heart be stopped to work on the arteries that are on the epicardial surface of the heart. To maintain adequate tissue perfusion, the patient needs to be on a heart-lung machine (cardiopulmonary [CP] bypass) when the heart is stopped.

Veins chosen are sewn from the aorta to the areas where the blockages are revascularizing areas that are ischemic or injured. CABG cannot revascularize dead or infarcted tissue. A minimally invasive technique can be used where the surgery is done without CP bypass. This is limited to patients with proximal disease of the left anterior descending or right coronary artery disease.

Some patients have inoperable disease and will need to be treated medically. These patients include those with very small coronaries distal to the blockage, severe aortic stenosis, and severe left ventricular dysfunction with other organ system disease.

After the patient is prepared, a midline incision is done (sternotomy) and the heart is stopped usually by an iced saline and potassium solution. The veins/arteries are procured and reimplanted. Then the heart is restarted by defibrillation.

Prognosis

CABG is done to increase the quality of life by decreasing anginal attacks and improve patient survival.

Interpreting Test Results Pre- and Postoperatively

CBC and electrolyte studies are done for baselines.

Nasal swabs for methicillin-resistant *Staphylococcus aureus* (MRSA) are completed to prevent contamination of the surgical field with a preexisting infection.

Baseline coagulation studies are done to prevent hemorrhage.

Renal and hepatic function tests are done to see if there are other preexisting conditions that might prevent the patient from tolerating the surgical procedure.

Pulmonary function tests are done as the elderly and patients with COPD are at greater risk for respiratory complications and need to be identified early.

Chest x-rays are completed to rule out a preexisting tumor, fluid accumulation, or infection.

Echocardiography is completed to determine ejection fraction, functioning of heart valves, and heart wall motion.

Nursing Diagnoses for CABG	Expected Outcomes
Impaired gas exchange due to malpositioned endotracheal tube, increased capillary permeability, increased fluids, pulmonary hypertension	The patient will have SaO$_2$ and baseline ABGs The CVP and PAP will be baseline
Decreased cardiac output due to stunned myocardium from sur-gery and/or cardiac dysrhythmias	The patient will have normal VS The patient will have normal PAP, PCWP, CO/CI The patient will be in normal sinus rhythm The patient will have a normal CVP, flat neck vein, and clear heart sounds
Fluid volume deficit due to bleed-ing from the incisional areas, chest tube sites	The patient will have a normal H&H, coag-ulation profiles, chest tube drainage

Interventions (Early)

Assess vital signs to determine if patient is stable and not going into cardiogenic shock and/or fluid volume deficit.

Assess airway and SaO$_2$ as the patient will be intubated and on the ventilator (see ventilator care; Chapter 2).

Plan for early intubation within 4 hours to decrease the chance of ventilator-assisted pneumonia.

Perform PA, CVP, PCWP, CO, and CI as per hospital protocol to determine if the patient is hemodynamically stable.

Assess urinary output every hour to determine if CO and fluid status is adequate, and also to see if renal status is impaired. The patient should have at least 30 cc/hr. The physician should be notified if this standard has not been met to prevent dehydration and early renal failure.

Measure chest tube output every hour until stable to determine if there is cardiac tamponade or hemorrhage. Observe surgeon's protocol for abnormal drainage, usually more than 100 mL/hr.

Monitor cardiac rhythm status as elderly patients can go into atrial fibrillation and may need to be treated with antiarrhythmic medications, anticoagulation, or cardioversion; PVCs are also frequent signs of ventricular irritability (see Chapter 4, Care of the Patient with Critical Cardiac Rhythm Disturbance Needs).

Rewarm (slowly) the patient if needed with warming blankets, by increasing room temperature, and/or using radiant heat to prevent hypothermia, which can lead to dysrhythmias, hypoxemia, and impaired coagulation.

Observe for pulmonary edema as a result of increased capillary permeability that occurs with third spacing after surgery.

Observe for PE and DVT as the patient is on bedrest and clots can be a complication of IABP, CP bypass, bedrest, and atrial dysrhythmias.

Monitor neurologic status using the Glasgow Coma Scale as patients are at increased risk for stroke. (see Chapter 5, Care of the Patient with Neurological Needs).

Assess bowel sounds as patients will have absent sounds initially, but they will return within a day of getting out of bed (OOB).

Monitor oral gastric tube and administer antiulcer medications to prevent stress ulcers.

Monitor IABP if patient needs counterpulsation to give the heart a rest after surgery.

Administer a hypertonic solution like D51/4NSS to reabsorb third-space fluids.

Have patient turn, cough, and deep breathe and administer percussion and incentive spirometry (when extubated) to prevent atelectasis and pulmonary infections.

Assist patient with getting OOB when medically cleared or according to protocols to prevent atelectasis and pneumonia.

Splint the incision when turning to prevent pulling on the sternotomy.

Administer vasoactive drips to maintain MAP greater than 80 mm Hg.

Administer pain medications to allow the patient to turn, cough, and deep breathe without undue pain.

Attach temporary pacemaker to the epicardial leads so they can be used immediately if the patient experiences bradycardias or heart blocks. Label leads clearly to prevent accidental attachment when pacer is needed. When manipulating wires, the nurse should wear gloves to prevent microshocks that can lead to ventricular fibrillation.

Give psychological support to significant others because when they visit the patient, the lines and equipment and physiological changes from edema can be overwhelming.

Interventions (Late)

Monitor for postpericardiotomy syndrome, which is a type of pericarditis (fever, malaise, dyspnea, chest pain, pleural and pericardial effusions, friction rub), as this is a common occurrence 4 days postoperatively.

Observe for cardiac tamponade as this can occur from fluid/inflammatory buildup (electrical alternans, increased neck veins, muffled heart sounds, hypotension).

Assess for wound infection associated with sternal infection (fever, increased WBCs, exudate and inflammation at the sternal incision).

Teach the patient regarding medications, mobility, rest, and pain relief to help give patient control over his or her situation.

Encourage patient to attend community support groups to help identify successful strategies and receive emotional support.

Heart Transplantation

What Went Wrong?

A heart transplant involves the removal of all or part of a patient's heart, replacing it with a donor's heart. A median sternotomy and CP bypass are completed as with CABG. An orthotopic technique is the most common and is performed when the recipient's right and left atria, pulmonary artery, and aorta are removed. The recipient's septum and posterior and lateral walls of the atria are left intact along with the SA nodes and inferior and superior vena cava. The donor's anterior walls of the atrial SA node, internodal condition pathways, and ventricles are attached. The left and right atria are connected as well as the pulmonary arteries and aorta. Pacing wires are attached.

Transplantation is usually performed when a patient has a cardiac structural defect or has lost so much myocardium due to myocarditis or MI that the heart cannot pump effectively, compromising CO. If greater than 40% of the left ventricle dies from an MI, the patient will swiftly succumb to heart failure without a transplant. The patient may be forced to severely restrict his or her activity or have lifesaving measures like the IABP instituted until a suitable donor is found.

Since both the donor's and the recipient's SA nodes are intact, the patient will have two "P" waves on an ECG. The recipient atrial depolarization cannot cross the suture line; therefore, the donor "P" wave depolarizes the heart. The donor "P" waves are denervated so they do not respond to vagal influences, thus the patient's heart rate will be slightly higher than normal around 90 to 110 beats/minute. Because of postoperative edema, the patient may need temporary cardiac pacing to maintain an adequate CO.

Prognosis

See section on open-heart surgery (OHS). The patient who requires transplantation usually has advanced heart disease. The likelihood of survival without a transplant in end-stage cardiac disease is less than 25% within 1 year. Patients with fixed pulmonary hypertension, unresolved pulmonary infarction, and advanced or poorly controlled diabetes are not candidates.

Interpreting Test Results

See tests for open-heart surgery (OHS).

HLA type to help decrease the likelihood of cardiac tissue rejection.

Nursing Diagnoses for Heart Transplantation	Expected Outcomes
See section on open-heart surgery (OHS)	

Interventions

See section on open-heart surgery (OHS).

Assess HR because the denervated heart rate does not respond as quickly as the normal heart.

Administer antirejection medications for life to decrease the incidence of graft-host rejection.

Attach and prepare for temporary epicardial pacing if the HR remains lower than normal to maintain CO.

Observe for right ventricular failure as this is the most common complication after transplantation (for unknown reasons).

Teach the patient about orthostatic hypotension and to rise slowly in the morning and during activity as the denervated heart does not respond as quickly as the normal heart.

Encourage the patient to attend cardiac rehabilitation programs to help strengthen the heart to respond to demands. The heart cannot respond to direct sympathetic nervous system stimulation; it must wait for circulating catecholamines, which may take more than 3 to 5 minutes. Exercise tolerance must be helped using warm-up and cool-down exercises.

Encourage the patient to keep annual stress test, angiography, or ultrasonography appointments as the denervated heart does not experience angina, so pain is not experienced and other quantitative means of heart function are needed to monitor progress.

Abdominal Aortic Aneurysm (AAA)

What Went Wrong?

An aneurysm is a weakening in the medial layer of the arterial wall that causes it to dilate. High pressure within the arterial system further weakens this area, causing it to balloon outward. Just like with an overfilled balloon, any more pressure can make it rupture or pop. When an AAA ruptures, the patient hemorrhages into the retroperitoneal space and quickly bleeds to death. Arteriosclerosis changes due to aging, hypertension, and smoking are risk factors associated with AAA. Genetics and race play an important part as AAAs tend to run in families.

There are two types of aneurysms: true and dissecting. A true aneurysm involves all three linings of the artery. It can be saclike, involving either side of the artery (fusiform), or one sided (saccular). Saccular aneurysms tend to rupture more frequently as the areas of weakness are concentrated into small areas. The problem with true AAAs is that they can rupture, causing death due to hemorrhage into the peritoneal cavity. A false or dissecting aneurysm is a tear that opens in the inner wall of the artery and is frequently associated with Marfan's syndrome.

Hallmark Signs and Symptoms

Most AAAs cannot be detected on physical examination, especially in obese patients. Usually they are found during a routine physical or x-ray. During the physical assessment the examiner may find a pulsating mass slightly left of midline in the upper abdominal quadrant. An associated bruit is often present as well. However, only 50% of patients with an AAA have a bruit present, so further diagnostic testing is necessary to confirm its presence. An AAA is not usually surgically corrected unless it is larger than 5 cm.

> **NURSING ALERT**
>
> *A pulsating abdominal mass should not be palpated aggressively as it could further damage or cause the rupture of an AAA. Auscultate any pulsating masses first! If the patient is experiencing pain, rupture may occur at any time! Notify the health care provider stat!*

The most deadly complication of an AAA is rupture. Rupture can be indicated by

- Sudden onset of severe, unrelieved back pain that radiates to the flank or groin
- Pulsating mass with bruit around the umbilicus
- Extreme abdominal tenderness
- Loss of pulses to the lower extremities

> **NURSING ALERT**
>
> *Severe, unrelieved pain in a patient with a history of AAA is a cause for activation of the quick response team as it can preclude imminent rupture.*

Prognosis

Over 1.5 million Americans have an AAA and the numbers are increasing. It is like a ticking time bomb as most patients are asymptomatic, but it is the 13th leading cause of death in America. It is a major cause of death in males over the age of 50.

If monitored closely and intervention is early to keep the BP down, prognosis is good. However, if one ruptures or dissects, even if the patient is in a health care setting when it happens, prognosis is very grave as death occurs due to an arterial bleed.

Lifestyle modification in terms of lowering blood pressure, smoking cessation, and cholesterol lowering are usually done. Diagnostic tests monitor the progress of the AAA.

Interpreting Test Results

Ultrasounds are a noninvasive way to assess for an aneurysm and monitor its growth.

CT scans can also look at whether clots are present in a dissecting or leaking aneurysm.

Arteriography and angiography must be done prior to surgery. Surgical intervention is rarely done on aneurysms smaller than 4 to 5 cm (see Table 3–18).

Nursing Diagnoses for AAA	Expected Outcomes
Pain, acute RT expansion of vascular mass	The patient will have pain controlled from 0 to +1/10
Tissue perfusion, alteration in (peripheral) due to expanding vascular lesions	The patient will have 0 expansion of vascular lesion

TABLE 3–18 Types of Surgeries for AAA		
Surgery	**Description**	**Postoperative Care**
Open repair with an endoaneurys-morrhaphy	Incision below xiphoid process to symphysis pubis Cross clamp above and below aneurysm Plaque and clots removed Graph is placed around AAA and sutured in place to aneurysm	Airway care—intubated Breathing—cough and deep breathing Incentive spirometry Circulation—monitor VS especially BP as graft can clot or leak if BP is too low or high Discharge planning—a longer hospital stay
Endovascular stent graft or endovascular aneurysm repair	Less invasive than open repair; decreased hospitalization and recovery time Bilateral groin incisions made. Contrast medium is injected so allergy to dye is assessment is critical Metal mesh stent inserted through femoral artery via fluoroscopy Graft is positioned by balloon inflation that bypasses the aneurysm Graft hooks on to intima of the artery; allows blood to flow through it to lower extremities	Airway care—intubated Breathing—cough and deep breathing Incentive spirometry Circulation—bilateral calf-high compression stockings applied. Observe for bleeding at the site Discharge planning—usually sent home very quickly

Nursing Interventions

Assess and continuously monitor VS, especially BP. HTN can increase the size of or rupture an AAA.

Assess and continuously monitor pain. Unrelieved pain can indicate an enlarging AAA or imminent rupture.

Assess for presence of thrill/bruit in lower abdominal area. This indicates a possible AAA.

Teach patient the possible surgical options, to help the patient make an informed choice.

Teach patient about keeping control of BP, cessation of smoking, and lowering cholesterol to prevent the AAA from enlarging.

Teach patient about the signs/symptoms of impending rupture/bleeding and seeking medical attention early.

Teach patient about keeping follow-up appointments. Lifelong monitoring is important.

CASE STUDY

❼ M.J., a 50-year-old African American, arrives at the hospital with complaints of frequent nocturia, a persistent cough, a 20-lb weight gain within 1 week, extreme fatigue, and shortness of breath while climbing his stairs at home and going outside to check his mail. He has a history of hypertension and sleeps with several pillows and his feet propped up since his "feet and ankles have become very swollen within the past week." As a nurse, you begin to suspect the onset of HF in M.J.

QUESTIONS
1. Identify probable causes of heart failure.
2. List assessment findings in M.J. that confirm the likelihood of HF.
3. Identify the diagnostic tools that might be used to support evidence of HF.
4. What side of M.J.'s heart is primarily affected in this scenario?
5. Develop several actual nursing diagnoses for this patient.
6. Describe nursing interventions that would promote the relief of some of M.J.'s persistent symptoms.

REVIEW QUESTIONS

1. Which isoenzyme most quickly reflects that a patient has suffered an acute and recent myocardial infarction?

   A. LDH

   B. CK–MM

   C. SGOT

   D. Troponin

2. A 75-year-old individual is admitted with a diagnosis of left-sided heart failure and is administered Lasix 80 mg by slow IV push. Which nursing assessment indicates that the Lasix (furosemide) is NOT having the desired effect?

   A. Oliguria

   B. Decrease in blood pressure

   C. Absence of crackles

   D. Polydipsia

3. A newly admitted patient, diagnosed with a myocardial infarction and left ventricular heart failure, might exhibit which of the following physical symptoms? Choose all that apply.

   A. Jugular vein distention

   B. Hepatomegaly

   C. Dyspnea

   D. Crackles

   E. Tachycardia

   F. Right-upper-quadrant pain

4. A patient is admitted to your telemetry unit with chest pain that has been increasing in intensity and duration. The critical care nurse can identify that this type of angina is called

   A. Stable

   B. Variant

   C. Predictable

   D. Unstable

5. A patient is admitted in acute distress with unrelieved back pain that radiates to his groin. This patient has a history of an abdominal aortic aneurysm (AAA). What additional signs and symptoms might the patient state?

   A. Midsternal chest pressure relieved with nitroglycerin paste

   B. Bruit to left of the midline in the abdominal area

   C. Extreme headache

   D. Numbness and tingling in the hands and arms

6. A nurse is monitoring a patient newly admitted with acute heart failure (HF). Which of the following laboratory/diagnostic results would indicate the presence of significant HF?

    A. BNP of 1000 pg/mL

    B. Sodium of 150

    C. Potassium of 5.7 mEq/L

    D. pH of 7.30

7. A patient is admitted with severe uncompensated pulmonary edema secondary to chronic heart failure. After diagnostic testing, it is found that the left coronary artery is blocked, which has led to his pulmonary edema. Which of the following signs and symptoms is consistent with this diagnosis?

    A. Elevated central venous pressure

    B. Elevated blood pressure

    C. Elevated pulmonary artery wedge pressure (PAWP) or PAOP

    D. Increased oxygen saturation

8. A patient is admitted with an ST segment myocardial infarction. The patient's wife overhears the physician talking about this and asks you, the nurse, what the physician means by this type of heart attack. The nurse's BEST response would include

    A. "Your husband has permanent changes that will stay on his ECG and the practitioner will always be able to tell he has had an MI."

    B. "Your husband has had a smaller MI that goes through only part of the wall of the heart and therefore causes small areas to stay elevated."

    C. "Your husband has had a rather large heart attack that has caused the death of the heart muscle through all of its three layers."

    D. " Your husband is lucky; his cardiac markers are not elevated but he has had a severe heart attack that we can take care of with medications."

9. The nurse is assessing the laboratory values for a patient with chronic heart failure before administering furosemide. Which of the following values would cause the nurse to withhold this drug and notify the primary care provider?

    A. Potassium level of 3.5 mEq/ L

    B. Digoxin level of 0.7 ng/mL

    C. Calcium level of 5 mg/dL

    D. Magnesium level of 1 mg/dL

10. **A patient is admitted to your acute coronary care unit with the diagnosis of ACS. The nurse has seen ECG changes that are indicative of an anterior wall infarction and is observing the patient for signs/symptoms of complications. The nurse has noted the following vital sign trends:**

Time	HR	RR	BP	Cardiac Rhythm
1100	92	24	140/88	NSR
1115	96	26	128/82	NSR
1130	104	28	102/68	ST
1145	120	32	80/52	ST with frequent PVCs

The nurse should be alert for which of the following complications? Choose all that apply.

A. Syncope

B. Pericarditis

C. Cardiogenic shock

D. Cardiac tamponade

E. Ventricular aneurysm

F. Acute respiratory failure

ANSWERS

CASE STUDY

1. HTN, MI, gender, and race.
2. Increased urination, persistent cough, 20-lb weight gain in 1 week, extreme fatigue and SOB with exertion, feet and ankle edema.
3. The BNP is the most definite, especially if it is greater than 400 pg/mL. Chest x-rays can show pulmonary edema but not the cause. ABGs can indicate respiratory alkalosis in the early stages and acidosis in the later stages. A decreased SaO_2 can confirm a drop in oxygenation, but ABGs are more specific. An ECG can show nonspecific ST segment elevation or MI changes (which can cause HF).
4. He has signs and symptoms of biventricular failure. His SOB and persistent cough indicate left (lung) involvement but his edema indicates right (peripheral).
5. Decreased CO RT effects of high systemic pressure, pulmonary pressures AMB greater than BP, cough, SOB, and peripheral edema. Ineffective gas exchange RT increased pulmonary capillary pressure AMB cough and SOB.
6.

Symptoms/Signs	Interventions
Nocturia Weight gain	Fluid restrictions especially after 6 p.m. Diuretic therapy Decrease intake of salt–laden foods
SOB Persistent cough	Elevate the HOB Rest on pillows on the over–the–bed table Oxygen Diuretic therapy
High BP	Antihypertensive medications like ACE inhibitors or ARBs, beta–blockers, calcium channel blockers Stress management therapy Weight reduction
Peripheral edema	Antihypertensive medications like ACE inhibitors or ARBs, beta–blockers, calcium channel blockers Diuretic therapy Stress management therapy Weight reduction Low sodium diet Elevate legs above the heart Periodic rest periods throughout the day

CORRECT ANSWERS AND RATIONALES

1. D. This enzyme is found in cardiac tissue and will rapidly increase with the onset of a myocardial infarction.

2. A. Furosemide (Lasix) is a loop diuretic, which should increase urinary output. Oliguria is scant or severely decreased urinary output.

3. C, D, and E are some of the signs and symptoms of left-sided heart failure, which backs up into the lungs. A, B, and F are indicators of right-sided heart failure, which is caused by systemic congestion.

4. D. Unstable angina increases in intensity and occurs more frequently with longer events. Stable angina is predictable; the patient can tell you when it is going to occur. Variant or Prinzmetal's angina is atypical and occurs at rest.

5. B. Bruits are associated with turbulence of blood flow and are auscultated in 50% of patients with an AAA. Otherwise the patient is asymptomatic. A is more associated with angina, and C is associated with stroke. Numbness and tingling in the lower extremities is usually due to a decreased blood supply to the lower extremities from hemorrhage into the peritoneal cavity.

6. A. The BNP is a significant diagnostic and monitoring tool for HF. Any value greater than 400 pg/mL indicates significant HF. Although all of the additional laboratory values may be elevated (sodium and potassium) or decreased (pH) in HF, BNP is the most accurate predictor.

7. C. An increased PAWP (PAOP) is consistent with fluid buildup in the lungs and inability of the left side of the heart to pump to the body. A would be correct if this patient had a right ventricular infarction causing right-sided heart failure. The BP and oxygen saturation are usually lower in left-sided HF.

8. B. An ST segment MI is one that is usually referred to as a smaller, less severe type where the enzymes are elevated but the depth of tissue death has not penetrated all three muscular coats. The ECG changes are not permanent; therefore, a trained practitioner would not see a "Q" wave that is permanent on the ECG.

9. A. Even though this potassium level is on the low side and it will go even lower without potassium supplementation. The other values are within normal limits.

10. C, D, and E. Because there is a progressive downward spiral in the BP and a dramatic increase in the HR and RR with rhythm disturbances, this patient could be experiencing cardiogenic shock and tamponade. In shock, the heart fails to keep the BP elevated to nourish the tissues, so the HR elevates causing tachycardias and tachydysrhythmias. The same sequela can occur when the heart is compressed and no blood can enter or exit as in a cardiac tamponade as well as an aneurysm, where the heart pumping can be compromised by lack of pumping in the ballooned out or weakened areas. Pericarditis is noted by a friction rub and elevated temperature with constant, dull chest pain. Syncope could look like the above but it is associated with activity, which this patient is not doing in an acute situation. Acute respiratory failure would look like the above if the BP were elevated.

chapter 4

Care of the Patient With Critical Cardiac Rhythm Disturbance Needs

LEARNING OBJECTIVES

At the end of this chapter, the student will be able to:

1. Identify nursing assessment skills needed to monitor rhythm strips and ECGs.

2. Tell how cardiac monitoring works.

3. Use an organized format for rhythm strip interpretation.

4. Label lead placement on the patient for a 12-lead ECG.

5. Identify medications commonly used to care for a patient with complex rhythm disturbance needs.

6. Compare uses and functions of cardiac pacemakers and implanted defibrillators.

7. Discuss nursing care required in a cardiac arrest, defibrillation, cardioversion, and ICD.

KEY WORDS

ACLS – Advanced Cardiac Life Support
Asynchronous pacing (fixed)
Atrial kick
Baseline
BLS – Basic Cardiac Life Support
Cardiac monitor
Depolarization
Dual-chamber pacing
ECG calipers
Ectopic beats
Electrode
Escaped beats

ICD – implantable cardioverter
    defibrillator
Isoelectric line
Lead wire
Nonconducted P wave
Pacemakers: transthoracic, epicardial,
    permanent, and transvenous
Premature beats
Repolarization
Supraventricular
Synchronous pacing (demand)
12-lead ECG

Assessment Skills

❶ Assessment of cardiovascular status is a vital skill set for critical care nurses. Good, solid experience with basic medical-surgical patients is required in many institutions prior to jumping into the critical care setting, because many of the signs are subtle and experience is necessary so that nothing is omitted. Not all of the rhythms you will learn in this chapter cause a serious drop in a patient's pulse and BP, but many of them do. The addition of complex cardiac monitoring and equipment the nurse is challenged to learn and master is no replacement for sound, organized, thorough nursing judgment. This is best acquired by exposure to a wide variety of patients and situations.

Whenever cardiac output is in question, many body systems are involved. We covered many of these in Chapter 3, but because these are essential skills, a bit of repetition might be, a very good thing. In Table 4–1, refresh yourself with what those signs and symptoms might be using the body systems approach. These are not written in the order that the nurse would perform the skills, because nurses are very good at multitasking and many of these might be done simultaneously.

TABLE 4–1 Symptoms of Decreased Cardiac Output

Body System	Method	Symptoms
Neurological	Inspection	Change in the level of consciousness or Glasgow Coma Scale; dizziness, anxiety, distress, confusion; sense of impending doom; dilated pupils
Cardiovascular	Inspection	Pale or bluish coloration
		Pulsations in the pericardial area lateral and inferior to the point of maximum impulse (PMI)
		Cool, clammy skin
		Diaphoresis
		Jugular venous distention (JVD)
		Peripheral edema
		Syncope (fainting)
	Palpation	Thrills/bruits
		Weak, thready pulses; full and pounding pulses
	Percussion	Not generally done as x-rays are readily available
	Auscultation	Orthostatic hypotension; hypotension, hypertension
		Bradycardia, tachycardia
		Pulse deficits; skipped beats
		S3, S4
		Muffled heart sounds; pericardial friction rubs
Pulmonary	Inspection	Productive cough; pink or blood–tinged sputum
		Use of accessory muscles of respiration (intercostals, abdominals); nasal flaring
	Auscultation	Diminished breath sounds
		Crackles (rales), gurgles (rhonchi), wheezes
GU	Inspection	Oliguria; concentrated amber urine
GI*	Auscultation	Decreased or absent bowel sounds
	Inspection	Nausea, vomiting; anorexia

NURSING ALERT

Remember your basic assessments; the order of physical assessment is changed here so that palpation/percussion will not alter auscultated bowel sounds.

Cardiac Electrophysiology

Electrophysiology of the heart (depolarization and repolarization) is much like electrical conduction along a wire for an electric light. Transmission of an electrical charge occurs because of the exchange of positive and negative ions from outside to the inside of the cell. In the heart this process is called depolarization. *Depolarization* occurs when a charged cell membrane is altered by the exchange of positively charged electrolyte sodium. Sodium is allowed into the cell, changing the membrane from the negative resting state to a positive, excited state. This excited state is transferred from one cell to another.

Repolarization happens when strong pumps return the positive electrolyte outside the cell and a resting state returns the cell back to a more negative condition. This starts with special cells in the SA node creating a rolling wave from one cell to the next until the entire heart has depolarized. Only after this electrical event occurs does the mechanical event or heart contraction happen. So the spark occurs first and then the pump next.

Let us review briefly the electrical conduction system of the heart by returning to Chapter 3 and looking at Table 3–1 and Figure 3–2, cardiac conduction system components. What is the normal pacemaker of the heart? What is its normal or native rate? What takes over if the SA node pacemaker fails? If you can answer these questions without looking, please proceed. If you cannot, review the information because it provides the basis for what we do when we perform rhythm monitoring and analysis.

How Does Cardiac Monitoring Really Work?

❷ So how does this electricity get captured so the critical care nurse can make some sense of it all? It requires special equipment to convert tiny amounts of electricity made by the heart during the electrical cardiac cycle. Although systems are extremely sophisticated today, the basics of cardiac monitoring require some standardized equipment no matter what kind of system is used. See Figure 4–1.

If we follow that all-important patient back to the system, we first need something to take the tiny amounts of electricity from the patient's heart and change them into something we can interpret. The conductor of electrical signals from the patient's heart is called an *electrode*. An electrode can come in many shapes and sizes from a simple tab that looks a lot like duct tape that is used to perform a 12-lead ECG to a disc that looks like a medication patch. No matter what it looks like, this electrode conducts millivolts! That is right! Millionths of

FIGURE 4–1 • A cardiac monitoring system.

a volt of electricity through a wire to the receiving unit *(monitor)*. So it is important that these have firm contact to the patient's skin in order to do their work. Also, the disc electrodes have a tendency to dry out from constant contact with a patient's warm body temperature, so periodically they need to be changed with fresh electrodes to ensure a really good picture (rhythm) of the patient's heart.

NURSING ALERT

Proper placement of electrodes is important for a good electrical "picture of the heart." They should not be placed over boney areas, scar tissue, or hair. These interfere with electrical conduction. If need be, wash the area with warm, soapy water and dry thoroughly. Hair may need to be clipped for closer contact. If respirations interfere, move electrodes closer together.

Next, a *lead wire* is attached to the electrode. This is done in many different ways. Sometimes it is clipped on to the electrode by an alligator clamp. Yes, again you are correct! It is called an alligator clamp because its jaws look just like an alligator. Be careful not to pinch the patient's skin when attaching these! Sometimes it is snapped on to the electrode. If you use this type of system, try to snap the electrode onto the lead wire before placing the electrode on the chest—attaching the lead to an electrode already on the chest might cause the patient pain.

The next step is to connect the lead wire to a cable, which finally attaches to the monitor or telemetry unit. So all of these pieces—the electrode, lead wires, and cable—are just conductors! No real work has been done yet to "see" the rhythm, but it is vital that these are checked periodically for proper attachment to the patient, to see whether they are frayed or damaged, and to ensure that the connections are tight.

The *monitor* does the real work of rhythm detection. It takes the electrical energy in the form of those millivolts and converts it to mechanical energy that we can analyze to tell if there are rhythm changes in the heart. That is essentially how it all works.

Following is a summary of the jobs done by a cardiac monitoring system:

- Electrode – the conductor
- Lead wires – further conductor
- Monitor – ultimate conversion tool

Not to confuse the issue when you think you have gotten it, but there are different kinds of monitoring devices: hardwire, telemetry, and Holter monitors. Table 4–2 describes the basic differences between these three systems.

These are not to be confused with a 12-lead ECG. (More on this later in the chapter when you have got some analysis under your belt!) So get ready for more experience with what happens.

So What Do These Systems "See"?

These systems pick up a series of small waveforms that we can analyze on special paper called ECG paper. When the heart depolarizes and repolarizes, those positive and negative charges cause waveforms to go up and down from the flatline, which is called the *baseline* or also *isoelectric line*. It is very logical and not hard at all. Positive electrical charges cause waveforms to go up and negative charges cause waveforms to go down (see Table 4–3).

When the waveform is traveling toward the positive electrode, it is positive; when it is traveling toward the negative electrode, it is negative; and when it is traveling toward neither or in the middle of the road, it is baseline or flat.

TABLE 4–2 Types of Monitoring Systems

System	What It Does	Where It Is Used
Hardwire monitoring	Patient is physically attached to a cable that leads to a monitor Little mobility; patient can be assisted OOB	ICU/CCU/ECU/PACU and OR First responders; ALS units
Telemetry	Small transmitting unit on chest Patient more mobile; can ambulate	Cardiac and intensive care recovery units (post OHS); less intensive care needed Cardiac stress testing Cardiac rehabilitation
Holter monitor	Continuously monitors and records patient's heart rhythm while patient wears it over 24–72–hour period.	Capture stubborn, periodic rhythm changes while patient resumes normal activity Patient wears like a larger iPod; cardiologist survey's any changes in patient rhythm with patient diary Patient keeps diary of signs/symptoms/events

So here is a real thinking question. If we had electrodes on the patient and placed the negative one on the left shoulder and the positive one on the lower right chest and placed the heart in the middle, where would the wave of depolarization in the heart be normally going? If it were traveling normally from the SA node to the AV node, the waveform would be upright and positive. If we

TABLE 4–3 Types of Baseline, Negative, and Positive Waveforms

	Where Electricity Is Traveling	What It Looks Like
Baseline waveforms		
Negative waveforms		Negative complex
Positive waveforms		Positive complex

reversed the electrodes, the waveform would be negative. That is not so hard. So the first thing is that we are looking at these waveforms created by the heart and looking for positive, negative, or baseline forms.

The ECG Paper

Next, we examine the ECG paper. It runs out of the monitor in grids that have little tiny squares on them. Each square (horizontal axis) across means time, but it is in small amounts of time—0.04 seconds. Each up and down square or vertical square is in measurements of voltage or strength. Each tiny box up or down is 0.1 millivolt. WOW! That is really small, is not it?

Look at Figure 4–2. You will need to commit those values to memory. Since we will spend most of the time on the horizontal axis you will get really good at

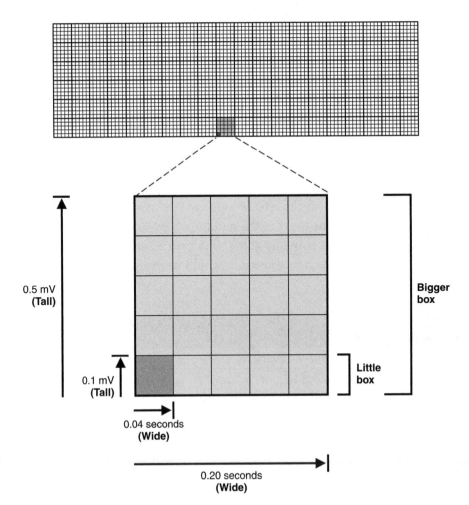

FIGURE 4–2 • Those little and bigger boxes.

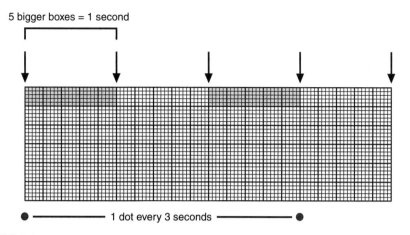

FIGURE 4–3 • Easier time measurements across the top of the rhythm strip.

multiples of 0.04 as each tiny box is this many seconds. If your eyes are getting a bit crossed looking at all the little boxes, do not fear. There are also bigger boxes that are reference points. Five bigger boxes across are 0.2 seconds and are marked a bit darker than the rest. Five boxes vertically are 0.5 millivolts and are a bit darker than the smaller boxes. So we will be counting the boxes and using them as part of our detective work, sort of like forensic detective work. Move over CSI!

You will also see marks across the top of the ECG paper as second references. You can go really batty or cross-eyed by counting all of those little and bigger boxes to determine the amount of time, so the ECG paper folks thought you might like some longer time references across the top. These will be helpful later on when we talk about counting heart rates. Companies are different, but if there are little dots every inch, they indicate 1 second; if there are dots every 3 inches, they indicate 3 seconds (see Figure 4–3).

So what do these little boxes have to do with depolarization and repolarization? Well, we look at the waveforms on this ECG paper and analyze them. What waveforms do we look at, you ask? The waveforms created as the wave of depolarization travels from the SA node to the AV node and into the ventricles. These all create unique but easily identifiable wave patterns that you can learn with guided practice.

The Heartbeat: Electrically, That Is!

The normal heartbeat contains

- P wave
- PR interval (PRI)

- QRS
- ST segment
- T wave
- QT interval

Now let us talk about what these mean and what they look like (see Figure 4–4A and 4–4B and Table 4–4).

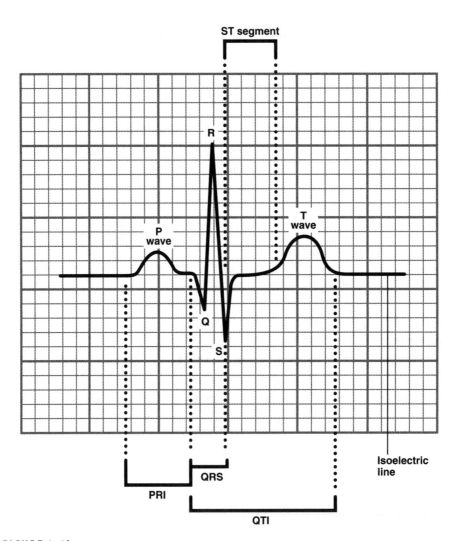

FIGURE 4–4A • ECG waveforms.

P wave   = Not measured: Upright
rounded, symmetrical

PRI   = Measured: .12 – .20 seconds

QRS   = Measured: .06 – .10 seconds

ST segment   = Should be isoelectric (flat)

QTI   = Measured: Rate related
.36 – .42

FIGURE 4–4B • Measuring ECG waveforms.

TABLE 4–4   The Waveforms of the Heartbeat

Waveform	What It Means	How It Is Measured	Its Normal Value
P wave	Two things happen here: SA node firing AND atrial depolarization	From the beginning of the first upstroke of the heartbeat to the end of that upstroke Usually not measured, but we look at the configuration of the wave	Upright rounded and symmetrical Usually smaller than T wave There are two atria but one little hump! They depolarize together
PR interval (PRI)	Three things happen here: SA node firing, atrial depolarization, AND the message getting down to the AV node	Beginning of the P wave including the isoelectric or flat line after it and ending where the baseline goes up or down (QRS complex) Do not include any of the QRS in this one or you will be including ventricles!	From three to five little boxes horizontally OR from .12 seconds to .20 seconds
QRS complex	This is ventricular depolarization: a bit tougher as this complex might have three waves!	Can include three different waveforms The Q wave is the first negative deflection after the PRI The R wave is the first positive deflection after the PRI The S wave is the first negative deflection after the R wave When the R wave comes back to the isoelectric line, then the QRS stops	From 1.5 to 2.5 little boxes OR .06 to .10 seconds Amazing, even though the ventricles are bigger, they take less time to depolarize!
ST segment	Time between ventricular depolarization and repolarization	Distance in between where the S wave stops and at the point the T wave starts upward Not usually measured for rhythm detection, but important in determining ischemia	Usually isoelectric but abnormal in 12–lead ECG in consistent leads may indicate an impending MI Bad if more than one box up or one box down!

TABLE 4–4	The Waveforms of the Heartbeat (*Continued*)		
Waveform	**What It Means**	**How It is Measured**	**Its Normal Value**
T wave	Ventricular repolarization	First positive wave after the QRS After the ST segment Usually bigger than the P wave	Rounded and symmetrical Watch to see if the T wave flips over or inverts. Abnormal in 12–lead ECG in consistent leads may indicate an impending MI
QT interval (QTI)	Two things happen here: total time of ventricular depolarization and repolarization OR total ventricular activation time	From the beginning of the Q wave to the end of the T wave	Very rate related If the heart rate speeds up, the QT shortens; if it slows down, the QT lengthens Usually ½ the R–to–R interval. Normally around .36 to .42 seconds. Used to look at drug influences on the heart rhythm Textbooks vary on normal values

---

NURSING ALERT

It is important to memorize and store the normal values of these waves, especially the PRI, QRS, and QT interval. With lots of practice they will become almost automatic for you, but it does take practice! And the help of a good mentor!

So How Does a Nurse Do Detective Work on These Rhythm Strips?

Forging an Organized Format for Rhythm Analyses

❸ In the previous chapter, we suggest that the nurse use an organized pain assessment so he or she can forward pertinent patient information without missing the main points. With analyzing a cardiac rhythm, we suggest the same thing. What you will be measuring falls into three categories:

1. Rate
2. Rhythm
3. Conduction

The rate can tell you whether the rhythm is fast, normal, or slow and where the pacemaker is. For instance, if the pacemaker is the SA node, the rate is usually between 60 and 100. But if the heart rate is 30, it may be coming from the ventricles. The rhythm can be regular, irregular, or regularly irregular. The conduction tells you about how long it took for this rhythm to go down through the normal conductive tissues. It involves using the norms we talked about before: the PRI, QRS, and QT intervals. Rhythm analysis involves looking at what we find using rate, rhythm, and conduction findings.

Using the eight-part organized detective work format can help you to be thorough and not miss any of the clues the heart is giving you. The eight-part format is

1. Count the atrial rate.   (RATE)
2. Count the ventricular rate.   (RATE)
3. Determine the atrial rhythm.   (RHYTHM)
4. Determine the ventricular rhythm.   (RHYTHM)
5. Measure the PRI.   (CONDUCTION)
6. Measure the QRS duration.   (CONDUCTION)
7. Measure the QTI.   (CONDUCTION)
8. Analyze what the patient's dysrhythmias is and continue to monitor OR take action

Wow! Again, this is a lot for the novice critical care nurse, but you will get lots and lots of practice with this from other nurses, your preceptor/mentor, or class work. But let us back up and do this slowly, so you see the way it is done.

NURSING ALERT

Rhythm interpretation is only another tool of assessment. No matter what, always look at the patient to see what he or she is telling you. What assessment data do you see, feel, hear, and touch? Always go by the patient's symptoms, not necessarily the ECG rhythm strip. Patient assessment FIRST, rhythm strip analysis AFTER assessment!

Step One: Rate—Counting the Atrial Rate

To do this, take the number of "P" waves in a 6-second strip and multiply this by ten (see Figure 4–5). Why? There are ten 6-second periods in a minute. You

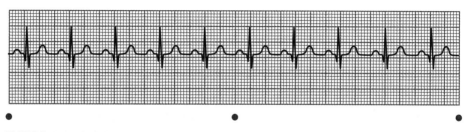

FIGURE 4–5 • Rhythm strip.

can get a rough estimate using this method of what the rate is which will help identify the heart's pacemaker. This example is slightly on the tachycardic side with a rate of 100. In the above rhythm strip the number of P waves in a 6-second strip is 10; so 10 times 10 = 100. So the atrial rate is 100.

Step Two: Rate—Counting the Ventricular Rate

You can use the same method as above, but this time count the number of QRS complexes in a 6-second strip. There are more complicated methods, but for now, let us stick with simple. In the rhythm strip above, the number of QRSs is 10, so 10 times 10 = 100. Okay, there were a lot of similarities in the last two, as you will see in the next two steps. With a rate of 100, the nurse can identify the location of the pacemaker, which is in the SA node as its natural rate is between 60 and 100.

Step Three: Rhythm—Determine the Atrial Rhythm

Determining the rhythm means you need to use some type of measuring tool. You can use a blank piece of paper to make marks OR you can use a pair of *ECG calipers*, which is a very accurate tool to measure tiny features from electrical stimulation of the heart.

If you are using a blank piece of paper, place it underneath the ECG rhythm strip along the isoelectric lines of the rhythm. Place a tiny mark at the beginning of the P wave on the blank paper and another one at the P wave of the next heartbeat. Then move the marks to the next P wave in the strip; this is sometimes called the P-to-P interval. It is also called "Marching out the P waves!" Do they all come regularly? If so, your rhythm is regular.

Now, if you are fortunate enough to have a pair of calipers, take the left caliper point and place it firmly at the beginning of the P wave and place the right caliper point or tip at the beginning of next P wave. That is right, now you are right on top of the ECG paper. Now lift the calipers and compare the distance between each P wave. If the P waves all track out evenly from one caliper tip to the next, the rhythm is regular. The atrial rhythm in Figure 4–5 is regular.

Sometimes you have early or late beats that can make the rhythm irregular. These are called *ectopic beats* as they are usually generated from outside the normal nerve conduction system of the heart. There are two types of ectopic beats: premature or escaped beats. We call early beats *premature beats* as they come before we anticipate them, just like a premature baby comes before those nine months that the parents had anticipated him or her. In this case, the P wave will be before the second caliper point. Interestingly, premature beats can come in an organized pattern but throw the rhythm off. We have words to describe these as well. They include

- Bigeminy – a normal beat, a premature beat (pattern of 1:1)
- Trigeminy – two normal beats, a premature beat (pattern of 2:1)
- Quadrigeminy – three normal beats, a premature beat (pattern of 3:1)
- Couplets – two premature complexes in a row

Occasionally, when the rate is very slow, another lower pacemaker can take over, then your beats will come in later than anticipated. There will be a slowing down of the rhythm because these beats come late. These we call *escaped beats*. Because any cardiac cell can become a pacemaker, it makes interpreting the rhythm a bit complicated. If you do not know exactly what you are seeing, the best advice is to describe it as best you can.

NURSING ALERT

No one is perfect, and if you give a strip to three different nurses, you might get three different answers. The important thing is if you do not know what it is, go through the organized assessment, using it to describe what you are seeing.

Step Four: Rhythm—Determine the Ventricular Rhythm

The ventricular rhythm is very similar to step three except now we see if the QRS complexes all come in a regular pattern. This time we measure from one QRS to another. This is sometimes called the R-to-R interval. The ventricular rhythm in our strip in Figure 4–5 is regular.

Okay, we have now completed rate and rhythm; time to go on to conduction, for which we will continue to use our paper OR calipers to determine time in seconds.

Step Five: Conduction—Measuring the PRI

Okay, we are almost done, and you have been really patient. We now have three more steps to do and they all include using the calipers or paper to measure time across the horizontal axis. After determining the numerical value, you will be comparing your results to what the normal value is for that conduction interval/complex.

The PRI is completed by taking your left caliper point, placing it at the beginning of the P wave, and stopping it at the beginning of the QRS. Do not measure just one; try to get an average of them for each heartbeat across your strip. If these measurements fall between .12 and .20 seconds, then this beat or rhythm comes from the SA node and has been conducted to the AV node in a normal fashion.

The PRI in Figure 4–5 is 0.16 seconds or normal.

Step Six: Conduction—Measuring the QRS

Next, we will measure ventricular depolarization by measuring the QRS interval. Start at the beginning of the Q wave and end where the S wave returns to the baseline. Having a bit of trouble with this one? That is okay because sometimes there is only a Q or an S. Or there also can be an RS and no Q. So we have to fine-tune this measurement by defining each one of these waves. It is important because you really want to be accurate with this tiny measurement—if it is off, it means you miscalculated those all-important ventricles. So use the following definitions and Figure 4–6 to help.

- Q wave – first negative wave after the P wave
- R wave – the first positive wave after the Q wave
- S wave – the first negative wave after the R wave

The QRS in Figure 4–5 is 0.1 seconds or normal.

Step Seven: Conduction—Measuring the QTI

The QT interval is important when it comes to monitoring the results of drugs the patient is receiving. The QT interval does not a rhythm make, but we want to make certain it does not prolong beyond one-half the R-R interval. QTs are measured from the beginning of the QRS complex to the end of the T wave. The QTI in the strip in Figure 4–5 is 0.32 seconds or on the shorter side.

NURSING ALERT

Some medications like sotalol (Betapace) or amiodarone (Cordarone) slow the heart rate down and prolong depolarization for so long that a nasty rhythm called torsades de pointes takes over. This is a cardiac arrest rhythm, so always measure the QT in relation to the R-R before you start these medications AND monitor it periodically after starting these medications.

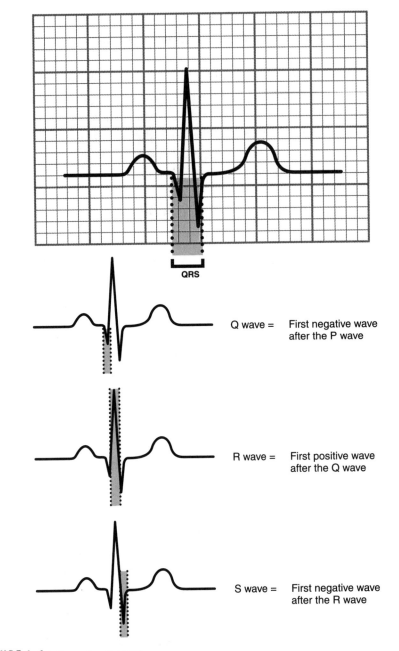

Q wave = First negative wave after the P wave

R wave = First positive wave after the Q wave

S wave = First negative wave after the R wave

FIGURE 4–6 • Measuring the QRS.

Step Eight: Analysis

The last step is taking all of the previous seven steps and putting them together to determine what the rhythm is and whether you need to do something about it!

Recounting a True Story

It was a very busy evening in the telemetry unit with six admissions in the 26-bed unit. All of the patients were finally settled in and all the admission assessments were completed, as well as preliminary treatments. We had just settled in to write up our nurses' notes when the alarm bells went off on bed number 10, a 35-year-old male who had been admitted with unstable chest pain for 23-hour observation. The monitor tech said the rhythm looked like ventricular tachycardia.

Running to check the patient, another very pregnant young nurse ran to get the defibrillator and was having trouble bending down to unplug it from the wall socket. When I went into the room, the man was vigorously brushing his teeth in the bathroom. His biggest scare was when the very flustered and red-in-the-face pregnant nurse ran into the room with the defibrillator. "What is that for?" he shouted, beginning to get nervous.

We settled him in a chair and told him what was happening and apologized for scaring the "living daylights out of him." The young, very nervous pregnant nurse learned that night that you always assess your patient first. Every time the alarms go off now, we look at each other and are reminded of this story.

Types of Basic Rhythms

Sinus Rhythms

A common theme about the rhythms in this group is that they all come from the SA node pacemaker. There are three types of sinus rhythms. You probably already know some information about them as you have been calling pulses by some of these terms since nursing school. They include sinus bradycardia, sinus tachycardia, and normal sinus rhythm. Let us start with the simplest first: normal sinus rhythm (NSR) or sinus rhythm.

Normal Sinus Rhythm (NSR)

In NSR, all the characteristics we used to forge a format are normal.

- RATE: Atrial/ventricular rate = normal
- RHYTHM: Atrial/ventricular rhythm = normal
- CONDUCTION
  - PRI = normal
  - QRS = normal
  - QTI = normal

This is an expected outcome for patients. We want to see them in this rhythm, especially if this is their baseline or normal rhythm.

Sinus Bradycardia (SB)

In sinus bradycardia, the SA node pacemaker slows to a rate of less than 60. The problem with this is that the vital organs may not get needed oxygen with a heart rate this low. So a symptomatic bradycardia is nothing to ignore. Sometimes people with very athletic hearts are in bradycardias. This is normal as their hearts hypertrophy and become much more efficient when they exercise. Sometimes people have an asymptomatic bradycardia when they sleep because their metabolic demands are low. The idea is, if they are not having symptoms, we do not treat this rhythm.

In an SB, all is normal except for the HR; it is less than 60.

- RATE: Atrial/ventricular rate = less than 60.
- RHYTHM: Atrial/ventricular rhythm = regular.
- CONDUCTION: All intervals are normal except the QTI may be prolonged.

NURSING ALERT

A patient should not be treated unless he or she has signs/symptoms of decreased cardiac output or a symptomatic bradycardia. Find the underlying cause and treat it! If the patient is digitoxic, give digoxin immune Fab (digibind); if the patient has been given Lopressor (metoprolol), hold the drug. If the patient is symptomatic, consider atropine, epinephrine, and possible transcutaneous or transvenous temporary pacing.

Sinus Tachycardia (ST)

In a sinus tachycardia, the SA node pacemaker speeds up so the heart rate goes above 100. This is a problem for the heart because it increases the energy needed for fast contraction. Unrelieved, it can cause undue stress and strain on the heart, increasing metabolic needs, which can cause an MI and heart failure. Any unexplained ST needs to be evaluated for the cause. Fever, hypoxia, and anxiety are some of the causes of tachycardias and need to be treated to reduce the heart rate. Figure 4–6 was sinus tachycardia.

- RATE: Atrial/ventricular rate = greater than 100.
- RHYTHM: Atrial/ventricular rhythm = regular.
- CONDUCTION: All intervals are normal except the QTI may be shortened due to decreased diastolic filling time.

NURSING ALERT

An unexplained tachycardia should always be investigated; what is causing it and why? Once determined, treat the underlying cause. If hypoxic, give oxygen; if feverish, give antipyretics; if anxious, give sedatives. If you can not find the cause, notify the health care provider.

Atrial Rhythms

In the rhythms covered previously, all of the pacemakers came from the SA node; now you have a rhythm where the pacemaker changes. It is no longer in the SA node; the pacemaker is in atrial tissue. Since the atrial pacemaker takes over, you can see very distinct changes in the atrial heart rate and shape of the P waves. Atrial rhythms we will explore include premature atrial contractions (PACs), paroxysmal atrial tachycardia (PAT), atrial flutter, and atrial fibrillation. Following are descriptions of what the nurse would analyze in each one.

Premature Atrial Contractions (PACs)

Premature atrial contractions, as their name suggests, are early contractions that come from the atria. Because they come early from an irritable, cranky area of the atrium, they cause the rhythm to fall out of synch. They can fall in any type of underlying rhythm. You will see the following on a rhythm strip.

- RATE: The underlying rate can be anything from SB to NSR to ST. Sometimes the P wave will be upside down or different looking from the patient's SA node P waves. Since these do not come from the SA node, they might look different than the native P waves.
- RHYTHM: The PAC throws the rhythm off because this beat is premature or early.
- CONDUCTION: The other conduction intervals should be normal. Occasionally, if the PAC originates close to the AV node, the PRI can be shorter than normal.

Paroxysmal Atrial Tachycardia (PAT) and Atrial Tachycardia

Paroxysmal atrial tachycardia occurs when a very irritable and cranky focus in the atrium takes over as the pacemaker of the heart. If the rhythm starts abruptly and ends just as suddenly, it is paroxysmal; if the rhythm is sustained and does not break, it is atrial tachycardia. Either way, it strains the heart by increasing oxygen and decreasing diastolic filling time. Diastolic filling time is important; it is here that the atria fill the ventricles. If the diastolic filling time is decreased due to a fast tachy rhythm, there is a decrease in *atrial kick*, which comprises 20% of the cardiac output.

- RATE: Atrial/ventricular rates are very fast; usually around 180 to 220.
- RHYTHM: Very regular. PACs can herald the onset of PAT.
- CONDUCTION: PRI sometimes is very short with P waves being difficult to see. The QTI can be short as this is a tachy dysrhythmia.

Atrial Flutter

Atrial flutter is a sustained, regular rhythm where the atrial tissue is the pacemaker of the heart. The rates are very fast but the P waves are each countable. However, since they are in the 200 to 400s, the ventricles can not beat that fast, so there are sometimes two, three, or four atrial beats to one ventricular beat. The ventricles just can not keep up with all of those multiple regular P waves.

- RATE: Atrial rate – 200 to 400 beats per minute. The configuration of the P waves is like a sawtooth pattern and are called flutter waves. The big difference between atrial flutter and fibrillation is the countable P waves. In atrial flutter you can count each and every P wave as they fall in a very regular pattern.

  Ventricular rate – 2:1 (2 Ps to 1 QRS), 3:1 (3 Ps to 1 QRS), and 4:1 (4 Ps to 1 QRS) conductions, which can be very regular or erratic.
- RHYTHM: The P-to-P interval is regular and the R-to-R interval depends on the ratio of Ps to QRS complexes (2:1; 3:1 etc.)
- CONDUCTION: Once the stimulus gets to the AV node, the conduction times are usually regular.

Atrial Fibrillation

Atrial fibrillation is a rhythm where the atrial tissues contract in an irregular, chaotic, disorganized way. It is estimated that atrial tissues are beating anywhere from 300 to 600 times per minute. Some say they are twitching, so the P waves are in a "now you see them, now you do not" pattern. Again, since the large ventricular muscle masses can not beat that fast, the AV node slows and filters the P waves but in a grossly irregular fashion. So just like in "Where is Waldo," it is hard to find the P waves and they are not always countable. Since the P waves are indeterminate, you can not count atrial rates, atrial rhythm, or the PRI.

- RATE: Atrial rate is uncountable; ventricular rate is very countable.
- RHYTHM: Since the P waves are uncountable you can not determine an atrial rate, but QRS intervals can be counted.
- CONDUCTION: You can not get a PRI but you can measure a QRS, which may be normal or short depending on the rate. Once the stimulus gets to the AV node, the conduction times are usually regular.

NURSING ALERT

In atrial fibrillation/flutter, the patient needs to be monitored for heart failure. Eddies and currents around the AV valves can set up systemic and pulmonary emboli, so anticoagulation is necessary to prevent blood clot formation. Also, if the ventricular response is less than 60 or greater than 100, we call it uncontrolled. The underlying cause must be found and treated or the patient will have too low of a cardiac output.

Junctional Rhythms

Okay, now the pacemaker is traveling again. The pacemaker for this rhythm is the AV junction, thus the name "junctional" rhythms. We will explore the characteristics of premature junctional contractions (PJCs) and a junctional rhythm in this section. One of the discriminating factors in junctional rhythms is their absent P waves and slow rates. The P waves are absent because the atria do not contract, and because there is no atrial contraction, voila—no P waves.

Premature Junctional Contractions (PJCs)

Like the PAC, these beats fall on some type of underlying rhythm like NSR or SB. The words in their names tell what they are—premature in that they fall early from the junction.

- RATE: Atrial rate—no P waves. Ventricular rate usually slow but can be normal.

- RHYTHM: Irregular at the PJC as it comes early.
- CONDUCTION: Other conduction intervals are normal except there is no PRI.

Junctional Rhythm

Think of a junctional rhythm as PJCs strung together creating a sustained rhythm coming from the AV junction.

- RATE: No atrial rate as no P waves; ventricular rate is 40 to 60.
- RHYTHM: The rhythm of the ventricles is normal.
- CONDUCTION: No PRI but the QRS and QT are within normal ranges. The QT interval can be prolonged.

> **NURSING ALERT**
>
> *Sustained junctional rhythms have the capacity to slow the cardiac output down. So look for an underlying cause but monitor the patient closely for decreased cardiac output signs/symptoms.*

AV Blocks

Think of any type of atrioventricular block as a roadblock between the atria and ventricles. Just like with road construction, the car will get there, but it will take longer depending upon the type of roadblock. There are three types of AV blocks: first degree, second degree (with two types: Wenckebach [Mobitz I] and Mobitz II), and third degree. These roadblocks in the heart affect the PRI primarily but can have consequences for the other characteristics as well.

First-Degree AV Block

A first-degree AV block affects the conduction between the atria and ventricles by simply prolonging the PRI.

- RATE: This is usually superimposed on an underlying rhythm.
- RHYTHM: Normal.
- CONDUCTION: PRI is prolonged beyond .20 seconds. Everything else is normal. The problem is above the ventricles or *supraventricular.*

Second-Degree AV Block—Type I (Wenckebach or Mobitz I)

A second-degree AV block has two types and is a bit more complicated to learn. It involves changes in the PRI as well. Wenckebach is sort of like a weight lifter doing reps. As the time gets longer and the muscle gets more and more fatigued, the time to complete the rep gets longer until the will is there but the weight cannot be moved. In Wenckebach, the PRI gets longer and longer with each heartbeat until you get a P wave that does not conduct to the ventricles. We often call this a *nonconducted P wave*.

- RATE: Depends on the underlying rhythm. There are missing P waves so the ventricular rate is slower than the atrial due to blocked P waves.
- RHYTHM: Atrial is irregular; ventricular is irregular.
- CONDUCTION: PRI gets longer and longer until a P wave occurs but no QRS or a nonconducted P wave (blocked P wave). The QRS and QTI are normal.

Second-Degree AV Block—Type II (Mobitz II)

A second-degree heart block or Mobitz II involves some P waves that are conducted and some that are not. These are usually in a 2:1, 3:1, or 4:1 conduction where there are more Ps than Qs. So you need to mind your Ps and Qs here!

- RATE: Atrial rate is usually 60 to 100; ventricular rate is slow as not every QRS is conducted.
- RHYTHM: Atrial is regular; ventricular is irregular.
- CONDUCTION: PRI is normal or prolonged but the P-to-P interval is constant. In other words, you can march out the P waves as they fall on time. The QRS is normal and the QT might be prolonged due to the slow rate.

NURSING ALERT

Watch the ventricular response on this rhythm as a slow heart rate can cause a dramatic drop in BP, causing decreased cardiac output. This can occur with ischemia or MI. You might need to prepare for temporary or permanent cardiac pacing with a sustained Mobitz II.

Third-Degree AV Block (Complete Heart Block)

This is the most severe of the four heart blocks, and it is now time to consider a pacemaker as cardiac output falls with this one quickly. In this rhythm the SA node pacemaker fires at its native rate and the ventricular pacer fires at its rate as well, but there is no communication between the two.

- RATE: Atrial rate of between 60 and 100; ventricular rate of 30 to 40.
- RHYTHM: Regular in atrium and ventricles but they beat independently of each other. The P does not cause the QRS as they are not communicating with each other.
- CONDUCTION: PRI varies from beat to beat. QRS are wide and bizarre and may have P waves imbedded in them.

NURSING ALERT

Watch the ventricular response on this rhythm as too slow a heart rate can cause a dramatic drop in BP, resulting from a decreased cardiac output. This can occur with ischemia or MI. You need to prepare for temporary and/or permanent cardiac pacing with this condition as most patients can not tolerate it for long.

Ventricular Rhythms

Along with the advanced heart blocks, ventricular rhythms must be identified and follow-up care rendered. Rhythms can be one or two beats or sustained rhythms. We will describe several of these bad actors, including premature ventricular contractions (PVCs), ventricular tachycardia (VT), ventricular fibrillation (VF), and asystole. The last three rhythms are seen in a cardiac arrest or Code Blue.

Premature Ventricular Contractions (PVCs)

A premature ventricular contraction is an irritable beat that fires the ventricles before the SA node can repolarize. The beat is early; the QRS is wide and bizarre with a T wave often in the opposite direction of the QRS. Frequently a pause after the PVC, called a compensatory pause, occurs because the heart received a wallop of a stimulus too early and needs a longer time to recoup. This sets the rhythm into an irregular pattern.

- RATE: Underlying rhythm could be anything.
- RHYTHM: Irregular at the PVC; it fires the ventricles early.
- CONDUCTION: PRI not present as no atrial conduction is associated with a PVC. The QRS is wide and greater than 0.1 seconds, and it is very different from the patient's normally conducted QRS.

Patterns of PVCs PVCs can come in a regularly irregular fashion. There can be

- Bigeminy – 1 normal beat; 1 PVC
- Trigeminy – 2 normal beats; 1 PVC
- Quadrigeminy – 3 normal beats; 1 PVC

They can also be named according to what they look like. There can be

- Unifocal or uniform – all looking alike
- Multifocal or multiform – all looking different
- Couplets – two in a row
- R on T phenomena – PVCs falling on top of the T wave

NURSING ALERT

PVCs can cause decreased cardiac output and multiple PVCs per minute, those falling on the T wave and multifocal PVCs can cause advanced irritability, watch out for their occurrence. Advanced irritability leads to more lethal rhythms where there is no cardiac output.

Ventricular Tachycardia (VT)

This rhythm is one that can lead to cardiac arrest. VT occurs when there are more than three PVCs occurring in a row. VT can have a pulse but may not have one, so it important to assess the patient when you see this on the cardiac monitor.

- RATE: No atrial; ventricular is 100 to 250.
- RHYTHM: Ventricular rhythm is regular.
- CONDUCTION: PRI is absent; QRS is wide and bizarre. QT is there but difficult to measure.

NURSING ALERT

Always assess the patient for a pulse or the absence of a pulse in this rhythm; the treatment depends on this. Check the electrolytes for imbalances, too.

Ventricular Fibrillation (VF)

Ventricular fibrillation occurs when there is electrical activity but with no regular form. The rhythm is chaotic with no discernible wave forms that occur. It is often caused by a large MI and is the most frequent cause of cardiac arrest. Clinically, without a cardiac monitor, the critical care nurse cannot tell VF from asystole. There is no pulse or breathing with VF, so the protocol for cardiac arrest is initiated with defibrillation as soon as possible.

- RATE: Atrial rate is not countable; ventricular rate is chaotic or has no characteristics of ventricular depolarization.
- RHYTHM: Extremely irregular with no discernable rhythm.
- CONDUCTION: No conduction intervals measurable.

> **NURSING ALERT**
>
> *Always assess the patient first. VF can be mimicked by the patient brushing his or her teeth or a loose electrode. Since there is no circulation, early defibrillation is important!*

Asystole

This is another type of code rhythm, but as the name suggests, it is known by the absence of systole. There is an extremely poor prognosis with this rhythm; so finding the cause and treating it is important. Asystole is known by its flatline appearance.

- RATE: There are sometimes P waves but they are not associated with anything and will disappear. No QRS complex is seen.
- RHYTHM: None.
- CONDUCTION: None.

> **NURSING ALERT**
>
> *Since there is no rhythm, consistently administered, high-quality CPR and identifying the cause is important. Causes can include hypoxia, hypovolemia, hypothermia, acidosis, electrolyte imbalance, drug overdose, cardiac tamponade, tension pneumothorax, and pulmonary emboli.*

Where Do 12-Lead ECGs Enter the Picture?

❹ A 12-lead electrocardiogram (ECG) is a noninvasive diagnostic tool that the critical care nurse and health care providers use to look at the major surfaces of the heart. Its limitation is that it is only a small space in time we are "seeing," so to analyze evolving changes in the heart, ECGs need to be done at spaced-out time intervals, so evolving changes are not missed. Baseline ECGs are also done as part of a routine physical, before surgery and any time the patient has a dramatic change in cardiac status like chest pain or hypotension.

Although only ten electrodes are placed on the chest and limbs, the ECG machine changes around the polarity (– and + poles) of the electrodes to "see" 12 different views of the heart. This diagnostic tool tells us much more about what is going on in the heart. It is similar to a car sitting in a valley; if you only see one view you might not be able to tell about the make/model or color of the car. But if you took a picture of 12 different views from all sides, then you know much more about that car.

An ECG can help the knowledgeable practitioner identify

- Ischemia, injury, or infarction in the heart
- Hypertrophies
- Right and left axis deviation (is the heart tipped to the left or right?)
- Electrical alternans with cardiac tamponade
- The rhythm the patient is in at the time ECG is done

How to Do It–Performing a 12-Lead ECG

1. Tell the patient what you will be doing and that no pain is involved.

2. Obtain the ECG machine and input patient data so the ECG is identified with that patient.

3. Have the patient take off any clothes and jewelry above the chest.

4. Clip hair on the chest if electrode contact is questionable.

5. Place electrodes on the right arm (RA), left arm (LA), right leg (RL), and left leg (LL). These are the frontal plane leads. A little jingle is worth learning here to identify the color-coding system used in an emergency: white (snow) on the right (RA = white), snow over grass (RL = green); smoke (LA = black) over fire (LL = red). These are the limb leads.

6. Place electrodes over the left chest starting from V1 (see Figure 4–7) to V6. V leads, also called the precordial leads, travel across the heart in the horizontal plane looking at the right but primarily the left ventricle.

7. Make sure all electrodes make good contact.

8. Run the ECG looking to see if all waveforms look straight without any respiratory interference. This will cause the waveform to ride up and down from the baseline.

9. Document copies for the chart.

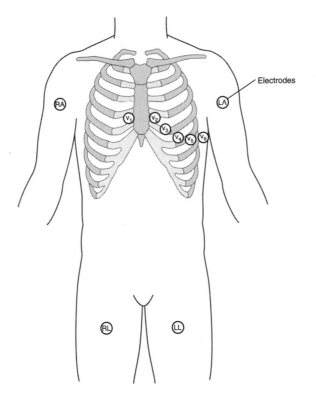

FIGURE 4–7 • Placement of ECG electrodes.

❺ Medications That Help With Rhythm Stabilization

TABLE 4–5 Cardiac Medications With Symptoms

Rhythm Disturbance	Treatment
Symptomatic bradycardias and heart blocks	Atropine
	Epinephrine
	Find the underlying cause
Tachycardias	Beta-blockers
	Calcium channel blockers
	Find the underlying cause
Ventricular tachycardia	If stable with a pulse, procainamide (Pronestyl)
	If unstable without a pulse, amiodarone and perhaps sotalol (Betapace)
	Electrolytes like potassium, magnesium, or calcium may need to be replaced

TABLE 4–5 Cardiac Medications With Symptoms *(Continued)*

Rhythm Disturbance	Treatment
Ventricular fibrillation	Epinephrine
	Vasopressin (one dose)
	Amiodarone
	Lidocaine
Asystole	Epinephrine
	Atropine

Special Cardiac Devices to Help Maintain the Patient's Rhythm

Cardiac Pacemakers: Transcutaneous, Epicardial, Transvenous, and Permanent Pacemakers

What Went Wrong?

❻ Pacemakers (pacers) are electrical devices that help the heart's electrical conduction by artificially producing a spark that captures the heart when the patient's SA node fails or there is a block in conduction in the heart. They can also be used to control very fast rhythms when medications are not effective because they can control the heart from an electrical charge greater than the heart can generate itself. So pacers are used for

- Heart block
- SA node dysfunction (sick sinus syndrome)
- Tachy rhythms (SVT, atrial fibrillation/flutter, VT)
- Cardiac arrest
- Open-Heart Surgery (OHS)
- Electrophysiological testing

All pacemakers include the following parts: generator box or power source, means of delivery (wires or catheter), and lead wires. The generator box or power source provides the power for the pacemaker and can be manipulated to increase the strength of electricity applied to the heart. This is especially helpful in fast rhythms where the generator box power overcomes the heart and commands the heart (takes over as an external pacer). The more permanent pacers have lithium batteries that must be replaced about every 6 years.

TABLE 4–6 Types of Pacers

	Description	Placement	Invasive?
Temporary Pacers			
Transcutaneous	Large electrode pads attached to chest in anterior and posterior position	Anterior and posterior chest	No: Used in emergency until more invasive mode/permanent type of pacing can be instituted. Activates heart from electrical stimulus from outside to inside chest.
Epicardial	Wires that exit the chest inserted surgically	Above mediastinal chest tubes	Yes: Placed on the atria, ventricles during OHS and removed before discharge.
Transvenous	Catheter inserted venously. Distal wires attached to positive and negative pole of external generator box.	Inserted through vein (subclavian, antecubital) or a part of a PA catheter that can pace the heart from inside the right atrium or right ventricle	Yes: Usually inserted through a central line access site but can be inserted peripherally.
Permanent			
Permanent	Implanted through surgical incision done under local anesthesia	Near the right pectoral muscle (subclavian space)	Yes: Wires passed through a vein and attached to a generator box.

Table 4–6 summarizes the types of pacers, their descriptions, how they are placed, and how they are used.

There are programmable functions/terms of pacers that you need to know. First, some terminology that will help you understand:

- Rate – what you will set the pacemaker at to fire; usually around 60 to 80.
- Mode (demand) – synchronous is when the pacer only fires when it needs to; think of it like a thermostat for heat—it only comes on when the heat is below a preset level. Asynchronous (fixed) means the pacer will fire all

the time, so make sure the patient has no underlying rhythm that comes through.

- Capture – when the pacer causes the heart to beat; usually signified by a pacer spike and the chamber paced (i.e., pacer spike and P wave for atrial pacing; pacer spike and R wave for ventricular pacing).
- Threshold – the minimum amount of voltage (mA) needed to consistently capture the heart.
- mA – amount of electricity needed to capture the heart.

NURSING ALERT

An asynchronous pacing mode is only used when there is no chance that the patient's own rhythm will break through and compete with the pacer. If the pacer fires on the patient's own T wave, it could create electrical chaos and lead to ventricular tachycardia or fibrillation.

The Pacer Codes

The critical care nurse needs to know about the five pacing codes that tell about different pacer functions. These are divided into chamber paced, chamber sensed, response to sensed event, rate modulation, and multisite pacing. Table 4–7 helps identify the modes of pacing.

The first three letters of the code refer to the prevention of bradycardias in the pacemaker. The first letter indicates the chamber that is *paced* or where the

TABLE 4–7   Codes of Pacemakers

Chamber Paced (First Letter)	Chamber Sensed (Second Letter)	Response to Sensed Event (Third Letter)	Rate Modulation (Fourth Letter)	Multisite (Fifth Letter)
O – none	O – none	O – none	O – none	O – none
A – atrial	A – atrial	T – triggered	R – rate modulated	A – atrial
V – ventricular	V – ventricle	I – inhibited		V – ventricle
D – dual (both atrial/ventricular)	D – dual	D = T and I		D – dual
S – single (atrial/ventricular)	S – single			

electrode is placed. A is the atrial chamber, V is ventricular, D is both atrial and ventricular (dual-chamber pacer), and S is a single chamber that is paced.

The second letter tells which chamber is *sensing* the patient's own native rhythm with the same letter corresponding to the chamber paced. The third letter refers to what the pacer's response would be to a patient's own native activity. The T means the pacer would trigger on top of the patient's own activity. This would be used if the patient had a complete AV block. It would mean the pacer would be inhibited if the patient's own rate came in on top of the paced beat. So a VVI pacemaker is one that would pace the ventricles, and if the patient's own QRS occurred, it would sense it and inhibit the pacemaker from firing.

Rate modulation is signified by the fourth letter, referring to a pacer that can increase and decrease the heart rate according to demand. So if a patient needs an increased heart rate due to activity, this pacer would increase the rate if the patient walks a set of stairs. The last position or fifth refers to multiple pacing sites. An "A" here would refer to sites in both atria and "V" would refer to both ventricles being paced. This would most commonly be used in pacing to help with heart failure or biventricular pacing.

Nursing Diagnoses for Paced Patient	Expected Outcomes
Decreased cardiac output due to slow or fast dysrhythmias	The patient will have NSR or controlled atrial/fibrillation flutter
	The patient will have a stable mental status
Fluid imbalance, more than body requirements due to decreased effectiveness of the heart pump	The patient will have no signs/symptoms of fluid overload

How to Do It—How to Prepare a Patient for Transcutaneous Pacing

1. Attach monitoring electrodes to the patient's chest: one anterior just below the left of the sternum and one posterior to the left of the thoracic spine.

2. Clip any excessive body hair; hair will decrease conduction of electrodes.

3. Connect the electrode cables to the pacing device, usually a defibrillator machine with this capacity.

4. Administer sedation/analgesics.

5. Turn the power on and select the synchronous (demand) or asynchronous (fixed) pacing.

6. The pacing rate is usually selected at around 80. Dial this in.

7. Set the pacing current output by slowly increasing the mA (strength) on the machine at the minimum amount of voltage until you see a spike on the cardiac monitor before the chamber being paced. Set 10% higher as a safety precaution.

8. To ensure proper pacing, a pacer spike needs to immediately precede the R wave, the QRS is wide and bizarre, almost like a PVC.

9. Document a rhythm strip, the vital signs, sedation used, pacer settings, and how the patient tolerated the procedure.

Nursing Interventions for Transcutaneous Pacemakers

Prepare the patient for this emergency procedure to decrease anxiety and provide trust in the health care provider.

Reassure the patient that he or she will be treated for pain with analgesia/sedation as the external shock can cause uncomfortable muscle contractions.

Prepare the skin for electrode placement by cleaning, clipping hair, and applying the pads firmly to the anterior and posterior chest. Firm contact ensures proper capture.

Turn the mA up using only the amount of voltage needed to pace the heart as this will decrease pain from electrical shock.

Observe the QRS; it will appear wide with a sharp pacer line immediately before it due to its coming from a source outside the normal conduction system.

Teach the patient and family that the muscles will twitch with each beat.

Nursing Interventions for Epicardial Pacing

Note that the wires are labeled on the outside dressing once the patient comes from surgery; there can be atrial, ventricular, and ground wires. If they are not marked, the nurse could attach them to the wrong ports on the external generator box.

Attach the wires to the appropriate ports on the external generator box while wearing gloves. The nurse needs to be grounded by the gloves or electrical current can pass through the wires into the heart causing a lethal rhythm.

Redress the wires according to hospital protocols to prevent infection.

Assist the health care provider with removal before the patient goes home. The wires will be pulled out of the chest and a dry, sterile dressing will be applied.

Teach the patient signs/symptoms of wires site infection and how to redress them, to give the patient a sense of control and increase observation for complications.

Assure the patient that the wires will be removed prior to discharge, so the patient does not worry about care of the wires at home.

Nursing Interventions for Transvenous Pacing

Assist with insertion of the catheter. The physician will ask the nurse to inflate the balloon for proper placement.

Document the rhythm on the monitor to determine the patient's baseline rhythm.

Set the rate, mA, and mode of pacing to individualize the settings for the patient.

Redress the site, maintaining electrical safety as with the epicardial wires to prevent dysrhythmia from outside electrical energy traveling along the catheter to the heart.

NURSING ALERT

The nurse must always be aware that a pacing catheter or epicardial wires, unless grounded, can carry large amounts of energy into the heart. Always secure them away from electrical interference, make sure the ends of the wires are completely covered with protective devices (according to manufactures' directions), AND wear gloves when touching them!

Permanent Pacemakers

Permanent pacemakers are implanted surgically, usually beneath the clavicle in the right chest. The generator box is small, about the size of an Oreo cookie, and easily overlooked, so look for a telltale horizontal surgical incision in that area. The surgery is done under local anesthesia and does not take long. One end of the pacemaker catheter is implanted or screwed into the chamber(s) of the heart to be paced; the other end is tunneled to the generator box. Since this is a permanent device usually for heart blocks and SA node dysfunctions, it requires much more patient education.

Nursing Interventions for Permanent Pacemakers

Assess the site for bleeding and infection teaching the patient to do so as s/he will have to check the site at home.

Check for a subclavian pulse on the right to determine if circulation was compromised during the procedure.

Teach the patient to keep the affected arm in a sling and not to move it vigorously until the pacer wires have had time to implant.

Have the patient demonstrate taking his or her radial pulse to check for regular rhythm.

Remind the patient to keep regular checkups to see if the pacer is working correctly.

Teach the patient the signs/symptoms of decreased cardiac output, so s/he can seek medical attention early.

Teach the patient to avoid close contact with very strong electromechanical devices like high-tension wires and magnetic resonance imagers (MRIs) as their strong interferences can shut off the pacemaker. Home devices are not really an issue with newer pacers.

Encourage the patient to obtain a medical alert tag to wear to alert health care providers of the pacer's presence, especially in a cardiac arrest.

NURSING ALERT

Patients with permanent pacemakers should carry a medical alert card. Nursing staff should be vigilant not to defibrillate over a permanent pacemaker as the electrical charge will follow the implanted lead wires and cause damage to the chambers of the heart at their distal ends!

Implantable Cardiac Defibrillators (ICDs)

What Went Wrong?

An implantable cardiac defibrillators (ICD) is an electrical device that is surgically placed at about the same anatomic place as a permanent pacemaker. This device is used when a patient has had past episodes of ventricular fibrillation uncontrolled by medication and has had an episode of cardiac arrest unrelated to an MI. ICDs can also be programmed to be pacemakers to stop fast or slow rhythms. ICDs sense how long the patient's rhythm stays on the isoelectric line.

If there is no time on it, it assumes the patient is in ventricular fibrillation so a shock is delivered. It is also programmed to fire like a pacemaker if the heart rate becomes bradycardic or tachycardic. Care of the patient is not unlike care after placement of a permanent pacemaker.

Cardioversion

❼ A cardioversion is different from a defibrillation because

- It can be elective if the patent is in a nonthreatening rhythm.
- It is usually started at a lower energy level for depolarization.
- It is synchronized into the patient's heartbeat.

How to Do It–Preparing the Patient for Cardioversion

1. Explain to the patient what will occur.
2. Prepare the defibrillator by pressing the synch button and recording a rhythm strip. There should be a dot over the R wave that indicates this when the machine will fire.
3. Attach the defibrillator pads/paddles in the anterior to posterior position OR under the right clavicle and apex of the heart.
4. Prepare and check the functioning of suctioning equipment.
5. Prepare and check the functioning of oxygen equipment and a BVM.
6. Make sure the patient has a patent IV.
7. Administer the preordered sedative to the patient.
8. Call "all clear?"
9. Depress the paddles firmly against the chest. The machine will hold the charge until it senses the R wave, so there is a delay in the shock delivered.
10. Administer the shock and observe and record the rhythm.
11. Monitor and record the vital signs.

12. Check the patient's chest for burns.

13. Guard the airway until the patient is fully awake and the 6th cranial nerve (gag reflex) is intact.

14. Tell the patient the procedure is over.

15. Document the voltage used, a rhythm strip, and the patient's response to the procedure.

Defibrillator machine

FIGURE 4–8 • Paddle placement for cardioversion/defibrillation.

Cardiac Arrest: Your Worst Nightmare

Arrest in VT or VF

7 In a pulseless VT and VF, effective defibrillation is to be done as soon as the arrest occurs. Survival depends on early recognition and defibrillation. The theory behind defibrillation is that it depolarizes all cardiac cells at once, allowing the SA node pacemaker to try to regroup and capture the heart into an NSR.

Pads are applied to the chest under the right clavicle and in the left apex of the heart. A shock is delivered after calling "all clear?" Three shocks are delivered and if the rhythm is unchanged, CPR and drugs are initiated along with continued shocks. Drugs usually given include epinephrine or vasopressin; lidocaine, amiodarone, or magnesium could also be ordered. Epinephrine is commonly used in almost every arrest scenario, so it is one of the drugs the nurse can get ready right away. CPR and defibrillation continues until the patient reverts to NSR or CPR and defibrillation is stopped if the patient's heart cannot be revived. Sodium bicarbonate can be given but only after a set of ABGs indicates acidosis.

Arrest Including Asystole

Because there is no electrical discharge from the heart, effective CPR is the treatment for asystole. Treating the underlying cause is important, so every effort to identify this is important. After intubation and a patent IV is established, epinephrine is administered and can be repeated every 3 to 5 minutes. One dose of vasopressin can be given in lieu of the first or second dose of epinephrine, after which an IV push of atropine can be given. This continues until an external or temporary transvenous pacemaker is inserted to spark the heart from within. Asystole carries a high mortality rate, but resuscitation will continue until the patient's rhythm returns or resuscitation attempts stopped.

Induced Hypothermia

The American Heart Association advises inducing hypothermia for unconscious adults who receive CPR within 10 minutes of their down time (arrest). Mild hypothermia is induced with ice packs to the groin and axilla. Iced saline can also be administered via a nasogastric tube until a cool blanket can be obtained. While caring for the patient post-arrest, the nurse insures sedation and monitors cooling and neuromuscular paralysis. Complications of hypothermia include acid-base and fluid/electrolyte disturbances, hypotension, pneumonia, sepsis, further dysrhythmias, hyperglycemia, and coagulopathies.

CASE STUDY

June Carrier is a 68-year-old widow who has been struggling with recurrent bouts of heart failure (HF) and has been hospitalized at least three times this year for exacerbation of this chronic medical problem. At the local grocery store, Ms. Carrier is waiting in line when she passes out. EMS is notified and when they arrive, Ms. Carrier is groggy but answering questions. She does not know where she is or what time it is, but knows who she is. The cardiac monitor shows atrial tachycardia with a rate of 180 without ectopy. After oxygen and an IV, Ms. Carrier reverts back to a sinus tachycardia, where she remains until she reaches the ECU.

You admit her to the ICU for close monitoring. Suddenly she states, I "can not catch my breath." The monitor shows that she is back in an atrial tachycardia at 190. Thus far, none of the medications given are working to convert Ms. Carrier to a sinus rhythm. Since she is symptomatic, has increasing crackles that are ascending to midscapula, and her SaO_2 is dropping despite increasing her to a 100% nonrebreather, the physician tells you to set up for an emergency cardioversion.

After giving Ms. Carrier sedation and three shocks of increasing amplitude starting at 50 W/s, Ms. Carrier converts permanently to an NSR. Ms. Carrier's short stay in the hospital is uneventful, but she has a medication adjustment and has a home health nurse on consult to help with medications and diet.

QUESTIONS

1. What characteristics would confirm the presence of atrial tachycardia on the monitor?
2. What characteristics would confirm the presence of sinus tachycardia?
3. What would you anticipate as usual treatment for ST tachycardia in the ECU?
4. What laboratory values would be important to anticipate seeing?
5. What nursing care will you perform to be ready for the emergency cardioversion?

REVIEW QUESTIONS

1. A patient is suspected of having a decreased cardiac output due to dysrhythmias. Which of the following assessments would be included in a decreased cardiac output? **Select all that apply.**

   A. Elevated jugular venous distention
   B. Polyuria
   C. Full and bounding pulses
   D. Diaphoresis
   E. Constricted pupils
   F. Crackles and gurgles
   G. Muffled heart sounds

2. A nurse is analyzing a patient's rhythm and counts a heart rate of 46. There are no "P" waves at all in this rhythm and the other components are normal. This rhythm is most likely

   A. A normal sinus rhythm
   B. A junctional rhythm
   C. Atrial fibrillation
   D. A ventricular rhythm

3. Good conduction of electricity from the patient's heart to the monitor requires that the critical care nurse

   A. Periodically change electrode pads for good conduct.
   B. Place electrodes over the ribs as they are excellent conductors.
   C. Place electrodes with contacts on their anterior and posterior surfaces.
   D. Place electrodes further apart if they pick up respiratory movement.

4. A nurse is describing one of the waveforms to a novice critical care nurse. S/he describes this wave as being upright rounded and symmetrical and occurring after the QRS. The nurse is describing the

   A. P wave
   B. QRS
   C. ST segment
   D. T wave

5. A nurse is measuring a waveform of the ECG strip and determines it is normally around 0.06 to 0.1. The waveform s/he is measuring is the

   A. P wave
   B. PRI
   C. QRS
   D. QT interval

6. A patient has multiple saw-toothed P waves at a rate of 300 beats per minute. This patient's rhythm is most likely
   A. Paroxysmal atrial tachycardia (PAT)
   B. Premature atrial contractions (PACs)
   C. Atrial flutter
   D. Atrial fibrillation

7. A patient has a VVIR mode pacemaker. The nurse knows that this pacemaker is characterized by which of the following?

Pacing	Sensing	Response to Sensing	Rate Modulation
A. Atrial	Atrial	Triggered	None
B. Atrial	Ventricular	Inhibited	Rate modulated
C. Ventricular	Atrial	Triggered	Rate modulated
D. Ventricular	Ventricular	Inhibited	Rate modulated

8. A patient is being taught how to care for his pacemaker site by the critical care nurse. Which of the following indicates that this patient understands safe care of the device?
   A. "I will not handle the pacemaker leads at the same time as the toaster."
   B. "I will obtain a medic alert tag as soon as I can."
   C. "Since it was implanted in the OR I do not have to worry about infection."
   D. "I must not be around a home microwave."

9. Which of the following pacemakers is usually used in an emergency and attached by the critical care nurse to the patient?
   A. Transcutaneous pacer
   B. Epicardial pacer
   C. Transvenous pacer
   D. Permanent pacer

10. A nurse is preparing drugs for a cardiac arrest victim. Which of the following drugs is used in almost all cardiac arrest scenarios?
    A. Atropine
    B. Epinephrine
    C. Adenosine
    D. Sodium bicarbonate

ANSWERS

CASE STUDY

1. An atrial and ventricular rate of 180; sometimes P waves may not be seen, so this can be confused with junctional tachycardia. Junctional tachycardia does not have this fast a rate, though. Atrial and ventricular rhythms should be regular. If P waves are seen, the PRI would be shorter than normal. The QRS should be of normal duration and the QTI might be short.

2. Sinus tachycardia is confirmed by an atrial and ventricular rate above 100 but below 160. Both atrial and ventricular rates should be regular. All intervals should be normal but sometimes they can shorten, especially the QT.

3. Ms. Carrier's medications should be reviewed to see what she is taking and when she took them last. IV beta-blockers, calcium channel blockers, and digoxin can be administered to control her ST.

4. It is important to check her digoxin level and her potassium, before administrating digoxin to her. Also be sure that baseline chemistries are drawn and note the sodium, potassium, calcium, and magnesium levels. Replace these if needed.

5. An emergency cardioversion is very much like a regular one but items must be set up quickly. First, make sure you have a patent IV line and working suction equipment. A functioning BVM is needed, and she is already on oxygen. Next, request sedation if none has been ordered. Delegate checking the defibrillator but make sure before it is used that there is a dot above every "R" wave, so the machine avoids the T wave. After the procedure follow the ABCs, keeping an open airway and monitoring her breathing. Montior VS every 15 minutes or according to protocol for the first hour. Check the chest area for burns and provide care if they occur. Keep close cardiac monitoring, remembering to document rhythm strips before/after and any time she has a rhythm change. Teach her all of the above and reassure her that the procedure went well.

CORRECT ANSWERS AND RATIONALES

1. A, C, D, and F are associated with fluid buildup in the body from a lack of pumping (cardiac) action. Patients have oliguria due to poor kidney perfusion, dilated pupils due to sympathetic activation, and do not usually have muffled heart sounds, which is associated with cardiac tamponade.

2. B. A junctional rhythm is known by a rate of between 60 and 40. Junctional rhythms are started in the AV junction, so they are not caused by atrial depolarization, hence no "P" waves. Everything else about them is normal. Atrial fibrillation is very fast and the P waves can not be counted. A ventricular rhythm is known by a ventricular rate of around 30.

3. A. Electrodes dry out rather quickly, so replace them periodically, especially if the patient is febrile. They are placed anteriorly over intercostal spaces with all surfaces

making good contact. To avoid respiratory movement, place the electrodes closer together.

4. D. The T wave is after the ST segment and is upright, rounded, and symmetrical. The P wave is upright, rounded, and symmetrical but it is after the T wave and is smaller. The QRS is after the P wave and can have three phases. The ST segment is after the QRS and before the T wave.

5. C. The QRS is around 0.06 to 0.1 seconds. The P wave is not usually measured but we look to see that it is upright, rounded, and symmetrical. The PRI is from 0.12 to 0.2 seconds, and the QT is rate related but is around 0.36 to 0.42 seconds.

6. C. Atrial flutter is detected by its multiple, saw-tooth-patterned P waves that are fast, countable, and regular. PAT is fast but has only one P wave/one QRS. PACs can fall on any underlying rhythm, but they are limited to one or two beats with premature P waves. Atrial fibrillation has uncountable P waves.

7. D. This is the most common mode for permanent ventricular pacing. V = ventricular, I = inhibited, and R = rate modulated.

8. B. The patient needs to get a medical alert tag as health care providers need to avoid the generator box site during defibrillation. There are no external wires, so electrical safety is not an issue. All surgical sites need to be monitored for infection, and home microwaves do not interfere with newer permanent pacers.

9. A. Transcutaneous pacers are placed on the anterior and posterior chest via electrodes by the critical care nurse. All other pacers are inserted by the physician.

10. B. "Epi" or epinephrine is used in almost all cardiac arrest scenarios. Atropine is reserved for asystole. Adenosine might be given for fast tachydysrhythmias. Sodium bicarbonate is reserved for after a set of arterial blood gases are obtained if the patient is in acidosis.

chapter 5

Care of the Patient With Neurological Needs

LEARNING OBJECTIVES

At the end of this chapter, the student will be able to:

1 Prioritize needs of the individual with complex neurological deficits.

2 Perform accurate components of the neurological assessment.

3 Identify changes in neurological status of the individual experiencing neurological compromise.

4 Provide comprehensive nursing management of the individual with neurological deficits.

5 Define key diagnostic tools used to collaborate neurological trauma or debility.

6 Use a case study scenario to apply learned skills while caring for a patient with complex neurological needs.

Introduction

The brain and nervous system has often been compared to a computer; they both rely heavily on one's knowledge of the diverse, intricate functioning and integration of internal circuits. Computers, just like the nervous system, function to obtain, analyze, and transmit innumerable signals and responses to the correct recipients. Numerous issues that can lead to computer meltdowns can also in the human being lead to compromises in neurological functioning, such as cerebrovascular accidents (CVAs), seizures, and traumatic injuries or incidents. Much is also expected of critical care nurses who are required to be computer literate as well as knowledgeable about the nervous system and accompanying neurological disorders.

Anatomy and Physiology of the Nervous System

The Neuron

The most basic cellular structure of the nervous system is the neuron. The organ that most predominantly affects the nervous system is the brain. The neuron consists of axons, dendrites, neuroglia, synapses, and a myelin sheath. Axons carry impulses away from the cell body and dendrites conduct impulses toward the cell body. Neuroglia is the "glue" or supportive tissue that binds nerve cells and fibers together. This glue also provides nourishment and protection of the neurons. Spaces where impulses hop scotch from one neuron to another are called synapses. Neurons make contact with other target cells through synaptic spaces. A synaptic transmission is described as a chemical process that can only occur with the release of excitatory and inhibitory neurotransmitters such as dopamine, norepinephrine, acetylcholine, serotonin, glycine, glutamic acid, and γ-aminobutyric acid. The myelin sheath is a membranous covering of lipid protein and white matter that is formed in the central nervous system (CNS) and it surrounds and protects the nerve fibers.

The nervous system is divided into the

Central nervous system – composed of at least 12 billion neurons including the brain and spinal cord

Peripheral nervous system – contains the cranial and spinal nerves

The Central Nervous System

The central nervous system includes the brain, meninges, blood-brain barrier, and cerebrospinal fluid (CSF). Table 5–1 reviews the components of the brain and Figure 5–1 shows the sections of the brain.

The Protecting Layers

The brain is surrounded by three tough layers that protect it and the spinal column. They are called the meninges and they help circulate cerebral spinal fluid (CSF) from the ventricles of the brain to the spinal column. They include

Pia mater – The inner layer of tissue that lies directly next to the brain.

Arachnoid – This middle layer contains a large vascular supply of oxygen and nutrients that are provided to the brain cells.

Dura mater – Sometimes nicknamed the "the tough mother" because it is durable. The thickest layer of the three membranes, the dura mater lies in the outermost layer adjacent to the bones that surround the CNS.

The subarachnoid space is positioned between the pia and arachnoid layer. It contains CSF supplying nutrients to the CNS, but not oxygen. This space also serves as a protective function to cushion the brain and spinal cord.

The blood-brain barrier is another method of protection that prevents many undesirable elements or substances from being exchanged between the blood and the brain due to an extremely tight connection between the endothelial and astrocyte cells. Lipid-soluble materials easily cross the blood-brain barrier, while larger, heavier proteins like molecules cannot cross the blood-brain barrier. The blood-brain

TABLE 5–1 Components of the Brain		
	Location	**Function**
Cerebrum (largest portion)	Divided into left and right hemispheres. Connected by band of white matter called corpus callosum. Each hemisphere of the cerebrum has four lobes: frontal, parietal, temporal, and occipital.	Hemispheres work together to produce the coordinated functions of written and verbal communication as well as thoughts that need to be appropriately communicated. Frontal (thoughts and emotions), parietal (movement, sensation, and speech), temporal (hearing), and occipital (balance and sight)
Cortex	Most superficial layer of the cerebrum	Responsible for all levels of higher mental functioning such as judgment, memory, language, creativity, and abstract thinking. Interprets all sensations and governs all voluntary motor activities.
Basal ganglia	Cell bodies in the peripheral nervous system that work with lower brain parts	Circuitry for basic and subconscious body movements such as muscle tone and coordination for walking and balance. Lesions of the basal ganglia can produce clinical ataxic abnormalities such as Parkinson's disease and Huntington's chorea.
Diencephalon	Lowest structure of the cerebrum. Lies below the cerebral hemispheres, directly above the brainstem. Paired on each side of the 3rd ventricle. Crucial areas of the diencephalon include the thalamus, reticular activating system (RAS), hypothalamus, pituitary gland, and the 1st and 2nd cranial nerves.	Thalamus functions as a sensory motor relay center for sight, sound, touch, and pain. The thalamus is also involved with the RAS. RAS is responsible for wakefulness, consciousness, and attention. Hypothalamus controls the regulation of body temperature, appetite, sleep, and water via the antidiuretic hormone (ADH). Pituitary controls hormonal secretions.
Midbrain	Connects the pons and cerebellum with the cerebral hemispheres	Contains centers for hearing and visual nerve stimulation. Relays impulses in response to these stimuli. Involved in voluntary motor movement of body and flexor muscle tone.

TABLE 5–1	Components of the Brain (*Continued*)	
	Location	Function
Pons	Between midbrain and medulla	Responsible for respiratory regulation. Contains two control centers: apneuistic and pneumotaxic. Apneuistic controls length of inspiration and expiration. Pneumotaxic center controls the respiratory rate.
Medulla	Between the pons and the spinal cord	Regulates vital functions of breathing and heart rate as well as reflexes such as sneezing, vomiting, and gagging.
Brainstem	Located in the inferior surface of the brain	10 of the 12 cranial nerves originate from the brainstem. The brainstem also regulates respirations.
Cerebellum (little or hind brain)	Known as "little brain" or "hind brain" because it is 1/5 the size of the brain. Located in the posterior/inferior head region. Composed of a cortex of gray matter and a core of white matter	Coordinates skeletal muscle actions, maintains balance, and controls posture. Involved in motor learning. Cerebellar disturbances can produce tremors, ataxia, and equilibrium problems.

FIGURE 5–1 • Brain.

barrier prevents some chemotherapeutic medications from entering the CNS, so those medications require another route of administration such as intrathecal.

The CSF is a clear, odorless, and colorless fluid that forms in the ventricles of the brain and flows in the ventricles of the brain, the subarachnoid space, and the spinal cord. Table 5–2 reviews the components of the brain. CSF is a great shock absorber, preventing injury to the spinal cord. CSF also exchanges nutrients between the cells and the plasma but, as previously stated, not oxygen, because it does not contain red blood cells (RBCs), which are needed for oxygen transport. CSF must travel to the arachnoid space for reabsorption. Daily reabsorption prevents the development of hydrocephalus as well as increased pressures in the CSF due to an excessive amount of fluid buildup. Obstructions to the reabsorption of CSF can be caused by meningitis, brain tumors, and blood clots from a subarachnoid hemorrhage or congenital anomalies.

The peripheral nervous system is composed of the spinal cord, somatic nervous system, autonomic nervous system, the cranial nerves, and the spinal nerves. The spinal cord lies within the neural canal of the vertebral column. It is long, ropelike, and composed of both gray and white matter. It exits at the base of the medulla through the foramen magnum and ends at the lumbar spinous process 1-L1. Also exiting from the spinal cord are 31 pairs of spinal nerves.

The somatic or voluntary nervous system is also known as the sensory division. It includes neurons that innervate the skin, skeletal muscles, joints, and viscera. Sensory information from the outside environment and conditions within the body are delivered to the CNS via afferent or sensory fibers such as visual, auditory, and tactile information.

TABLE 5–2 Components of CSF	
Colorless/odorless	Clear
Rate of production	20 mL per hour or 500 mL per day
Circulating volume	135–150 mL
pH	7.35–7.45
White and red blood cells	0
Glucose	50–75 mg/mL
Specific gravity	1.007
Lymphocytes	0–10
Protein	25–55 mg/mL
Lumbar puncture pressure	70–200 mm/H_2O
Ventricular pressure	3–15 mm Hg

The autonomic or involuntary nervous system (ANS) is also known as the motor division in which motor neurons connect the CNS with smooth muscle and cardiac muscle, as well as the glands and internal organs. The ANS regulates functions of the heart, respiratory, and gastrointestinal activity. The ANS division includes the sympathetic and parasympathetic branches. Motor fibers are known as efferent fibers that transmit CNS responses to the appropriate organs, muscles, or glands. The transmission of both sensory (afferent) and motor (efferent) information in the CNS is conducted by internuncial fibers.

There are 12 pairs of cranial nerves that originate in the brainstem with the exception of 1 and 2, which arise from the diencephalon. Motor and sensory sensations are supplied to the head, neck, and upper back except cranial nerve number 10, the vagus nerve, which supplies the viscera. The cranial nerves are described in Table 5–3.

TABLE 5–3 Cranial Nerves

Number	Cranial Nerve	What It Does
I	Olfactory	Smell
II	Optic	Vision
III	Oculomotor	Pupillary constriction and accommodation, elevation of upper eyelids, and extraocular movements (EOMs)
IV	Trochlear	Downward, inward movement of the eye
V	Trigeminal	Muscles of chewing, opening jaw; tactile sensations to the facial skin, cornea, oral, and nasal mucosa; and eardrum tension
VI	Abducens	Lateral deviation of the eye
VII	Facial	Tears, salivation, taste sensation, facial expressions, closing of eyes
VIII	Acoustic/auditory or vestibulocochlear	Equilibrium and hearing
IX	Glossopharyngeal	Salivation, swallowing, speech, and gag reflex
X	Vagus	Laryngeal control of voluntary swallowing and phonation. Involuntary activity of the heart, lungs, and digestive tract
XI	Spinal accessory	Control of movements of the head and shoulders or of the sternocleidomastoid and trapezius muscles
XII	Hypoglossal	Tongue movements

The spinal nerves are attached to the spinal cord by a dorsal and a ventral root. The dorsal root is an afferent pathway that carries sensory impulses from the body into the spinal cord. The ventral root is an efferent pathway that carries motor information from the spinal cord to the body. Spinal nerves are attached to the spinal cord in pairs (see Figure 5–2). There are 8 cervical, 12 thoracic, 5 lumbar, 5 sacral, and 1 pair of coccygeal spinal nerves. Now that we have had a brief overview of the neurological anatomy and physiology, a neurological assessment is much more understandable.

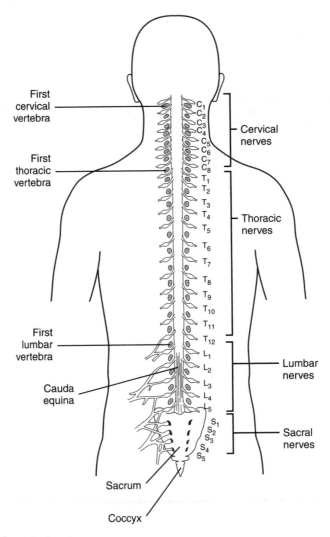

FIGURE 5–2 • Spinal cord.

Neurological Needs: Assessment

It is far too easy for the health care provider to miss the most minor change in a patient's neurological status. The slightest change can be an initial sign that the patient's condition is deteriorating and can rapidly worsen. Therefore, it is paramount that a thorough clinical assessment be completed especially in patients with a neurological problem.

History

In obtaining a comprehensive neurologic history, it is necessary to identify the patient's associated signs and symptoms, statements of concern, onset, severity, and duration of clinical manifestations that describe a neurological disturbance, such as confusion and other behavioral changes, slurred speech, seizures, loss of consciousness, abnormal balance and loss of motor coordination, weakened musculature, pupillary abnormalities, localized or generalized paralysis, visual changes such as blurred vision, diplopia or double vision, or even partial visual field blindness. Determine if the patient has sustained any recent falls or injuries that would contribute to his or her onset of illness. A drug history is also essential to determine if neurological deficits can be attributed to particular medication combinations, over the counter or street drugs. The patient's past medical history should also be well known and documented by the health team.

Inspection

This is the major component of a thorough neurological assessment. The nurse spends most of her or his time in baseline observation, trending of data, and communicating this information to other nurses and members in the health care team.

It consists of evaluating major components such as the level of consciousness (LOC). The AVPU scale, general terms for LOC description, and the Glasgow Coma Scale are ways the critical care nurse can evaluate and track the patient with neurological issues. A quick and easy way to perform LOC without the use of charts or graphs is the AVPU scale:

A – Alert

V – Verbal response

P – Pain

U – Unconsciousness

Many other terms are used to describe the LOC and the critical care nurse must be familiar with these terms. Table 5–4 describes commonly used general terms for LOC.

TABLE 5–4 General Terms Used in LOC Description		
Arousal	Lowest level of consciousness that focuses on the patient's ability to respond to verbal commands or painful stimuli appropriately, repeat the task when asked again	"Open your eyes" or "Squeeze my hand." The successful response is that the patient will be able to perform simple tasks on command and repeat the task when asked again. The nurse can also use the blunt end of a pen or pencil to apply firm pressure to the patient's nailbeds to elicit an appropriate withdrawal response.
Awareness	Higher-level function of consciousness concerned with the patient's orientation to person, place, and time. Full orientation is documented as A + O × 3	Ask the patient who he or she is, where he or she is, and what time it is. The patient must give correct responses and appropriate answers to a series of non-trick questions. Changes in these answers can indicate increasing levels of confusion, irritability, and disorientation, further demonstrating signs of neurological deterioration.
Lethargic	A state of drowsiness and inaction that requires an increased amount of stimulus to awaken the patient	Call the patient loudly or bang on their door. Shake the patient gently.
Obtunded	Barely responds to and minimally maintains a reaction to external stimuli.	Tapping on the patient's face or lightly pinching the inner aspect of the patient's arm or leg.
Stuporous	Patient arousal can only be achieved through vigorous and continuous external stimuli.	Sternal rub by using the nurse's knuckles of one hand to rub the patient's sternum, trapezius squeeze, firm nail bed pressure.
Comatose	The patient remains unresponsive and vigorous stimulation fails to produce any reaction.	

Recounting a True Story

As a Medical/Surgical Administrative Supervisor, I always made visiting rounds of my patients to determine their levels of care, safety, and satisfaction of care received. On report, I learned of a young, married man and father of two children who returned with his family to the area from Mississippi to visit his parents. On a hot and humid summer day, he frivolously and without looking dove backwards into his parents' empty swimming pool and sustained a serious head injury. Hospitalized, he was maintained on a general medical/surgical unit because according to staff members, he was oriented to person, place, and time. (A + O × 3.) His level of consciousness, vital signs, and motor and pupillary responses were all within normal limits. As I looked in on the patient, there was something about his "gaze," that bothered me, so I decided to introduce myself and began to ask him the standard questions of his name, date, and current location. The patient seemed to be a tad agitated with my inquiries, so I ended it by asking him if he knew the name of the hospital he was in and he answered correctly. However, when I asked him where the hospital was located, he angrily replied, "Why in Mississippi of course!" Perhaps to a less seasoned nurse, this response could have been viewed as a small sign of a communication error. However, coupled with what I believed was an out-of-focus facial stare or gaze, I knew then that this patient's neurological status was not up to par and perhaps deteriorating. He was immediately transferred to ICU for more in-depth care and observation. A subtle additional question by a concerned nurse probably saved this man's life and provided interventions to prevent further neurologic disaster.

The Glasgow Coma Scale or GCS is the most widely recognized international scale and assessment tool used to determine a person's level of consciousness. It is a SCORED SCALE that evaluates the categories of eye opening and verbal and motor responses. Also, awareness of the environment, cognition, and demonstrating the ability to perform tasks and understand given directions are evaluated. The ideal GCS score is 15; the worst is 3. A score of 7 or less generally indicates that the patient is in a comatose state.

? How To Do It—Glasgow Coma Scale

Best Eye Opening Response	Score
Spontaneously	4
To speech	3
To pain	2
No response	1

Best Motor Response

Obeys commands	6
Localizes stimuli	5
Withdrawal from stimulus	4
Abnormal flexion (decorticate)	3
Abnormal extension(decerebrate)	2
No response	1

Best Verbal Response

Oriented	5
Confused and disoriented	4
Inappropriate words	3
Garbled sounds	2
No response	1

Assessing Motor Movements—Strength and Coordination

Each extremity is evaluated and its function compared to the opposite extremity. Sources describe muscle weakness as a cardinal sign of dysfunction in many neurological disorders.

Categories of motor movement assessments include

Romberg's test – Have the patient stand with feet together, first with eyes open and then closed. Observe the patient for signs of swaying or signs of beginning to fall, and if so, in what direction.

Finger-to-nose test – Have the patient touch one finger to the examiner's finger and then touch his or her own nose. The term for overshooting the mark is known as dysmetria.

RAM (rapid alternating movement) test – Have the patient perform rapid pronation and supination of each hand on each leg.

Heel-to-shin test – Moving from the knee to the ankle, have the patient extend the heel of one foot down the front or anterior aspect of the shin.

Pronator drift test – This is a quick test to detect upper extremity weakness. Have the patient hold his or her arms straight out with eyes closed and palms outward. The nurse observes for any downward drift or pronation of the patient's forearms.

Lower extremity weakness can be tested by having the patient raise one leg at a time off the bed against the examiner's resistance.

According to some authors, motor function for each extremity is reported as a fraction, such as

0/5 – No muscle contraction.

1/5 – A trace of muscle contraction.

2/5 – Movement, but cannot balance against gravity.

3/5 – Can resist gravity, but cannot overcome resistance of examiner's muscle strength.

4/5 – Can move with some weakness against the resistance of the examiner's muscle strength.

5/5 – The patient has normal power and strength.

These can often be documented as a stick figure (man) with the numbers written by each extremity.

> ### NURSING ALERT
>
> *Muscle strength can be further assessed by having the patient perform additional tasks such as shrugging the shoulders, raising the arms and legs, flexing or bending the knees and elbows, or by simply stretching or extending the extremities.*

Abnormal Motor Responses to Stimuli

A patient may also have abnormal motor responses to various stimuli. These responses include withdrawal, localization, decorticate and decerebrate posturing, opisthotonus, and flaccidity (see Figure 5–3.) These terms are described as follows:

Withdraws from pain – The patient normally flexes or withdraws an extremity away from the source of painful stimuli.

Localization to pain – Occurs when the extremity opposite to the one receiving the painful stimuli crosses over the middle of the body and tries to remove the painful stimuli from the affected limb.

Decorticate posturing or abnormal flexion – Spontaneous flexion occurs in response to painful stimuli in an unconscious patient. The arm, wrist, and fingers flex and the upper extremity adducts inward. The lower extremity extends, internally rotates, and exhibits plantar flexion. Associated with injury to the cortex (decorticate). See Figure 5–3A.

Decerebrate posturing/rigidity or abnormal extension – This is a spontaneous extension response to painful stimuli in an unconscious patient. When stimulated, the teeth clench and arms stiffly extend, adduct, and hyperpronate. The legs also stiffly extend with plantar flexion of both feet. Associated with injury to the cerebrum and is a worse injury than decorticate. Easily remembered by the number of "es" in decerebrate. See Figure 5–3B.

NURSING ALERT

While both conditions of decerebrate and decorticate rigidity are very serious, decerebrate posturing has a more significant detrimental prognosis as compared to abnormal flexion or decorticate posturing.

A. Decorticate

B. Decerebrate

C. Decorticate on right; decerebrate on left

D. Opisthotonus

FIGURE 5-3 • Decorticate and decerebrate rigidity.

Opisthotonus – Spasm where the head and heels are bent backward and the body is bowed forward. Seen in severe meningitis, tetanus, epilepsy, and rabies. See Figure 5–3D.

Flaccid – Absolutely no response at all to painful stimuli. Such a nonreaction can be caused by extensive brainstem dysfunction.

Pupillary function and eye movement – The critical care nurse must assess the patient's pupillary size, shape, and degree of reaction to light while equally comparing both pupils. Pupillary changes occurring during the nurse's examination could indicate increasing pressure and compression on the oculomotor nerve, which happens with increased intracranial pressure. The nurse should check papillary size and reaction to light accommodation, EOMs, oculocephalic reflexes, and oculovestibular reflexes. The latter two reflexes are usually done by the neurologist in a patient who has severe brain damage and survival is questionable.

Normal Pupils

A normal pupil is round in shape. Each pupil should be of equal size and react briskly to light by constricting to protect the eye. A narrow-beamed light should be used and directed into each eye from the outer canthus of the eye and observed for the response of constriction. Also observe for a consensual response or pupillary constriction in one eye that occurs as a result of the light beam being shone into the other eye. Consensual response is necessary to rule out optic nerve dysfunction (see Figure 5–4).

A pupil that is suddenly bigger than the other and more sluggish to light along with vital sign changes could indicate an increase in intracranial pressure.

NURSING ALERT

The term for unequal pupil size is Anisocoria. Changes that occur in pupil size can result from the instillation of eye medications, which can cause large, dilated pupils. Constricted pupils can occur from narcotic overuse. Also, a nurse should recognize that on rare occasions a patient could have a prosthetic eye, in which case the size, shape, and reaction to light of the artificial eye will remain stationary and never change. To spare embarrassment on the part of the nurse, please determine if your patient does indeed have a fake eye. Having had other eye surgery such as an iridectomy will also affect pupillary size, shape, and reaction to light. Shining a light into a blind eye will not produce a direct light response in that eye, nor will it produce a consensual response in the other eye.

FIGURE 5–4 • Pupillary responses.

Accommodation

Nurses may also check for accommodation. The nurse should point to the far wall and assess the patient's pupils, which should dilate in an attempt to accommodate for distance. Then, using an object or the examiner's finger, have the patient focus on that as it is brought closer into the patient's field of vision. Normal pupils will constrict at this time.

NURSING ALERT

Normal pupillary responses to testing are recorded as PERRLA, which means pupils equal round and reactive to light accomodation. A change in pupillary size and sluggishly reactive to light may indicate increased intracranial pressure. This along with bradycardia, hypertension, and respiratory changes indicates increased intracranial pressure is highly suspicious. Call the neurologist stat!

Assessment of Eye Movements (EOMs) or Extraocular Movements

Extraocular movements are intact and coordinated in the conscious patient if both eyes move together through the full range of eye motions. The nurse instructs the patient to follow his or her finger (the nurse's) with the eyes as the finger is pointed upward, downward, and sideways.

Oculocephalic Reflex or Doll's Eyes Movements

This response can be observed in the unconscious patient. With the patient's eyelids held open, the nurse briskly turns the patient's head to one side and observes the eye movements. The eyes should deviate to the opposite direction from which the head is turned if the doll's eyes response is present and intact. Repeat the process by briskly turning the head to the opposite side and observing the response. The doll's eye response is absent and indicates brainstem injury when the eyes with head movement either remain midline, move with the head, rove about in circles, or move up and down. This is usually done in a patient with severe brain damage and a positive result can indicate brain death.

NURSING ALERT

Before proceeding with this reflex in the unconscious patient, it is necessary to make sure that the patient has not suffered a cervical neck injury, which, if provoked through excessive movement, can cause complete transection of the cord! Make sure the C-spine x-ray is negative before attempting this.

Oculovestibular Reflex or Cold Caloric Test

This is also a test to evaluate brainstem function and should never be conducted on a conscious patient. This test involves instilling 20 to 50 cc. of ice water into the external auditory canal of the ear. Brainstem integrity is confirmed when there is a normal eye movement response of a rapid rotary nystagmus toward the irrigated ear. A neurologist usually performs this test in a patient with severe brain damage . A positive result can indicate brain death.

An abnormal response is evident with dysconjugate eye movements or no movements whatsoever, which can progress to decorticate or decerebrate posturing in the comatose patient and the suggestion of an absence of brainstem function.

Respiratory Patterns

Since the medulla and the pons are the centers of the brainstem that control respirations, patterns of breathing must be assessed as they can be severely affected by brain injury.

> **NURSING ALERT**
>
> It is not unusual to observe hypoventilation in an individual with an altered level of consciousness. Therefore, the effectiveness of oxygen and carbon dioxide levels and gas exchange must be evaluated and maintained accordingly. Hypoxemia and hypercarbia can lead to further neurologic impairment and an increase in ICP or intracranial pressure.

Further physical examination includes assessing the patient's cough, gag, and swallowing reflexes, which may be absent or diminished as a result of brain trauma, anesthesia, or stroke. Airway protection in the vulnerable patient must be guaranteed and the dangers of aspiration prevented. With a tongue depressor, touch the far posterior surface of the pharynx. If the patient gags, his or her reflex is intact. The nurse must also assess the position of the patient's tongue and uvula. If they are deviated to the side within the patient's mouth, this can be an indication of paralysis of the hypoglossal and glossopharyngeal cranial nerves, wherein an absence of the cough, gag, and swallowing reflexes will be most likely. The nurse should observe a true cough and swallowing effort in the patient, which should be present if the gag reflex is intact.

> **NURSING ALERT**
>
> Always check the patient for a gag reflex, especially after anesthetic agents, stroke, or cerebral trauma. Checking the gag or the 6th cranial nerve helps decrease the likelihood of aspiration, especially before feeding a patient.

Additional Assessments

These should include the signs of CSF leakage from the nose and ears: otorrhea and rhinorrhea. Battle's sign and raccoon eyes—severe ecchymosis behind the ears and around the eyes. Inspect for further signs of physical trauma such as swelling, bruising, bleeding, lacerations, bodily areas out of alignment or paralyzed, and any indications of pain and discomfort on behalf of the patient.

Palpation

The critical care nurse should gently palpate areas of the patient's body that have created pain and distress for signs of fractures, deformities, lack of functioning capabilities, and dislocations.

Percussion—Deep Tendon Reflexes

Critical care nurses must develop delicate and refined methods of assessing individual responses to various stimuli in an effort to determine a person's level of neurological functioning or deficits that could identify specific injuries. Such examinations consist of the nurse testing deep tendon or stretch reflexes for degrees of muscle contraction in response to direct or indirect percussion of a tendon. Reflexes generally occur without conscious thought and are responses to sensory impulses placed on tendons and muscle groups. Sensory impulses consist of sensory, CNS, and motor neuron components that comprise the three-neuron reflex arc. An example of the three-neuron reflex arc is the withdrawal reflex where a body part will withdraw from painful stimuli.

How to Do It –Deep Tendon Reflexes (DTRs)

1. Gently support the tendon and allow it to relax.

2. Use a flick of the wrist when tapping the tendon.

3. Note that the muscle group should contract when tapping with the reflex hammer.

4. Compare the muscle groups bilaterally. Commonly elicited groups are shown in Table 5–5.

5. Record your responses by writing in the chart or making a stick man with numbers by each group.

6. Grades include the following: 0 = no response; 1+ = hypoactive, a sluggish or diminished response; 2+ = normal or an expected active response; 3+ = a slightly hyperactive or very brisk, more than normal response, however, not necessarily pathologic; 4+ = an abnormal, intermittent clonus or repetitive and brisk hyperactive reflex action usually associated with neurological disease.

TABLE 5–5 Commonly Assessed Deep Tendon Reflexes

Reflex	Procedure	Results
Patellar or knee jerk	Patient should be sitting with the legs hanging downward, knees flexed at 90 degrees. Strike the patellar tendon with the pointed tip of the reflex hammer just below the knee.	The quadriceps muscle should contract causing extension of the lower leg.
Achilles tendon reflex	Hold the bottom of the patient's foot in one hand and use the flat end of the reflex hammer to strike the Achilles tendon at the heel or posterior ankle area of the foot.	The gastrocnemius muscle should contract causing plantar flexion of the foot.
Triceps reflex	The patient's relaxed arm should be placed over the nurse's arm. The patient's elbow should be flexed at 90 degrees and held by the nurse who strikes the triceps tendon just above the elbow with the reflex hammer.	As the triceps muscle contracts the elbow will extend.
Biceps reflex	Position with the elbow flexed at 90 degrees and the arm relaxed. The nurse places his or her thumb over the biceps tendon in the antecubital space and fingers over the biceps muscle. The nurse uses the pointed end of the reflex hammer and strikes his or her own thumb instead of directly striking the tendon.	The biceps muscle should contract causing flexion of the elbow.
Brachioradial reflex	The nurse holds the patient's slightly pronated and relaxed arm in his or her hand and strikes the brachioradial tendon about 1–2 in above the wrist	The expected response is pronation of the forearm with flexion of the elbow.
Babinski's reflex	The handle of the reflex hammer can be used to stroke the side of the sole of the foot from heel to ball, curving across the ball of the foot.	A normal or negative response should elicit plantar flexion of the toes. Abnormal or positive response is evident when the great toe dorsiflexes and the remaining toes on the same foot fan outward indicating upper motor tract neuron disease.

Other Responses

Blink Reflex and Corneal Response

Normal blinking is frequent, bilateral, and involuntary, averaging 15 to 20 per minute. To assist in determining brainstem function, this response is tested by passing a wisp of cotton either from the side of each eye toward the sclera or over the lower conjunctiva of each eye to cause blinking. There is no blink response in the unconscious patient.

Signs of Meningeal Irritation

It is important to mention signs of meningeal irritation that the patient might be experiencing such as nuchal rigidity, fever, resistance to neck flexion, headache, and photophobia. Two specific signs of meningeal irritation that the nurse should become familiar with are

Brudzinski's sign – involuntary flexion of the hips when the patient's neck is flexed toward the chest.

Kernig's sign – pain in the neck is evident when the thigh is flexed onto the abdomen and the leg is extended at the knee.

Auscultation

Neurological examination relies heavily on frequent, accurate vital sign assessments. Slight trends can signal worsening degrees of neurological impairment. Auscultation includes assessment of respirations, temperature, pulse, blood pressure, and bruits.

Respirations

A patient may have difficulty maintaining a patent airway as a result of increasing intracranial pressure, a partially obstructed airway, a high cervical spinal cord injury, a decreasing level of consciousness, or progressive diaphragmatic paralysis. Respiratory distress can range from the crescendo- decrescendo pattern of Cheyne-Stokes respirations interspersed with periods of apnea, to hypoventilation and respiratory acidosis or hyperventilation, which can lead to respiratory alkalosis. Assess for status of lung sounds, provide for adequate gas exchange, monitor gas exchange levels, avoid aspiration difficulties, and promote a patent airway.

Temperature

Increases in body temperature with neurological trauma could be evident and resistant to antipyretic therapy. In these cases, patients might benefit from being placed on cooling blankets to create mild hypothermia, prevent increases in intracranial pressure, and decrease cellular metabolism.

NURSING ALERT

Remember that temperature regulation is controlled by the hypothalamus of the brain. Any time a severe trauma like stroke/brain injury occurs, the temperature can soar to high levels! Change in temperature increases metabolism and can lead to further increases in intracranial pressure.

Pulse

Variations in cardiac rate and rhythm can occur from increases in intracranial pressure leading to bradycardias and other dysrhythmias. Extreme bradycardia can be viewed as a sign of impending death.

Blood Pressure

Blood pressure is controlled by the medulla. Hypertension is most commonly seen with a neurological injury because cerebral blood volume and blood flow increase dramatically, resulting in an increase in intracranial pressure (ICP).

The normal ICP is 0 to 10 or 0 to 15 mm Hg. Increases of 20 mm Hg for periods of 5 minutes or longer is life threatening. Causes of increased intracranial pressure are brain disorders such as hematomas, tumors, infection, CVA, hydrocephaly, head trauma, cerebral hemorrhage, and edema. The body attempts to compensate for ICP by displacing CSF into the spinal canal or by absorbing it into the venous blood system.

Classic symptoms of an increase in intracranial pressure include Cushing's triad or syndrome. This is a classic response to an accompanying brain lesion or injury and is a life-threatening event. There is an increase in the systolic blood pressure with an increased and widening pulse pressure, decreased pulse (bradycardia) and respiratory rate (bradypnea), decreased levels of consciousness, diminished reflexes, projectile vomiting, unequal pupil size and decreased pupillary reaction to light, and respiratory changes. The patient may also assume the posturing of decerebrate (abnormal extension) or decorticate (abnormal flexion) as his or her condition deteriorates.

> ## NURSING ALERT
>
> *Close trending of vital signs is a must to prevent increased intracranial pressure and resultant brainstem herniation. Impending herniation is signified by elevated temperature, bradycardia, widening pulse pressure, and respiratory changes. Make sure the patient is on oxygen and the head of the bed is elevated 45 degrees. Administer Mannitol or Lasix as per order to decrease ICP. Call the MD stat!*

Bruits

These are abnormal or adventitious high-pitched, vascular blowing sounds, which, if heard over the carotid arteries, can be indicators of obstruction, stenosis, or vessel narrowing and can be associated with intracranial aneurysms. The sounds vary in volume, resulting from either blood flow through a tortuous or partially occluded vessel or increased blood flow through a normal vessel.

Collaborative Diagnostic Tools

A variety of tools are used to monitor and trend a patient with a neurological problem. These diagnostic tools include cerebral spinal x-rays, lumbar punctures, magnetic resonance imaging (MRI), intracranial pressure monitoring, and ventricular drains. The following is a summary of these tools.

C-Spine and Cerebral X-Rays and Scans

Routine x-rays are still performed as initial screening tools on the skull and spine to identify specific traumatic injuries or abnormalities. However, routine x-rays are frequently replaced by the more reliable diagnostic tools of the CAT scan (computerized axial tomography), MRI (magnetic resonance imaging), and PET scans (positron emission tomography). The CAT scan and MRI provide detailed outlines of bone, blood, and tissue structures of the body, and the CAT scan is a safer procedure to verify a subarachnoid hemorrhage in the patient. The PET scan is a superior technology in that it measures not only image structure but also the physiological and biochemical processes and functions of the nervous system, thus aiding in the diagnosis of tumors and vascular disease as well as cerebral metabolism and blood flow. However, the PET scan is complex and high priced, making it impractical to use clinically as compared to other diagnostic modalities.

Spinal Tap or Lumbar Puncture

This is an invasive procedure done to detect blood in the cerebrospinal fluid and to assess for infection or autoimmune disorders. After skin preparation and providing a local anesthetic, a sterile needle is inserted into the subarachnoid space at the L3-4 or L4-5 vertebral level. Ten milliliters of obtained fluid is analyzed for culture and sensitivity, cell counts, chemistry, and microbiologic examination. CSF pressure readings are also obtained. Remember that normal CSF pressure is 70 to 200 mm H_2O. Also, one-half to 1 hour prior to a spinal tap, a blood glucose sample is drawn and used as a comparison with the CSF glucose level of 50 to 75 mg/dL or 60% of serum levels. Patient positioning for a spinal tap is very important to allow for the maximum separation of the vertebrae. Patients are positioned on their sides, curled up into a ball with their head and feet as close to each other as possible. In other words, the patient assumes the fetal position.

Complications from a spinal tap include a post-procedure headache that can last for 24 hours or longer, nuchal rigidity, fever, and dysuria. The patient may be instructed to remain flat in bed for a few hours post procedure to prevent spinal headaches. Further treatment includes the injection of a "blood patch" or blood into the dura mater to stop the CSF leak.

Magnetic Resonance Imaging (MRI)

An MRI produces computerized cross-sectional images of finely detailed anatomical slices of the body. It is most useful in the early diagnosis of cerebral infarction, multiple sclerosis, and tumors and hemorrhages that might not be identified on CAT scan. The use of an MRI is limited in that it cannot be performed on patients with pacemakers, surgical clips, and prosthetic implants made of ferrous metal, including life support mechanical ventilators.

Intracranial Pressure (ICP) Monitoring

To maintain a normal ICP, the following three brain components need to be regulated to maintain a fixed intracranial volume. As long as the total intracranial volume remains the same, ICP remains constant at 0 to 15 mm Hg = normal. Parts that compose the total intracranial volume are CBF or cerebral blood flow = 3% to 10%, cerebrospinal fluid circulation = 8% to 12%, and intravascular plus the volume of semisolid brain tissue, which is more than 80% H_2O.

A constant perfusion pressure to the brain is needed to supply oxygen and nutrients to the cerebral neurons and to prevent excessive pressure leading to brain herniation. In order to do this, cerebral perfusion pressures need to be monitored via an intracranial monitoring device. An intracranial monitoring device records the ICP, which is used to calculate the cerebral perfusion pressure (CPP).

CPP is calculated by taking the mean arterial BP (MAP) minus the ICP. Normal CPP is between 70 and 90 mm Hg. Let us see an example of this calculation.

How to Do It–Calculation of Cerebral Perfusion Presure (CPP)

1. Take the MAP of 120 mm Hg.

2. Record the ICP from the monitor as 80 mm Hg.

3. MAP – ICP = CPP: 120 – 80 = 40

4. Analysis: This is too low of a CPP to sustain life. Nursing action is required! Usually this involves decreasing the BP since the MAP is high.

NURSING ALERT

According to the Monro-Kellie doctrine, when there is an increase in volume of the brain, blood, or CSF properties, the pressure within the brain will increase unless one or more of these components decrease.

Intracranial Pressure Monitoring Devices

Before the patient can be attached to a monitoring device to monitor his or her ICP, a measuring device must be inserted by a neurologist. These can be inserted into the intraventricular, subarachnoid, or epidural spaces or into the brain parenchyma itself. Following is a brief description of each site.

Intraventricular catheter	Small catheter inserted directly into the ventricle through the skull. Neurologist inserts the catheter through a small hole in the brain called a burr hole. Used primarily for the removal of CSF for diagnostic or therapeutic purposes.
Subarachnoid bolt	A small, hollow bolt or screw is inserted into this space. It does not penetrate the brain and it cannot drain CSF. Inserted through burr hole.
Epidural sensor	A small, fiber-optic sensor is placed into this space. It is the least invasive of the catheters, easier to insert, and has a low risk of infection. It does not penetrate the brain or the dura and does not drain CSF. Inserted via burr hole.
Parenchyma	A small, fiber-optic catheter that is inserted approximately 1 cm into the parenchyma through a subarachnoid bolt. It cannot drain CSF.

A popular, more versatile type of ICP monitoring system is the fiber-optic small-transducer-tipped 4 Fr. catheter. However, this type of catheter is fragile and vulnerable to kinks and pulls, which could then block or occlude the function of the catheter. Figure 5–5 shows an ICP monitoring catheter and system.

How to Do It–Setting Up an ICP Monitoring Device

1. Verify that the patient is a candidate for ICP monitoring, which is usually indicated by two or more of the following:

   Age greater than 40

   Motor posturing, bilateral or unilateral decorticate or decerebrate

Systolic BP less than 90 mm Hg

Diagnostic studies indicative of edema, distortion, or hydrocephalus

2. Check that a consent form has been signed.

3. Time out to verify the identity of the patient.

4. Premedicate the patient with a sedative to prevent movement.

5. Position the patient in a high Fowler's with the bed controls locked out.

6. Set up and maintain a meticulous sterile field; all personnel near the patient must wear sterile gloves, mask, and hat at all times when assisting with insertion and anytime during care of the site, drainage bag, or obtaining a CSF specimen.

7. Set up an airless unprressurized monitoring system, priming the tubing according to manufacturer's directions without heparin. This system is similar to an arterial line or pulmonary artery line setup but without a pressurized bag.

8. Check that all IV lines are tight.

9. Position the transducer at the foramen of Monroe and the top of the transducer by using a level or laser level.

10. If there is a drainage bag, check for order of level to be maintained so that CSF fluid does not drain excessively or flow back into the brain causing increased ICP.

11. Make sure all stopcocks are closed to air and open between the monitor and patient.

12. Record the ICP once hooked to the transducer by the neurologist.

13. Calculate the CPP.

14. Document the initial pressures, characteristics of the CSF, height of the drain, and leveling of the transducer.

This procedure is a bit tricky and it takes several times to really get comfortable with insertion and readings. An experienced critical care nurse and a teaching neurologist help make this experience beneficial for the new nurse and the patient.

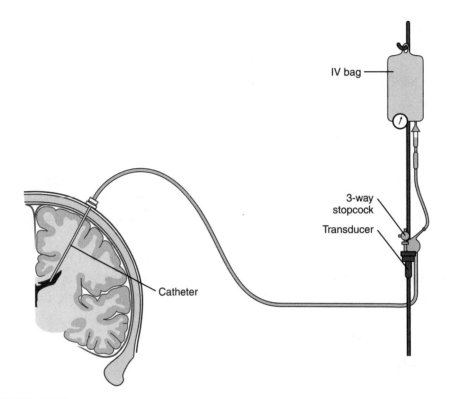

FIGURE 5–5 • ICP monitoring catheter and system.

With the monitoring devices in place, critical care nurses have the advantage of observing the ICP monitoring system at work. Data is provided regarding neurological assessment results, patient progress, and responses to interventions and treatments by monitoring these continuous waveforms. All of these results are seen as ICP waveform patterns on a monitoring system. The normal waveform has three main peaks that decrease in height and correlate with the arterial pulse waveform (see Figure 5–6). These peaks are as follows:

P1	Signifies blood being ejected from the heart and is affected by extremes in blood pressure such as hypotension or hypertension. P1 represents arterial pulsations.
P2	Represents intracranial brain bulk. If the P2 is equal to or higher than P1, it means that the brain tissue has decreased in compliance and there is an additional risk of an increase in ICP.
P3	Identifies closure of the aortic valve of the heart. P3 represents venous pulsations.

The nurse should also look for trends in waveforms to identify changes in the intracranial pressure waves, which are further described as follows:

Plateau wave (A wave) – between 50 and 100 mm Hg	Identifies advanced intracranial hypertension on a trending strip, which is crucial for the nurse to observe because the wave will not change on the monitor and the actual rise in ICP will only be evident for a short time. Opportunities for rapid interventions to reduce ICP can be missed.
Saw-tooth wave (B wave) – <50 mm Hg	Represents respirations and blood pressure and warns of risks of increased ICP and impaired intracranial compliance.
C wave – 16-20 mm Hg	Small, rhythmic waves that correlate normal blood pressure and respiratory changes. Its clinical importance is not really understood.

All of the information provided from the waveform monitoring system will determine if changes in the types of interventions are necessary to achieve the best patient outcomes for a successful recovery.

NURSING ALERT

Plateau waves indicate increased ICP. Protocols and orders to reduce ICP should be instituted immediately or brain death can result!

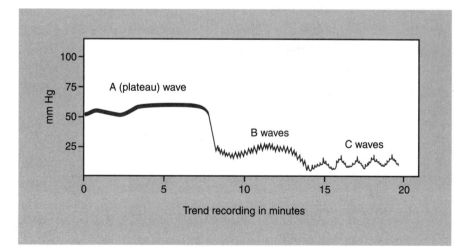

FIGURE 5–6 • ICP waveforms.

Nursing Care of the Patient to Decrease ICP

Nursing Diagnoses for the Patient With Increased ICP and ICP Monitoring	Expected Outcomes
❹ Tissue perfusion, altered, cerebral	The ICP will be <90 mm Hg
	The CPP will be <14 mm Hg
❹ Risk for infection	The patient will have a normal temperature
	The CSF will be clear, colorless

Nursing Interventions

1. Assess baseline vital signs to observe for signs of increased ICP, which include hyperthermia, bradycardia, respiratory changes, and widening of the pulse pressure.

2. Balance the transducer at the level of the foramen of Monroe by using the tragus of the ear and the top of the transducer to make trending readings consistent.

3. Calibrate the transducer according to manufacturer's/hospital protocols to ensure consistency in trended readings.

4. Monitor and record the MAP, CPP, and ICP, especially in response to nursing care to determine early signs of increased ICP that can occur with patient procedures like suctioning.

5. Consult neurologist if abnormal changes occur to treat the patient early and prevent complications.

6. Monitor the system for air bubbles; disconnect and purge if needed. Air bubbles could enter the brain, creating an embolism, and can dampen waveforms.

7. Monitor the insertion site for bleeding, edema, leakage of CSF, and infection to prevent complications.

8. Perform baseline and ongoing neurological assessments.

9. Position the patient with the head of the bed elevated at least 30 degrees, keeping the bed in lock-out to ensure this. This promotes cerebral venous drainage by gravity.

10. Keep the patient's head and neck midline to decrease ICP by promoting drainage from the head through the jugular veins.

11. Prevent hips and chest flexion to prevent intraabdominal and intrathoracic pressure, which in turn will increase ICP.

12. Avoid placing the patient in the prone position, which can also increase ICP.

13. Administer sedatives and analgesics. Consider the use of propofol or barbiturate coma if restlessness increases ICP. This keeps the patient comfortable and decreases energy demands, which increase ICP.

14. Plan nursing procedures to space them apart to decrease external stimulation, which can increase ICP.

15. Teach the patient and family about ICP monitoring with results, duration, and complications in mind. This decreases fear of this complex device.

16. Apply cooling blankets and antipyretic medications to reduce and control episodes of hyperthermia, which will increase body metabolism leading to increases in ICP.

Medications That Help With Symptoms

A variety of medications are used in the care of a patient with neurological deficits. These include seizure medications, medications to induce barbiturate coma, and diuretics (see Table 5–6).

Medical Conditions Requiring Complex Care

Status Epilepticus (SE)

What Went Wrong?

Neurological disorders such as trauma, epilepsy, electrolyte imbalances, hypoxia, and brain tumors can lead to seizures, which are abnormal and repetitive electrical discharges within the brain. These are caused by hyperexcitability of neurons due to changes in the flow of ions across the cell membranes.

SE is diagnosed when seizures are unrelieved with treatment. It is generally defined as constant generalized seizures lasting between 5 and 30 minutes or two or more seizures during which the patient does not return to his or her previous level of consciousness. These repetitive seizures occur so frequently and repeatedly that brain function cannot return to normal between attacks. Also, increased metabolic demands cannot be met or achieved, resulting in permanent neurological damage.

TABLE 5–6 Commonly Used Medications for the Neurologically Impaired Patient

Medication	Action	Use	Precautions
Dilantin (Phenytoin)	Alters ion transmission to prevent seizure activity	Seizures	Incompatible with all solutions except NSS. Monitor the patient for suicidal thoughts. Observe hypersensitivity reactions such as fever, skin rash, and enlarged lymph nodes; can lead to renal failure, hepatic necrosis, rhabdomyolosis, all of which can be fatal. Monitor VS and ECG continuously during IV administration. Monitor CBC for agranulocytosis and aplastic anemia. Monitor serum albumin and liver enzymes before and during therapy at least once per month.
Furosemide (Lasix)	Nonosmotic loop diuretic	Decreases cerebral edema and removes excess Na and H_2O from edematous areas and injured neurons. Used in an effort to decrease ICP.	Can cause hypokalemia. Monitor the serum potassium level prior to administering. Monitor BP for hypotension due to volume depletion. Increased risk of digitoxin toxicity if concurrently taking digoxin. Assess hearing; can cause ototoxicity with high IV doses
Mannitol (Osmitrol)	Hypertonic crystalloid solution. Reduces blood viscosity, increases cerebral blood flow and oxygen metabolism. Decreases diameter of cerebral arteries	First-tier therapy for reducing ICP after brain injury	Must insert indwelling urinary catheter to monitor output. Used in early trauma in tandem with IV crystalloids to correct hypovolemia. Transient volume expansion can occur. Monitor VS, UA, PA pressures before and hourly throughout administration. Observe for signs of fluid overload as in an increased CVP reading, crackles, and dyspnea. Observe for signs of dehydration such as dry skin and mucous membranes, low CVP, and tented skin turgor.

TABLE 5-6	Commonly Used Medications for the Neurologically Impaired Patient (Continued)		
Medication	**Action**	**Use**	**Precautions**
Pentobarbital (Nembutal) Thiopental (Sodium Pentothal)	To induce barbiturate coma and decrease ICP. Second-tier therapy used when other methods of sedation do not control restlessness or increased ICP. Also used as an anticonvulsant.	Helpful in reducing ICP because they slow down cerebral metabolism, which in turn decreases the oxygen and glucose demands of the brain.	Totally dependent upon the nurse for respiratory and circulatory support. Requires mechanical ventilation for oxygenation, BP support through the use of pressor therapy such as dopamine and Levophed usually with an arterial line; requires PA pressure monitoring tapered off gradually. Monitor for DVT, PE, pneumonia, and infection. Do not confuse with phenobarbital.
Propofol (Diprivan)	General anesthetic. Sedative for seizure control after use of a benzodiazepine has been unsuccessful.	Sedation of mechanically ventilated patients	Observe for bradycardia and hypotension. Monitor vital signs for respiratory depression; can cause apnea lasting more than 60 seconds. Must have intubation equipment available if not vented. Monitor for metabolic acidosis, hyperkalemia, rhabdomyolosis, and liver, cardiac, and renal failure. Change IV lines every 12 hours in ICUs due to support of bacterial growth on tubings and vials. Use larger veins of forearms since burning and stinging can occur at the site of administration. Do not use if solution separates; it should be milky and opaque in appearance.
Valium (Diazepam) Ativan (Lorazepam)	Sedative. Depresses CNS by potentiating an inhibitory neurotransmitter. Also promotes skeletal muscle relaxation by decreasing spinal afferent pathways.	Seizures. Decreases restlessness in patients with increased ICP or if fighting mechanical ventilation.	Provide respiratory support if giving it IV. Monitor VS frequently. Use cautiously in severe renal impairment. Can lead to physical and psychological dependency if used long term. Can be severe with flumazenil.

If the SE shows no signs of diminishing, propofol (Diprivan), a general anesthetic, can also be administered to provide continuous sedation.

Prognosis

Recurrent seizures can be prevented and controlled with medication therapy. Occasionally, surgery is done to remove an epileptic focus in the brain if the problem is difficult to manage medically. The impact of epilepsy is reduced by 75% postoperatively.

Interpreting Test Results

Electroencephalograms (EEGs) can tell if seizure activity is present. These can be done continuously at the bedside.

ECG – to monitor for dysrhythmias and cardiac failure.

Hallmark Signs and Symptoms

Generalized seizures can be grand mal (tonic-clonic) with loss of consciousness and rhythmic twitching and jerking.

Partial seizures may involve simple (no loss of consciousness) or complex with altered consciousness.

❶ Nursing Diagnoses	Expected Outcomes
Ineffective airway clearance	The patient will have clear breath sounds
Tissue perfusion, alteration in	Vital signs will be within normal limits
	The patient will have absent seizure activity

Nursing Interventions

Maintain a patent airway to promote adequate air exchange and ventilation to control SE.

Monitor vital signs for abnormal changes that might need to be treated to control seizure activity.

Provide continuous EEG monitoring. More than 50% of seizures go undetected due to unwitnessed motor activity. More accurate assessment of patient's response to treatment is indicated.

Administer first-line drugs like a benzodiazepine such as Ativan (lorazepam), as well as Valium (diazepam) to decrease brain activity to external stimuli. Sedative hypnotic qualities of Ativan and Valium work by depressing the subcortical areas of the CNS.

Prepare to administer other antiseizure drugs like Dilantin and phenobarbital. Propofol (Diprivan), a general anesthetic, can also be given to provide continuous sedation if seizures continue.

Prevent complications like DVT, ventilaton-assisted pneumonia, and paralytic ileus, which are common issues due to mechanical ventilation and sedation.

Guillain-Barré Syndrome (GBS)

What Went Wrong?

This syndrome is a rare but rapidly progressive paralytic disorder of the peripheral nervous system. It is believed to develop after a previous viral infection, usually upper respiratory or gastrointestinal. It might be caused by an immune response to infectious antigens that create a local inflammatory reaction that triggers further inflammation.

Hallmark Signs and Symptoms

Motor weakness, especially in the lower extremities, has an abrupt onset that progresses to flaccidity and ascends through the body over a period of hours to days until the person's mobility is absent and breathing, swallowing, speech, and cough status is impaired to the point where approximately one-third of such patients require intubation, mechanical ventilation, and a critical care environment. Pain in the hips, back, and thighs are common symptoms. The loss of motor function can occur in as little as a few days up to 2 to 3 weeks.

Interpreting Test Results

Clinical diagnosis is based on actual symptoms, CSF analysis, and nerve conduction studies. Nerve conduction studies demonstrate a significant reduction of nerve impulses. The CSF analysis will initially show a normal protein level that elevates within the 4th to 6th week of illness.

Prognosis

This situation is reversible, but there is no curative treatment and the disease must simply run its course. During its acute phase, the patient must be maintained in a critical care environment. Medical management focuses on the prevention of complications and supporting bodily functions. The use of steroids such as Decadron (dexamethasone) or Solu-Medrol (methylprednisolone) might be beneficial because of their anti-inflammatory effects. Steroids also protect the neuromembrane from further destruction and promote healing and tissue repair by improving blood flow to the site of injury. Patients with rapidly progressing paralysis can also benefit from plasmapheresis, which involves plasma exchanges to wash away or remove the antibodies that cause GBS. The administration of immune globulin (IVIG) is also beneficial as a treatment modality. Full muscular strength does eventually occur in cases of Guillain-Barré, but recovery could take many months up to 1 year, in which case extensive physical therapy and rehabilitation are required.

❶ and ❹ Nursing Diagnosis	Expected Outcomes
Impaired mobility related to muscle flaccidity and paralysis	Patient will have increased muscle strength
	Patient will regain full level of mobility

Nursing Interventions

Provide passive range of motion exercises several times daily within the patient's level of tolerance.

Provide massages alternating between heat and cold applications to maintain muscle tone.

Initiate gentle stretching and active assisted exercises.

Teach the patient a sequence of stretching and active range-of-motion exercises as patient's condition stabilizes.

Closely monitor and control episodes of pain with appropriate analgesic therapy.

Assess and prevent signs of skin breakdown through frequent change in position and adequate nutrition.

Gradually increase patient's level of mobility and exercise as patient's condition strengthens.

Monitor for signs of muscular atrophy and contractions.

❶ and ❹ Nursing Diagnosis	Expected Outcomes
Fear and anxiety related to uncertain status of recovery	Patient will understand the concept of the disease
	Patient will have a positive outlook regarding the outcome of his or her illness

Nursing Interventions

The nurse will address all patient concerns honestly and compassionately.

Patient misconceptions about his or her illness will be clarified.

Explain all procedures to the patient to reduce anxiety prior to and during treatment.

Provide reassurance as it pertains to prognosis.

Teach patient and family health care resources available to them to enhance recovery.

Cerebrovascular Accident (CVA)

What Went Wrong?

A stroke or brain attack is a form of neurologic damage caused by an occlusion or interruption of normal blood circulation to the brain. The two types of strokes are ischemic and hemorrhagic. Hemorrhagic strokes are further subdivided into subarachnoid and intracerebral hemorrhage.

An ischemic stroke usually results from a clot that occludes a blood vessel and creates a loss of blood supply to the brain. Clots can develop from an accumulation of fatty or atherosclerotic plaque in the blood vessels. Risk factors include hypertension, obesity, smoking, elevated blood lipids, stress, diabetes, and a familial history of cardiac and other vascular diseases.

Interpreting Test Results

A CAT scan is the initial step in identifying the cause of a stroke as clear images of the brain structures are outlined to reveal offending blood clots, active bleeding, or aneurysms. The results of an EEG, laboratory, and arterial blood gas analysis are valuable in measuring the patient's total baseline profile for comparison.

Hallmark Signs and Symptoms

A sudden onset of symptoms usually indicates an embolism as the incriminating offender to an ischemic stroke. Symptoms are classic and include hemiparesis, aphasia, and hemianopsia (which is blindness in one-half of the visual field).

At times individuals may experience TIAs or transient ischemic attacks, which are brief episodes of strokelike symptoms that disappear within a short period of time after onset and are precursors or warning signs to an actual stroke event.

Medical management of an ischemic stroke includes treating complications such as cerebral edema or seizure activity. Certain patients may be eligible to receive thrombolytic therapy if it can be provided within a 3-hour time frame from the onset of symptoms and if a CAT scan is negative for hemorrhage. t-PA is given initially as an intravenous bolus over 1 minute and the remainder of the maximum dosage of 90 mg is infused over 1 hour. The recommended dosage is 0.9 mg/kg. Thrombolytic therapy acts by degrading the fibrin that is present in clots. Therefore, a complication of thrombolytic therapy can be active internal bleeding and an increase in CNS hemorrhaging. Other treatment modalities might include carotid endarterectomy, embolectomy, or angioplasty. Medications such as steroids, barbiturates, and antihypertensives can be used to treat stroke victims.

Prognosis

The degree of recovery varies according to the amount of stroke insult suffered by the individual. Residual damage such as paralysis and difficulty speaking may forever alter the quality of life and lifestyle of the patient.

❶ and ❹ Nursing Diagnosis	Expected Outcomes
Risk of aspiration related to dysphagia	Patient will be able to cough, chew, and swallow unimpeded Patient will maintain clear lung sounds

Nursing Interventions

Assess lung sounds.

Turn and position frequently.

Maintain patient in an upright position at mealtimes.

Monitor oral secretions.

Provide adequate hydration to promote moist secretions.

Maintain a patent airway and provide suctioning if needed.

Provide good oral hygiene.

Assess for adequate chewing, swallowing, and pocketing of food.

Provide a mechanical soft diet for easier chewing, swallowing, and digestion.

Allow sufficient time to complete meals in an unhurried manner.

Hemorrhagic Stroke

What Went Wrong?

Six to seven percent of all CVAs occur as a result of an SAH or subarachnoid hemorrhage, which is bleeding into the subarachnoid space usually from rupture

TABLE 5–7 Medications Used to Treat Stroke Victims

Medication	Action	Use
Nimodipine (Nimotop)	Calcium channel blocker that crosses the blood-brain barrier and acts as a potent peripheral vasodilator. Binds with cerebral tissue and has a high lipid solubility.	Improves neurologic deficits due to spasm following subarachnoid hemorrhage. Also used to treat migraine headaches and ischemic seizures. Use with care with liver impairment.
Labetalol (Normodyne and Trandate)	Beta-blocker effects. Reduces BP through vasodilation, decreases peripheral resistance.	Reduces blood pressure. Take apical pulse prior to giving and withhold if <60. Baseline VS and laboratory evaluation of liver and kidney function. Monitor for skin rash, edema, and tachycardia. Assess for dizziness and hypotension.
Naloxone (Narcan)	Narcotic antagonist reverses effects of opiates	Reverses CNS and respiratory depression. Used for narcotic overdosage or when nature of respiratory depression is unknown.
Adderall XR	Amphetamines that function as the brain's main excitatory neurotransmitter. Increases synaptic release of norepinephrine and dopamine in the brain. Releases norepinephrine from nerve endings	Stimulates respirations and the CNS by direct action on the cerebral cortex and the RAS. Results in increased motor activity, less fatigue, mood elevation, alertness, and wakefulness. Useful to treat narcolepsy.

of a cerebral aneurysm or an AVM (arteriovenous malformation). Hypertension, smoking, alcohol, and stimulants are risk factors. An SAH may result in coma or death. A cerebral aneurysm is a weakened outpouching of a blood vessel wall that can be congenital or a result of a traumatic injury that stretches and tears the middle layer of an artery. An AVM is a tangled mass of arterial and venous blood vessels that become connected and "shunts" blood away from normal cerebral circulation from the arterial side to the venous side and bypasses the capillary system. AVMs are primarily congenital and can also be found in the GI tract, spinal cord, and renal and integumentary systems. On the skin, it is seen as a small port-wine stain. AVM is supplied by "feeders" of one or more cerebral arteries. These feeders enlarge over time, become engorged, and tend to rupture. An AVM can also cause chronic ischemia and cerebral atrophy because of the abnormal blood flow, which is directed away from normal blood circulation.

Hallmark Signs and Symptoms

An unruptured AVM may only reveal symptoms of headache, dizziness or even syncope.

With an SAH, the patient may have had what are described as "warning leaks," such as sudden onset of headaches and vomiting several weeks prior to experiencing a major SAH. With a warning leak, small amounts of blood will ooze from a cerebral aneurysm into the subarachnoid space. The blood irritates the meninges causing headache, stiff neck, and photophobia. However, the patient does not seek medical advice believing the symptoms to be temporary and not especially severe.

Interpreting Test Results

Diagnosis of the cause of the SAH, an aneurysm, or an AVM is made by CAT scan, patient symptoms and a lumbar puncture. A CAT scan will detect bleeding or a clot in the subarachnoid space where an MRI cannot. If, and only if, the CAT scan is negative will a spinal tap be done to measure the CSF for RBCs. The CSF will be bloody in appearance after an SAH and the RBC count will be greater than 1000 mm. Once diagnosed, a cerebral angiogram is indicated to identify the cause of the SAH. Surgery may be done to control the bleed. The decision to operate depends on the size and location of the problem, which can be so deep in the cerebral structures that attempts at removal could create even more severe neurological deficits. The patient's age, overall condition, and history of prior hemorrhage and injuries are all considered when deciding whether or not to operate. If surgery does occur, a craniotomy is performed to expose and locate the area of the aneurysm or an AVM.

If the problem is an aneurysm, a surgical clip is placed over its neck or stem to isolate it and eliminate and completely destroy the weak area. It is recommended that surgery take place within the first 48 hours after rupture. SAH patients who are within the Grade 1 or 2 categories of the Hunt and Hess Classification System of Subarachnoid Hemorrhage have a better postoperative outcome as compared to the more serious grades on the scale.

A description of the Hunt and Hess Classification System of Subarachnoid Hemorrhage is as follows:

Grade I	Asymptomatic, with a minimal headache and slight nuchal rigidity
Grade II	Moderate to severe headache, nuchal rigidity, no neurologic deficit other than cranial nerve palsy
Grade III	Drowsiness, confusion, or mild focal deficit
Grade IV	Stupor, moderate to severe hemiparesis, possible early decerebrate rigidity, vegetative disturbances
Grade V	Deep coma, decerebrate rigidity, moribund appearance

A major complication postoperatively is rebleeding caused by hypertension. The mortality rate increases substantially when rebleeding occurs. Generally, an elevated blood pressure is a normal response to maintain adequate cerebral perfusion after a neurologic insult. Hypertension does, however, contribute to the complication of rebleeding. Medications are required to maintain a systolic blood pressure no greater than 150 mm Hg. The patient may also receive anticonvulsant therapy as a prophylactic to prevent seizures.

Additional Blood Pressure Maintenance Medications

Medication	Action	Use
Nitroprusside sodium, Nitropress, Nipride	Antihypertensive—acts directly on vascular smooth muscle to produce peripheral vasodilation	Lowering of BP. Useful to rapidly reduce BP during a hypertensive crisis. Also used to produce controlled hypotension during anesthesia to reduce bleeding. Monitor laboratory enzymes and use cautiously in patients with liver impairment.
Hydralazine (Apresoline)	Antihypertensive—directly affects vascular smooth muscle causing vasodilation	Reduces blood pressure
Inderal (propranolol)	Antihypertensive beta-blocker	Decreases blood pressure

An intracerebral hemorrhage bleeds directly into cerebral tissue usually from a small artery, again caused by an aneurysm or AVM rupture, trauma, or a hypertensive hemorrhage. Cerebral tissue is destroyed and cerebral edema and ICP are increased.

❶, ❷, and ❹ Nursing Diagnoses	Expected Outcomes
Discomfort associated with head-aches, stiff neck, and photophobia	Patient will be relieved of neurological symptoms
	Discomfort will be reduced to within acceptable levels

Nursing Interventions

Ask patient to rate his or her level of discomfort on a scale of 0 to 10.

Provide frequent neurological assessments to detect signs of improvement or deterioration.

Administer analgesic medications as prescribed to reduce discomfort.

Provide distraction measures such as guided imagery.

Reduce levels of environmental stimuli.

Provide a quiet, relaxed atmosphere for patient recovery.

Surgical Conditions Requiring Complex Neurological Care

The purposes of surgery for head trauma victims are to control hemorrhaging; remove blood clots, bone matter, and tumors; repair torn and severed blood vessels; prevent a shift in brain tissue; and ultimately to prevent brain herniation.

Brain Tumors

What Went Wrong?

These are abnormal growths occurring in the brain as either a benign or metastatic lesion. Causes of why or what precipitates their growth is unclear. The most common type of brain tumor is identified as the glioblastoma multiforme. Astrocytomas and meningiomas fall within the glioblastoma category.

Hallmark Signs and Symptoms

If a brain mass is large, papilledema will be present upon assessment in 70% to 75% of all brain tumor cases caused by increased intracranial pressure due to the tumor pressing on the optic nerve. Severe headaches and blindness may rapidly result if the pressure is unrelieved.

Interpreting Test Results

Usually diagnosed via CAT scan.

Prognosis

Glioblastomas are clinically very aggressive with a rare survival rate of no greater than 2 years.

Benign, well-defined brain lesions are usually removed surgically and successfully. Invasive, poorly defined brain tumors are not totally 100% removed via craniotomy. However, surgery will decrease or debulk the tumor, which in turn will reduce pressure on the surrounding structures and slow the tumor growth process.

Radiation may be used to treat tumors of the brainstem, thalamus, and hypothalamus instead of surgery, because if surgery is attempted in these difficult-to-reach areas, severe neurologic deficits can result. The goal of radiation therapy is to slow down or destroy the growth of tumor cells without damaging normal brain tissue.

Stereotaxic radiation is a process in which radioactive loaded catheters are implanted into the tumor bed as a form of radiosurgery. Intracranial catheter placement is done in the operating room and the patient stays overnight in the critical care unit. The following day, a single high dose of ionizing radiation, or radionuclide seed implantation, is directed via a Gamma Knife toward a small, well-defined brain lesion. A Gamma Knife is an external high-energy photon beam that is directed from a linear accelerator.

Radiosurgery is performed under local anesthesia and without a surgical incision. As such, it is a good form of alternative treatment for the elderly, the medically challenged and infirm, and for those who refuse microsurgical removal.

Steroids, as described previously, are used to eliminate cerebral edema associated with brain tumors pre- and postoperatively.

Apparently, regional hyperthermia is another considered avenue of treatment to destroy brain tumor cells. The inner regions of many brain tumors are hypoxic, have an acidic pH and poor blood flow, making them ultrasensitive to the benefits of hyperthermia.

Chemotherapy

It is thought that the benefits of chemotherapy are in question because many of the drugs are unable to cross the blood-brain barrier. Therefore, the brain tumor mass might not be 100% sensitive to specific chemotherapeutic agents.

For Those Hard-to-Reach Places

An advance in scientific technology is that of Robotics. This is a method of using computerized or automated devices along with microsurgery and laser surgery to perform procedures or surgical functions that are too difficult or too obscure to reach and perform manually. These are delicate devices that can improve the control of surgical instruments by the physician such as scalpels and laparoscopes. Robotics as a method of microsurgery is becoming increasingly more popular for use by neurosurgeons to reach difficult and deep lesions of the brain for repair and excision. Formerly inoperable and invasive tumors can now be reached and more successfully eliminated.

Cerebral Aneurysms

What Went Wrong?

Aneurysms are usually small, berrylike sacs that are localized, abnormal dilatations of an artery due to a weakness in the wall of the vessel.

Hallmark Signs and Symptoms

The patient might complain of specific symptoms such as nuchal rigidity, headache, vomiting, photophobia, pain behind the eye with a dilated pupil, and ptosis of that area. However, the patient might just have a sudden unresponsive collapse, in which case the success of surgical intervention is questionable.

Interpreting Test Results

Aneurysms can be identified via CAT scan along with sudden onset of patient symptoms.

Prognosis

Surgical repair of a cerebral aneurysm through surgical clipping can be very successful if identified and reached prior to the patient experiencing an actual rupture of the aneurysm. A bypass graft replaces the segment that was the aneurysm.

Head Trauma

TBIs or traumatic brain injuries are injuries that range from mild to severe.

What Went Wrong?

Head injuries can occur in many ways such as by force or a blunt, penetrating trauma or missile injury. These are known as primary injuries because they happen at the time of impact, for example, gunshot wound, baseball bat, MVA. Secondary injuries are those that occur after the primary injury insult.

The more severe injuries may require surgery to remove bone fragments or to evacuate hematomas via burr holes or a craniotomy.

> ### NURSING ALERT
>
> *There is always a high risk of patients with penetrating head wounds developing infections and brain abscesses as secondary injuries. The injured brain must always be protected.*

Specific Types of Head Injury

Can be open where the brain dura is torn, or closed where the brain dura remains intact. Open skull fractures require surgery to close the dura and remove bony fragments.

Hallmark Signs and Symptoms

Assessment findings might demonstrate CSF leakage through otorrhea or rhinorrhea and ecchymosis over the mastoid process (bruising behind the ears—Battle's sign) as well as raccoon eyes (ringlike ecchymosis around the eyes).

Concussion

What Went Wrong?

A brain injury in which there is a loss of consciousness that lasts from a few seconds to 1 hour.

Signs and Symptoms

The victim might experience confusion, irritability, disorientation, and have a period of posttraumatic amnesia. Patients may complain of headache, fatigue, dizziness, inability to concentrate, and impaired memory. Despite the loss of consciousness with functional impairment, the brain remains structurally intact.

Interpreting Test Results

Diagnosis is confirmed based upon symptoms; length of time of unconsciousness, if it occurred; nature of the injury; and CAT scan.

Prognosis

Patients are generally admitted to the hospital for observation for a period of 24 hours with discharge instructions to seek immediate care if the post-concussion symptoms persist or worsen.

Contusion

What Went Wrong?

The patient sustains bruising of the brain with some superficial parenchymal bleeding mostly over the temporal area.

Hallmark Signs and Symptoms

Contusions can increase in size and severity several days after injury as further bleeding and cerebral edema occur, creating a worsening of symptoms and an increase in intracranial pressure. Extreme ecchymoses is evident at the injured site.

Interpreting Test Results

Diagnosis is made via CAT scan, presenting symptoms, and physical and neurological assessments.

Prognosis

These larger evolving areas of bleeding may require surgical intervention to reduce the ICP and cerebral edema and to evacuate the hematoma.

Specifically, there are three types of hematomas.

Epidural Hematoma

What Went Wrong? A collection of blood between the inner skull and the outermost layer of the dura, which has been pulled away from the skull. Frequently it occurs as a result of a fall, blow to the head, or MVA that causes a skull fracture and a laceration to the middle meningeal artery.

Hallmark Signs and Symptoms Classic symptoms include a brief loss of consciousness followed by a lucid period that can last up to 12 hours. Deterioration in the person's level of consciousness begins to occur with hemiparesis seen on the opposite side of the body from impact and a fixed, dilated pupil seen on the same side of the body as that on which the impact occurred. These are the characteristic qualifiers of an epidural hematoma. The patient may also complain of a severe, localized headache.

Interpreting Test Results A CAT scan reveals a collection of epidural blood.

Prognosis Surgery is required to evacuate the hematoma and cauterize the bleeding vessels. Postoperative recovery depends on how well the patient's level of consciousness returns and to what degree. Mortality rates vary and can increase according to how well the patient responds to the surgical intervention.

Subdural Hematoma

What Went Wrong? Bleeding occurs between the dura and arachnoid membranes probably caused by a rupture of the veins between the brain and the dura mater.

Hallmark Signs and Symptoms Based on the time frame from injury to the onset of symptoms, subdural hematomas can range from acute (symptoms materializing within 48 hours) to subacute (symptoms occurring within 2 days to 2 weeks) to chronic (symptoms occurring within 2 weeks to 2 months). Symptoms appear more gradually with each classification of subdural hematoma, but surgical intervention is still a must!

Intracerebral Hematoma

What Went Wrong? Occurs when there is actual bleeding within the brain tissue caused by depressed skull fractures and penetrating wound injuries. The rate of bleeding expands significantly and surgical intervention is necessary to control the bleeding.

Missile Head Injuries

Caused by objects such as a bullet that penetrates the skull but does not exit the brain. A missile injury can also be classified as perforating in that it enters and also exits the brain.

Head trauma is also classified according to degrees of injury as follows:

Mild	There is a loss of consciousness for up to 15 minutes with a Glasgow Coma Scale of 13–15. The patient is often released after being evaluated in the hospital Emergency Room.
Moderate	The Glasgow Coma Scale is 9–12 with a loss of consciousness for as long as 6 hours. Patients are hospitalized and treatment is initiated to prevent an increase in ICP and cerebral edema and to curb a deterioration in the patient's condition.
Severe	These patients are in critical care settings often requiring ventilatory support. Their condition deteriorates within 48 hours after admission and their Glasgow Coma Scale is often 8 or less even after resuscitation efforts.

Mechanisms of Head Injury

The ways in which head trauma occurs provide useful information in dealing with the challenges of neurological deficits. See Figure 5–7.

Acceleration injury	A moving object strikes the nonmoving head, for example, a baseball bat striking the head or a missile such as a bullet fired into the head (see Figure 5-7B).
Deceleration injury	Injury is sustained when the head is moving and it strikes a stationary object such as in a fall or MVA where the moving head strikes against a dashboard or a windshield (see Figure 5-7B).
Coup/ contrecoup injuries	When the head is struck, the brain moves or shifts inside the cranium bouncing back and forth. If the injury is sustained at the site of the initial blow or directly beneath the impact, this is known as a coup injury. If the injury is on the opposite side of the impact or on either side of the blow, it is known as a contrecoup injury (see Figure 5-7A).
Rotational	Occurs when the injured brain twists inside of the skull causing white brain matter and blood vessels to tear.

A. Coup/contrecoup

B. Acceleration/deceleration

FIGURE 5–7 • (A) Coup/contrecoup and (B) acceleration/deceleration injuries.

Types of Skull Fractures

Linear	This is the most common type of skull fracture. It resembles a line or hairline on the skull and is not too detrimental because it is not displaced and only becomes a problem if it extends into a sinus or an orbit or across a blood vessel.
Depressed	The outer skull is caved in and the bone is pressed into the dura. The dura can be bruised, torn, or remain intact. Surgery is often required to elevate the skull and remove pressure from the brain.
Comminuted	This type of fracture resembles a broken eggshell with multiple linear fractures spreading out in different directions and a depressed area at the site of impact.

NURSING ALERT

Drainage of CSF from the ear or nose indicates injury to the dura mater. Such drainage can also be mixed with blood. The nurse can apply a loose gauze dressing to the area of the ear or nose that is draining to determine the amount and character of the CSF. The drainage will appear as a yellowish ring of CSF on the gauze dressing. This yellowish ring is known as the HALO SIGN. Sometimes patients might report experiencing a sweet or salty taste in their mouths if CSF drips into the back of their throat. It is important to note if blood is indeed mixed with CSF. It will appear in the center of the loose gauze dressing.

❷, ❸ and ❹ Nursing Diagnosis	Expected Patient Outcomes
High risk for infection related to open skull fracture	Patient will be free from signs of infection
	Cerebral edema will be minimized

Nursing Interventions

Perform neurological assessments frequently within the critical care unit.

Observe for signs of infection at site of injury such as purulent drainage, odor, warmth, redness, and edema.

Provide absolute and total sterile techniques when providing care to the skull fracture.

Assess for signs of papilledema, which are indicators of ICP from cerebral edema and possible brain herniation.

Monitor vital signs for hypertension and hyperthermia and Cushing's triad.

Provide adequate amounts of fluid therapy to maintain hydration levels.

Administer appropriate antibiotic and steroidal therapy as ordered.

Assess results of laboratory and x-ray analysis to determine status of patient's condition.

Nursing Diagnoses	Patient Outcomes	Implementations	Evaluation
❷ and ❻ Ineffective cerebral perfusion	Level of consciousness will return to status of alert and aware. Ability to respond verbally and appropriately to questions and obey commands will improve. Patient will suffer no ill effects of ICP.	Assess patient responses to external stimuli, questions, and commands. Perform Glasgow Coma Scale q 15 minutes. Assess hypertensive status and Cushing's triad. Provide medications as ordered. Maintain adequate fluid and electrolyte balance.	Determine effectiveness of planned outcomes and interventions frequently throughout each shift.
Potential for impaired gas exchange related to hypoventilation (to correspond with Learning Objectives 1 and 4)	Gas exchange will remain within normal limits.	Promote adequate gas exchange. Maintain effective O_2 and CO_2 levels. Provide oxygenation of 2L/min. Assess status of lung sounds for signs of aspiration and fluid accumulation. Monitor arterial blood gas results. Maintain a patent airway through position changes and suctioning as needed.	Determine effectiveness of planned outcomes and interventions frequently throughout each shift.

CASE STUDY

⑤ An 84-year-old pleasantly smiling female arrives independently to the Emergency Room with the chief complaints of "double vision, severe and worsening headache for 1 week." She is awake, alert, and admits to no recent falls or injuries. She has been taking antihypertensive medications for the past 20 years. Vital signs are T: 100, P: 84, R: 16, and BP: 150/80. Within minutes of her initial assessment, the patient's condition begins to rapidly decline. Vital signs are now T: 101.8, P: 70, R: 12, and BP: 210/60. The patient's gaze is now dysconjugate and verbal responses to questions and commands are nonexistent. Vital signs indicate Cushing's triad, with a widening pulse pressure of 150. Her daughter arrives and provides the information that 1 week ago, as her mother was cleaning a chandelier, she fell off of her dining room table and struck her head on a corner of the table.

QUESTIONS

What additional nursing considerations and interventions would be indicated and why?

REVIEW QUESTIONS

WHAT HAS BEEN LEARNED?

1. A 59-year-old female is brought to the Emergency Room via ambulance and is pronounced DOA (dead on arrival.) She has sustained a TBI (traumatic brain injury) having been struck in the head with a baseball bat. This type of traumatic brain injury is an example of what kind of impact? Choose all that apply.

   A. Contrecoup
   B. Perforating
   C. Deceleration
   D. Acceleration

2. A nurse is evaluating a patient with a coup/contrecoup injury after the patient was rear-ended. Which areas of the brain would be most likely affected?

   A. Cerebellum
   B. Cerebrum: frontal lobe
   C. Cerebrum: temporal lobe
   D. Cerebrum: occipital lobe

3. The nurse knows that the reason for the flow of bodily CSF to be reabsorbed daily is to

   A. Maintain a high intracranial pressure level
   B. Increase hydrostatic pressure
   C. Impede cerebral circulation
   D. Avoid the development of excessive CSF buildup and hydrocephaly

4. The patient performs the finger-to-nose test and overshoots the mark. This is an example of

   A. Anisocoria
   B. Dysmetria
   C. Hemaniopsia
   D. Diplopia

5. Which ICP reading is considered to be at an acceptable level in your patient?

   A. 0–15 mm Hg
   B. 0–20 mm Hg
   C. 0–18 mm Hg
   D. 0–25 mm Hg

6. The nurse is assessing the patient for signs of meningeal irritation. Identify the responses that would indicate a positive Kernig's sign?

   A. Dorsiflexion of the toes.
   B. Knee-jerk response.
   C. Involuntary flexion of the hips as the neck is bent toward the chest.
   D. Sharp neck pain occurs when the thigh is flexed onto the abdomen and the leg is extended at the knee.

7. An accurate description of the Cushing's triad assessed in the patient can be summarized as

   A. Decreased systolic blood pressure, bradycardia, widening pulse pressure
   B. Increased systolic blood pressure, widening pulse pressure, bradycardia
   C. Hyperactivity, projectile vomiting, fever
   D. Unresponsiveness, narrowing pulse pressure, tachycardia

8. The nurse should instruct the patient to remain flat in bed for several hours post-spinal tap to prevent complications such as

   A. Severe headache and stiff neck
   B. Seizures, difficulty urinating
   C. Vomiting, sore throat
   D. Fainting, leg numbness

9. The nurse is aware that patients who have pacemakers or surgical clips and implants should avoid the following diagnostic study:

   A. CAT scan
   B. Myelogram
   C. PET scan
   D. MRI

10. Identify the areas that compose the total intracranial volume in the patient.

    A. Spinal fluid and lateral ventricles of the brain
    B. Parenchyma and semi-solid brain tissue
    C. Cerebral blood flow, cerebrospinal fluid circulation, and intravascular semi-solid brain tissue
    D. Basal ganglia, red blood cells, and internuncial fibers

ANSWERS

CASE STUDY

Continue to assess the widening pulse pressure of the Cushing's triad, which is a valid indicator of an increase in ICP.

Level of consciousness and responses to verbal questions and commands also need to be scrupulously observed for signs of improvement or deterioration as they are also clinically significant of an increase in ICP.

Laboratory analysis, blood work, and arterial blood gases need to be drawn and scrutinized to establish the patient's baseline chemistry profile.

Results of diagnostic studies such as a CAT scan will determine the extent of the head trauma and the relevance of the ICP.

Implement the Glasgow Coma Scale immediately and q 15 minutes, comparing each attached score. Rationale: To determine patient status of motor and verbal responses, and eye opening.

Maintain a patent airway and oxygenation through proper patient positioning, suctioning as needed, and mechanical ventilation if required.

Administer medications and intravenous therapy as ordered and monitor for outcomes as well as side effects. Rationale: Certain medications will prevent seizure activity, while others such as steroids will reduce inflammation and cerebral edema and promote cerebral perfusion.

Assess for onset of secondary injuries or problems such as respiratory or cardiac arrest, onset of seizure activity, or area of paralysis.

Continue to examine pupillary responses to light and accommodation as well as assessing the size and shape of the pupils, which could help to identify the site of brain trauma.

Performing reflex and motor response activities will also validate muscle strength and weaknesses as well as motor neuron tract disease.

Continue to assess for patient's reactions to external stimuli. Rationale: Reactions will indicate normal and abnormal levels of consciousness.

ICP waveform monitoring system is an effective tool for the nurse to use to ascertain changes in status of ICP.

Any ventricular drains in use must be assessed for patency and status of continuous or intermittent drainage.

Implement measures to decrease ICP such as pain control, quiet environment, relief of anxiety, and proper positioning. Avoid improper flexing of the head, neck, legs, and hips, all of which will increase intraabdominal and intrathoracic pressure, which in turn will increase ICP.

If possible, determine from the patient's daughter the name and dosage of the antihypertensive medication that the patient has been taking for 20 years. Also question if there is a family history of cardiac disease.

CORRECT ANSWERS AND RATIONALES

1. D. The victim was struck by a moving object while her brain was in a stationary position, which defines an acceleration injury.
2. A, B, D. If the patient is hit from the rear, the force of the collision will propel the brain forward first and then backward. This injury would result in cerebellar, frontal, and occipital lobe damage.
3. D. An excessive buildup of CSF can create obstructive difficulties leading to hydrocephalus.
4. B. Anisocoria means unequal pupil size, hemaniopsia is defined as blindness in one-half of the patient's visual field, and diplopia means double vision.
5. A. All other levels are high and considered to be life threatening to the patient with neurologic deficits.
6. D. The response A. identifies an abnormal Babinski's sign. B. signifies the patellar reflex, while C. identifies a positive Brudzinski's sign.
7. B. These are the classic characteristic signs of a Cushing's triad syndrome.
8. A. In order to avoid a post–spinal tap headache, it is recommended that a patient remain flat and on bedrest for several hours to re-equalize the volume and pressure of cerebrospinal fluid.
9. D. Any substances containing ferrous metal including ventilators will limit the safe use of an MRI due to the hazardous and magnetic pulling potential of the MRI against metal.
10. C. All of those elements compose the total intracranial volume.

chapter 6

Care of the Traumatized Patient

At the end of this chapter, the student will be able to:

1. Recognize the varied differences and types of trauma injuries.

2. Relate the statistics associated with the Trimodal Distribution Peaks of trauma deaths.

3. Use the appropriate standards of trauma triage in the care of the injured individual.

4. Recognize the six phases of trauma care and the need for a systematic approach in the management and care of the injured patient.

5. Identify medications commonly used to care for a traumatized patient.

6. Explain types of fluids that can be used in hypovolemic shock.

7. Identify commonly used intravenous access sites used in the traumatized patient.

8. Describe the nursing care of common traumatic injuries.

KEY WORDS

ABCs – airway, breathing, circulation	GCS – Glasgow Coma Scale
ACI – acute lung injury	Golden Hour
AVPU – awake, verbal, pain, unresponsive	MVCs – motor vehicular crashes
Circumferential burn	NIRS – near-infrared spectrometry
Colloids	PEA – pulseless electrical activity
Cricothyroidotomy	Primary injury
Crystalloids	Rapid IV infuser
DPL – diagnostic peritoneal lavage	RTS – revised trauma score
EMS – Emergency Medical System	Rule of Nines
Eschar	Secondary injury
Fasciotomy	Sublingual capnometry
FAST – focused assessment with sonography for trauma	3:1 rule
	Triage
	Trimodal Distribution Peaks

Introduction

In the background, one can hear the soft, musical refrains of "How Great Thou Art." Lily, who is 16, beautiful, and unresponsive, lies in her bed in the Neurological Intensive Care Unit surrounded by her loving parents. They have requested that their daughter remain on life support until their son, who is in the military, arrives home from Afghanistan in time to say goodbye.

Lily was on her way to the mall with a few classmates to shop for prom dresses. On a cold, rainy day, the car she was a passenger in hydroplaned on a wet patch and skidded into a tree. Her classmates were treated for minor injuries. Lily was not so fortunate, and after 3 days her condition remained critical and unchanged.

In yet another bed in the same Neurological Intensive Care Unit, a grief-stricken mother cries over her 16-year-old unresponsive son who was shot in the head, the victim of a drive-by shooting.

Too often, the critical care nurse encounters these heart-wrenching dilemmas and it never gets easier. However, as these two teens face the end of life, for all of the negative outcomes, positive outcomes in the care of trauma sufferers are also beginning to emerge. More lives are being saved, as the time from injury to definitive care has decreased and the methodology of care management has improved, so that the patient has an increased chance of survival.

Trauma can be described as an event or incident that severely impairs or disrupts an individual's ability to sustain life or to function in a reasonable manner. Accidents can be caused by numerous factors, incidental or otherwise, such as falls, MVCs (motor vehicular crashes), contact sports, diving, drowning, poisonings, overdoses, assaults and attacks, and forces of nature. In order to understand trauma, one must take a closer look at the mechanisms of injury, how traumatic injuries are classified, and evaluating reports from the field.

Mechanisms of Injury (MOI)

Mechanisms of injury means the types of injuries sustained and the amount of force utilized to create specific injuries. These mechanisms of injury were explained in Chapter 5 but are mentioned again as blunt, penetrating, and perforating types.

A blunt injury is a direct blow or impact that causes the greatest injury. The body surface and the injuring culprit are in direct contact. The most common causes of blunt, forceful trauma are the acceleration/deceleration injuries of head and neck trauma.

Penetrating injuries are produced by foreign objects such as knives, glass, and fence stakes that penetrate and impale. They cause internal damage to body organs and tissues. A bullet can also be included in this category in that it produces a missile injury that enters but does not exit the body.

Perforating injuries are injuries caused by items that enter and exit the body causing severe internal damage. Examples are bullets and knives.

Classification of Injuries

❶ Injuries can be classified as primary and secondary. Primary injuries are those that occur at the time of impact and include contusions or bruising, lacerations, shearing or tearing injuries, hemorrhage, and subluxations. Such injuries can be mild with minimal or absent neurologic damage, or severe with major organ (flail chest; cardiac tamponade) and/or neurologic damage.

Secondary injuries occur after the primary injury, such as infection or sepsis that leads to increased organ and tissue damage and even increases in intracranial pressure. These can be just as lethal as the initial or primary injury and cause the need for close nursing observation.

> **NURSING ALERT**
>
> *Secondary injuries can lead to death. The nurse needs to be vigilantly observant for signs of infection and respiratory failure after an initial injury has occurred.*

Evaluating Reports From the Field

❷ Deaths that occur as a result of trauma are said to take place in a trimodal distribution (Trimodal Distribution Peaks) that involves three peaks. The first peak includes victims who die immediately from the trauma insult before medical attention can be provided. The second peak is when death occurs within a few hours after injury. The third peak is when death occurs days to weeks after injury due to complications such as embolism, infection, or multiple organ dysfunction syndrome (MODS).

There is a 60-minute time frame or interval called the Golden Hour that can support and increase the individual's chances for survival if particular trauma measures can be implemented within that time frame after injury. These measures include the activation for help, responses, and communication of the EMS (Emergency Medical System), evaluation of what happened to the victim/victims (mechanism of injury [MOI]), prehospital stabilization and triage (which means the sorting out of the nature of injuries according to severity which is done to prioritize the urgency of treatment), transportation to the appropriate trauma care facility, rapid in-hospital resuscitation, and definitive care.

Sources describe two theories about the prehospital management of patients in the field. The first theory is the "Stay and Play" theory, in which time is spent and utilized to stabilize the patient's condition in the field prior to transport. The second theory is the "Scoop and Run" theory, where only the most life-threatening issues should be addressed in the field and immediate transport should take priority.

Trauma Center Levels and Classifications

❸ Trauma centers are categorized according to expected levels of care provided to injured individuals and the availability of support services (see Table 6–1).

TABLE 6–1	Levels and Classifications of Trauma Care
I	Most developed; total patient care. Magnet hospital. Usually the leading hospital in the region for trauma care. Has residency programs; does research and has specialty practices.
II	Care for emergent, complex needs but transport to Level I facility is required for more advanced/extended surgical care. Does not have research or residency programs. Fewer physician specialties.
III	Exists where there are no Level I or II facilities. Physicians, nurses in ECU required to have additional training.
IV	Provides advanced trauma life support but prepares patient for immediate transport to Level I center. Increases access to care for patients who would otherwise not receive it.

Six Phases of Trauma Care

❹ There are six phases of trauma care that start at the scene of an accident and progress to the patient's stay within critical care.

1. **Prehospital stabilization** – Achieved at the trauma scene, the ABCs of airway, breathing, and circulation are completed to ensure and maintain an effective airway. For example, foreign objects are cleared from the airway such as vomitus, blood clots, broken teeth, dirt, and gravel. Substantial bleeding is controlled. Neurological status is also quickly assessed such as level of consciousness and pupillary size and reaction. Until otherwise ruled out, a spinal cord injury is always suspected and the cervical spine is immobilized either manually or with a rigid cervical collar, with the patient's head, neck, and body secured to a spinal board or stretcher.

NURSING ALERT

A high spinal cord injury above the level of C5 causes paralysis of the diaphragm and vagus nerve. The result is a failure to breathe independently as the patient's airway and pattern of gas exchange will be severely compromised. The trauma victim will require ventilatory assistance.

2. **Hospital resuscitation** – When the patient arrives in the emergency room, a systematic and organized approach is implemented in the care of the trauma victim to discover and treat life-threatening injuries. Two surveys of patient assessment are conducted together and in concert with each

other and the next phase of care will not proceed until the current priority is satisfactorily managed. The first survey is known as the primary survey.

3. **Primary survey** – Five steps are involved in this process and include airway management, breathing support, circulatory support, examining for disabilities, and exposing other injuries. These are known as the ABCDE priorities of the primary survey.

A – Airway: A continued assessment of the patient's airway for clearance and removal of obstructions. Head and neck stabilization must be maintained until cervical spine x-rays rule out spinal cord injury.

B – Breathing: A balance between oxygen supply and demand must be ensured. Supplemental oxygen is provided to ease the efforts of breathing, particularly if the patient has dyspnea and discomfort from chest trauma.

C – Circulation: Circulatory status is assessed through skin color, temperature, mental status, and signs of hypothermia and hypovolemia. Cardiac monitoring with pulse oximetry is also initiated to identify cardiac dysrhythmias. An IV is inserted and the patient is monitored for shock.

D – Disabilities: A mini neurological examination is completed to determine motor strength and level of consciousness (LOC). Some sources use the AVPU method to describe levels of consciousness for its ease of memorization. For example: A – alert, V – responds to verbal stimuli, P – responds to painful stimuli, and U – unresponsive. A Glasgow Coma Scale is performed.

E – Exposure: The patient is undressed and each body region is examined for additional injuries. The patient's dignity must be maintained, and it is also important to keep the patient warm with warming blankets if available. Evidence for legal issues may be assessed, like bullets, drugs, or weapons. Try not to compromise evidence.

> ### NURSING ALERT
> *A rapid assessment of a traumatized patient with life-threatening conditions should take no longer than 60 seconds to perform.*

4. **Secondary survey/resuscitation** – A more detailed survey is conducted and starts at the patient's head and works down to the patient's feet. The patient needs to be log-rolled from side to side to inspect the

posterior parts of the body for injury. A more focused, thorough assessment of the area of pain or obvious deformity is conducted. An in-depth patient history is obtained as further information is forthcoming from the family and the EMS team as to the specifics of the trauma, medical history, and whether drugs and/or alcohol were involved. Diagnostic studies such as x-rays, CAT scans, EKG, hemoglobin, and hematocrit are performed. A chemistry profile and arterial blood gases are ordered and completed.

The most common type of shock is hypovolemic. Instances of hemorrhage must be identified and corrected with blood products to replace intravascular volume and the oxygen-carrying capacity of the blood. Fluid replacement is needed in the form of lactated Ringer's solution, which are crystalloids, or plasma and albumin, which are colloids. Intravenous fluids can be warmed and utilized along with warming blankets to correct and prevent hypothermia. Urinary catheters are inserted to monitor hydration levels through urinary output.

5. **Definitive care** – Specific injuries are taken care of during this phase such as surgical interventions, suturing of lacerations, jaw wiring, reduction of fractures, and cast applications.

6. **Critical care** – Seriously or critically ill patients are cared for postoperatively or directly admitted from the emergency room to the critical care unit as needed for intensive follow-through care.

Medications Used in Trauma Care

❺ Spinal Cord Injury (SCI)

Medication	Action	Nursing Actions
Histamine–2 antagonists	Reduces ulcer formation from traumatic stress	1. Usually administered IV
Methylpredni–solone	Suppresses the inflammatory response by decreasing spinal cord edema	1. Assess patient for adrenal insufficiency 2. Monitor I and O 3. Assess for headache or change in LOC 4. Monitor for signs/symptoms of infection

(Continued)

Medication	Action	Nursing Actions
Morphine sulfate	Used in pain control for major burns	1. Assess the patient's respiratory status for hypoventilation 2. Assess the patient's BP; do not give if BP is <100 mm Hg systolic
Tetanus toxoid prophylaxis if needed	Used to prevent tetanus from "dirty wounds"	1. Assess the last date of last tetanus toxoid 2. Check if patient is on steroids or is immunocompromised 3. Observe for drug reaction
Vasopressors	See Chapter 3	

Fluid Volume Replacement (FVR)

❻ One of the most frequent challenges a critical care nurse implements in the care of a traumatized patient is in the area of FVR. Replacement of body fluid with IVs and blood are the first-line treatments in hemorrhagic shock for almost all severely traumatized patients. The goal of FVR is to ensure that the tissues get oxygen and nutrients. Without FVR, the patient would quickly succumb to multiorgan failure.

Sites of FVR

IV access is of utmost importance, and multiple access with several different sites many be needed in severe fluid loss. Sites are accessed with the largest gauge needle possible (#14 and #16). Table 6–2 lists common IV access sites for FVR. The central venous site is most preferable.

To administer fluid quickly, a rapid infuser may be used. This piece of equipment warms a solution and can administer a liter over 2 minutes.

Preferred Solutions

There are many solutions that can be used for FVR in the traumatized patient. In deciding which solution to use, the cause of the volume loss and blood components that need to be replaced are two decisions that need to be made. The three main types of solutions are crystalloid, colloid, and blood products.

❼ TABLE 6–2 IV Sites for FVR

Sites	Rationale	Issues
Peripheral (antecubital or large forearm vein)	Easy Quick May be started at the scene of the accident by trained first responders	Infiltrates with rapid rates May not be capable of administering enough fluid in a short amount of time Collapses first with hemorrhage or cardiac arrest
Central venous catheter (CVC) (subclavian, internal jugular, femoral)	Larger volumes can be given Able to monitor response with CVP port Access for frequent venous blood sampling May be used later as PAC insertion site with guide wire	Requires special training and frequent practice for proficiency by those involved in insertion at the trauma site May result in pneumothorax, hemothorax, or hydrothorax if chest x-ray not done to confirm placement Time taken for placement confirmation
Pulmonary artery catheter (PAC)	Can use other ports for monitoring of Pulmonary capillary wedge pressure (PCWP), Cardiac output (CO), Cardiac index (CI) Pacemaker available on some PACs	Not needed initially Trained physician to insert Time required for setup, monitoring Risk of infection if going through burn tissue (eschar)

NURSING ALERT

A chest x-ray must be taken to verify any IV line that is inserted in the chest or neck area. If the nurse runs a solution fast into a CVC or PAC without placement confirmation the patient may develop a hydrothorax, which would need to be relieved with a chest tube.

Crystalloids include electrolytes (sodium, chloride, potassium, etc.). The two most commonly used to replace serum include lactated Ringer's (LR) and normal saline solution (0.9% NSS). Current ACS protocol recommends 3 mL of solution be replaced for each milliliter of blood lost. This is sometimes called the 3:1 rule. Crystalloids or blood replacement should also be done first prior to starting vasopressor therapy.

Table 6–3 shows commonly used crystalloids highlighting their benefits and precautions.

TABLE 6–3 Crystalloids in Trauma Shock

Solutions	Benefits	Precautions
Isotonic Solutions		
Lactated Ringer's (LR)	Restores intravascular volume Neutralizes an acidosis when lactate breaks down to bicarbonate	Liver damaged patients cannot metabolize lactate, possibly creating an alkalosis Can cause fluid volume overload especially with patient having underlying heart, renal problems Rapid infusion can dislodge clots formed in peripheral circulation leading to embolic phenomena
Normal saline solution (NSS)	Restores intravascular volume Can be used for fluid challenge to determine if hypovolemic	Rapid infusion can cause increase in chloride leading to loss of HCO_3 and creating an acidosis Can cause fluid volume overload especially in patient with underlying heart, renal problems Rapid infusion can dislodge clots formed in peripheral circulation leading to embolic phenomena
Hypertonic Solutions		
3% NSS (controversial; some studies confirm the benefit)	Pulls fluid from extravascular compartments More rapid fluid resuscitation with less volume Used to decrease increased intracranial pressure	Less fluid volume overload Watch in patients with heart and renal failure

The complications of intravenous therapy include

• Massive edema including pulmonary from fluid shifting to third space

• Hypothermia due to rapid infusion of room temperature fluid

• Coagulopathies due to rapid dilution of blood

Colloid Replacement Therapy

In addition to crystalloid solutions, colloids can also be used to help with FVR. Colloids are used to replace plasma proteins, which act like a magnet to hold fluid in the intravascular space by pulling fluid from the interstitial spaces.

Pulling of fluid into the intravascular space is known as an osmotic gradient or colloidal osmotic pressure. The benefit of colloid therapy is that it is longer acting, requires less volume to administer, and therefore is quicker.

Problems with colloids are similar to those of FVR with crystalloids. Use of colloids in burns can be controversial, as some believe that until the acute phase is over and capillary membranes are reestablished, vessels are permeable to colloids, therefore crystalloids should be used. Colloids are also more expensive and some are developed from blood products, which can cause an ethical dilemma in some instances. Common colloids that may be used include albumen, dextran, and hetastarch.

Blood Replacement Therapy

In addition to crystalloid and colloid therapy, blood can be administered to help improve fluid volume deficits especially from frank hemorrhage. Crystalloid

How to Do It–Administering a Blood Transfusion

1. Check that a consent form has been obtained from a physician whenever possible and the patient has been typed and crossed for blood.

2. Place a large-bore IV (16–18 gauge is preferred) with an NSS solution Y tubing and filter.

3. Perform baseline vital signs.

4. Obtain blood from the blood bank.

5. Two nurses need to check and sign that the type, screen, and patient ID are confirmed. Type O blood can be used if the patient needs packed red blood cells and time is of the essence.

6. Administer the blood slowly during the first 15 to 30 minutes, checking VS after the first 15 minutes and then every hour.

7. Observe for transfusion reactions, which can include acute hemolytic, febrile, and allergic reactions and circulatory overload.

8. If a transfusion reaction is suspected, stop the blood immediately. Preserve the IV line by infusing a bag of NSS. Call the laboratory and the ordering health care prescriber immediately. Anticipate the administration of fluids and corticosteroids, pressors if the BP drops to shocklike levels.

therapy is initiated first and blood and colloids are considered if the response of the heart rate, blood pressure, and baseline laboratory values do not improve. Blood replacement is usually determined by changes in the patient's hemoglobin and hematocrit levels. Although resources vary, when the patient's hemoglobin drops to 8 g/dL and the patient has other associated symptoms like unstable hemodynamic parameters, blood should be administered. Typically, packed red blood cells or whole blood is given in the traumatized patient, with whole blood being reserved for patients with coagulation problems like acute gastrointestinal bleeding from esophageal varices.

In an emergency, massive transfusions may be needed. Massive transfusions are defined as the total replacement of a patient's blood volume in a 24-hour period or half the patient's estimated volume within an hour. Complications of massive transfusions include those listed in Table 6–4.

TABLE 6–4 Complications of Massive Blood Transfusions

Complication	Cause	Signs/Symptoms	Treatment
1. Acid–base disturbances	Lactic acid buildup in stored blood	Headache, confusion, restlessness, nausea, vomiting, lethargy, weakness, stupor, coma, Kussmaul's respirations	Administer sodium bicarbonate according to the ABGs
2. Coagulation factor depletion	Unclear May be associated with DIC (disseminated intravascular coagulopathy) or loss of coagulation factors in stored blood	Bleeding from traumatized sites, IV sites, indwelling urinary catheters. Drop in H & H and platelets	Stop bleeding by pressure Administer clotting factors
3. Hypocalcemia	Each unit of blood contains citrate, which binds with ionized calcium	A drop in serum calcium Twitching and ticks, which can progress to tetany and seizures	Administer calcium IV
4. Hyperkalemia	Potassium concentration in stored blood is higher than normal	An elevation in the serum potassium Weakness and lethargy High-peaked T waves on ECG	Give glucose, insulin, and potassium, which will drive the K into the cell

TABLE 6–4 Complications of Massive Blood Transfusions (*Continued*)

Complication	Cause	Signs/Symptoms	Treatment
5. Hypothermia	Blood is kept stored in a refrigerator and when rapidly infused changes core temperature	Chills and shakes Core temperature drops	Blood warmer to infuse blood
6. Oxygen delivery changes	Stored blood binds more strongly with hemoglobin	Change in the level of responsiveness; tachycardia, tachypnea, and lower SaO_2	Monitor the O_2 level of the ABGs Administer higher FiO_2
7. Thrombocytopenia	Platelets do not store well in blood	Drop in thrombocytes	Administer platelets Stop bleeding by pressure

Care of the Patient With Specific Traumatic Injuries According to the ABCs of Trauma Assessment

Airway

Maxillofacial Injuries (MFIs)

What Went Wrong?

❽ MFIs are caused from blunt or penetrating objects that meet the cranium with force. Many MFIs are benign and heal without surgical intervention. Since the airway can be compromised all MFIs must be suspected of causing airway obstruction, breathing issues because the upper airway is a conduit for gases to the lungs, or circulatory problems because this area is very vascular. These can be life threatening if not detected early.

The face is largely unprotected, with soft tissues as well as bony structures that can be injured in traumatic incidents. MFIs often coincide with head and cervical spinal cord injuries. Obvious deformities may exist with maxillofacial injuries and can cause airway obstruction and death if airway and breathing mechanisms are not immediately and adequately established. Soft tissue swelling can obstruct the airway and occlude breathing. Because of the nature of the injuries, the patient may also be unable to see, smell, taste, or even speak. Nasal bones, the zygoma and mandibular condyle, are most susceptible to fracture.

The patient can be at risk for developing meningitis from fractures of the cranium and dura mater as oral bacterial flora can enter the CSF.

Prognosis

Some MFIs are minor, rarely resulting in increased mortality if treatment is rendered. However, high-impact facial fractures can be life threatening if involving the head, neck, and chest. Major soft tissue injuries may be more difficult to treat and have poorer outcomes. Severe hemorrhage and airway obstruction can result in death.

MFIs require multiple disciplinary coordinated team management as more than 50% of these patients have other multisystem trauma. The prognosis for severe facial injuries is improving as rapid treatment and transport to trauma centers that can evaluate and treat these injuries is improving.

Interpreting Test Results

Halo ring test should be done when inspecting the nasal and auditory canals for actual drainage of cerebrospinal fluid. A light yellow color at the edge of a spot of clear drainage or sanguineous CSF also has a high sugar content and can also be tested for the presence of glucose.

Specific facial and head/neck x-rays are also required for the accurate diagnosis of maxillofacial fractures.

CBC every 4 hours to follow hemoglobin and hematocrit if excessive bleeding or hemorrhagic shock is suspected.

Electrolyte panels.

Blood type and cross match.

Coagulation studies.

Hallmark Signs and Symptoms

Changes in breathing rate, rhythm, dyspnea, and stridor if airway is compromised.

Hemorrhage from torn facial arteries may be prevalent as well as epistaxis with any fracture that communicates with the nose.

Pain, swelling, asymmetry, and deformity in the location of the fractures/trauma.

Malocclusion, intraoral ecchymosis.

Periorbital edema/ecchymosis.

Crepitus with resultant air leak.

Lost or broken teeth.

TABLE 6–5	Types of Le Fort Fractures
I	Horizontal fractures in which the entire maxillary arch moves separately from the upper facial skeleton
II	An extension of Le Fort I that includes the orbit, ethmoid, and nasal bones
	CSF rhinorrhea with this and Le Fort III
	Extends nasal bridge through the frontal processes of the maxilla, through the lacrimal bones and inferior orbital bones; travels under the zygoma
III	Serious craniofacial disruption in which cerebrospinal fluid frequently leaks
	May follow impact to nasal bridge and extend through the nasolacrimal groove and ethmoid bone; the fracture continues through the floor of the orbit
	This type of fracture predisposes the patient to a CSF leak more than the other types of fractures

Change in the level of consciousness if head injury or hypoxemia.

Anxiety.

Fractures of the maxilla are diagnosed according to Le Fort's classification of three broad categories that depend on the level of the fracture (see Table 6–5 and Figure 6–1).

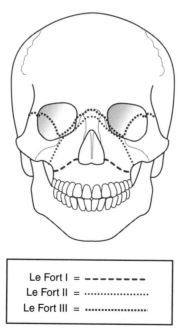

Le Fort I   = - - - - - - - -
Le Fort II   = ·····················
Le Fort III = ·····················

FIGURE 6–1 • Le Fort fractures.

Treatment

Le Fort fractures are reduced surgically by using direct wiring or fixation devices.

In any soft tissue injury there is always the possibility of contamination and infection.

Many facial wounds require tetanus immunization and a cleansing debridement to clear the area of dirt, grease, glass, and gravel.

Nursing Diagnoses for MFIs	Expected Outcomes
Airway clearance, ineffective	The patient will have a clear chest x-ray
	The patient will have clear breath sounds
Risk for infection	The patient's temperature will be baseline
	Surgical sites will be clean, dry, and intact
Risk for aspiration	The patient will have a clear chest x-ray
	The patient will have clear breath sounds
	The sputum will be clear
	Sputum cultures will be clear of organisms

Nursing Interventions

Assess bony structures and soft tissues for symmetry to determine the type of fracture.

Assess any open areas or surgical sites for signs of infection.

Monitor the patient's breath sounds, chest x-rays, and ABGs to look for symptoms of infection.

Keep the patient in a position of sitting up as this is the most comfortable and prevents blood or exudate from entering the airways.

If the patient needs a nasal gastric tube, insert it orally to prevent inadvertent intubation of the brain through the sinuses in a nasal approach.

Administer antibiotics to prevent infection from possible CSF leak.

Administer analgesics to help decrease pain.

Debride and cleanse the wound according to health care provider's protocol.

Instruct the patient what to do if he or she feels like vomiting.

Keep wire clippers at the bedside to remove surgically placed wires if an airway obstruction occurs.

> ### NURSING ALERT
>
> *Nasal intubation (pulmonary and gastric) is contraindicated in the presence of facial fractures because of the danger of passing the tube into the cranium.*

For more information on facial injuries, go to http://emedicine.medscape.com/article/434875-overview (last accessed July 10, 2010).

Tracheobronchial Injuries (TBI)

What Went Wrong?

The tracheal and bronchial areas are unprotected and can be injured in an MVC when these areas hit the dashboard or steering wheel. They are also associated with injuries like esophageal, spinal, and vascular damage.

The neck area where the tracheobronchial tree is located is highly susceptible to spinal cord injury from acceleration-deceleration injuries. The airway must first be monitored, as blunt or penetrating injury can cause airway narrowing and possible closure due to swelling from trauma to the area. Lacerations to the trachea can lead to massive air leaks into the subcutaneous tissues also causing swelling, with crackling felt under the skin upon palpation. The patient will need to be monitored for airflow, severe swelling, and subcutaneous emphysema.

As with the MFIs, tracheobronchial injuries can involve vascular damage leading to blood loss from the rupture of major vessels in this area. The patient will need to be monitored for blood loss leading to hypovolemic shock.

Prognosis

Severe injury to the tracheobronchial area results in an increased mortality rate.

Interpreting Test Results

Cervical spine x-rays must rule out fractures to the spinal cord.

Head and neck x-rays will show the extent of injury and bleeding.

MRI of neck will help show extent of injury and bleeding.

Chest x-ray will confirm diagnosis of subcutaneous emphysema.

ABG will assist with gas exchange difficulties.

Hallmark Signs and Symptoms

Often can be subtle and overlooked

Cough

Hemoptysis

Subcutaneous emphysema

Hoarseness

Anxiety and air hunger

Stridor

Treatment

Keeping the airway patent may require emergency tracheostomy, especially if swelling is severe and airway is compromised. Mechanical ventilation (MV) may be needed if gas exchange is comprised. Monitor and treat for shock if the patient is symptomatic.

Nursing Diagnosis for TBI	Expected Outcomes
Airway clearance ineffective	The patient will maintain a patent airway
Ineffective breathing pattern	The patient will have regular breathing patterns with normal breath sounds

Nursing Interventions

Observe for change in level of consciousness, increased respiratory rate, dyspnea, cough, and stridor, *which can indicate airway compromise.*

Ask patient if he or she has air hunger, which can be the first symptom of a tracheobronchial issue.

Palpate for the presence, location, and extent of subcutaneous emphysema, *which can indicate swelling and subsequent airway closure.*

Administer oxygen *to help load up hemoglobin molecule, getting oxygen saturation at optimum point.*

Prepare for intubation and MV if the patient's status deteriorates *to get oxygen more directly to the alveolus.*

Teach the patient *to report post-nasal drip, which could indicate bleeding or cerebral spinal fluid (CSF) leak.*

Breathing
Head Injury

See Chapter 5 (Care of the Patient with Neurological Needs).

Injuries to the Bony Thorax (Fractured Ribs, Flail Chest)

What Went Wrong?

Injuries to the bony thorax include rib fractures and flail chest (see Figure 6–2). Rib fractures may be located along the interior ribs and can be associated with trauma of the liver and spleen. Injury of the liver and spleen can cause hemorrhage and shock, as they are blood-filled organs. Fractures of the ribs higher up in the areas of the 2nd and 3rd rib can signify high-impact trauma, as they are usually protected by the shoulder girdle and surrounding musculature. Higher rib fractures are associated with many complications including pneumothorax, hemothorax, pulmonary contusion, and tension pneumothorax.

A flail chest is a specific pattern of rib fractures where two, three, or more adjacent ribs are broken in multiple places. Most commonly caused in MVCs, a flail chest can also be caused from falls in the elderly. Frequently a sternal fracture is also involved in a flail chest. Because these fractured ribs are separated from the chest wall, the injured part of the chest wall moves independently from the uninjured ribs.

A flail chest affects the dynamics of respiration. The fractured area will drop inward on inspiration and expand outward on expiration, thus the term "floating ribs." The inward fall is caused when the lung expands and the intrapleural pressures become more negative; outward expansion is caused when the more positive pressures occur in the lung during exhalation. This is also called paradoxical chest wall movement as the chest moves the opposite of how it normally moves during respiration. This paradoxical movement increases the work of breathing and, along with pain associated with the injury, can cause serious interference in blood oxygenation.

To see a flail chest in a traumatized patient visit http://www.medicalvideos.us/play.php?vid=1318 (last accessed July 12, 2010).

Prognosis

Underlying lung contusion causes respiratory failure in patients with a flail chest. A flail is one of the worse subsets of chest injuries and continues to be a leading cause of complications and death in trauma victims.

Interpreting Test Results

Chest x-ray will show flail but may not show underlying lung contusion initially; chest x-rays need to be repeated frequently to see the extent of the damage.

ABGs will show respiratory acidosis if condition is worsening.

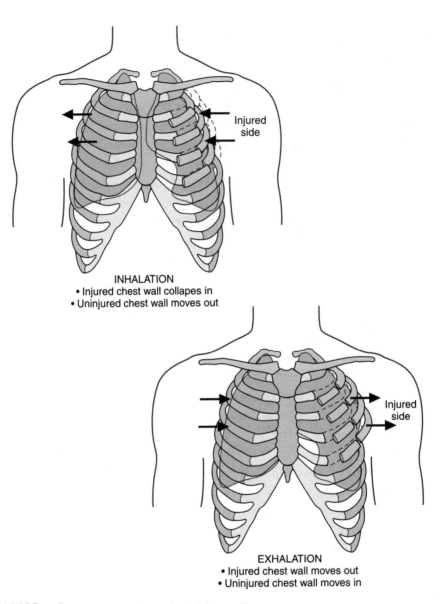

INHALATION
• Injured chest wall collapes in
• Uninjured chest wall moves out

Injured
side

EXHALATION
• Injured chest wall moves out
• Uninjured chest wall moves in

Injured
side

FIGURE 6–2 • Flail chest with paradoxical chest wall movement.

Hallmark Signs and Symptoms

Bruising around the areas covered by seat belts

Paradoxical movement in the area of flail

Crepitus in the chest areas

Severe chest pain in the location of the injury

Treatment

Pain control using intercostal nerve blocks, patient-controlled analgesia (PCA), epidural analgesia

Avoiding narcotics, which can lead to respiratory depression and hypoventilation

Intubation and mechanical ventilation (MV) using positive pressure to help stabilize a flail internally (see Chapter 2, Care of the Patient With Critical Respiratory Needs)

Nursing Interventions

Assess the patient for bruising around the chest and neck in the area of seat belts, *which can indicate traumatic injury associated with bony thorax.*

Palpate for subcutaneous emphysema (crepitus) in the chest area, *which is caused when air leaks from the lungs through the skin from trauma.*

Continuously monitor for other injuries like punctured blood vessels or lung contusion, *as a flail may not show up right away until the patient is working harder to breathe.*

Monitor for pneumonia by assessing temperature, lung sounds for crackles, and sputum cultures/sensitivities. *Pneumonia is the most common complication of a chest injury.*

Administer analgesics via protocol, which may include PCA and epidurals *to help control pain leading to hypoventilation.*

NURSING ALERT

A flail chest may not be diagnosed immediately! Check the mechanism of injury, the number and place of ribs fractures, and look for signs/symptoms of underlying lung contusion, which would lead to a high index of suspicion for a flail.

Acute Lung Injuries (ALIs)

What Went wrong?

Pulmonary contusion, hemothorax, pneumothorax, and tension pneumothorax are injuries to the lungs that can occur from multiple trauma. A pulmonary contusion is bruising of the lung tissue as a result of trauma. Damage to the capillaries in the lung tissue causes blood and other fluids to accumulate in the traumatized area, leading to hemorrhage, inflammation, and interstitial edema. The end result is hypoxemia. A pulmonary contusion is the most common potentially lethal chest injury.

A hemothorax is caused by blood building up between the lung and the pleural space from blunt or penetrating trauma. The hemothorax is usually limited in expansion due to the tight space where it occurs. Rib fractures, contusion, and venous injuries are usual causes of a hemothorax. If the hemothorax is large, hypoxia from blood preventing alveolar oxygenation, possible airway clearance issues, and hemorrhage can result.

A pneumothorax is a lung collapse due to either blunt or penetrating trauma. When the lung is punctured from a rib or blunt trauma, the negativity in the intrapleural space is compromised, resulting in either a total or partial collapse of the lung on the traumatized side. A pneumothorax may be closed where there is no connection to the outside environment, as with many blunt chest traumas, or it may be open where outside air is drawn into the lung during inspiration (sucking chest wounds). If unrelieved pressure enters the lung and it does not escape back out, a tension pneumothorax may develop. This is a life-threatening emergency. Whether open or closed, a pneumothorax leads to less functioning alveolar oxygenation in the area that has collapsed. The higher the percentage of pneumothorax, the more likely that hypoxemia can occur. For more information on a pneumothorax please consult Chapter 2.

A tension pneumothorax is created when air becomes trapped in the chest with no avenue of escape. As pressure builds up, the highly moveable structures in the mediastinum become pushed away from the affected side. The compromised lung cannot participate in oxygenation, leading to hypoxemia. The heart and great vessels become compressed, preventing blood from entering and leaving the heart. Profound drops in cardiac output result. (See Table 6–6 for signs/symptoms of the lung injuries)

Prognosis

The prognosis of all lung injuries is dependent on how quickly the patient is diagnosed and treated. Pulmonary contusion plays a very large role in whether an individual will succumb or suffer serious effects. It is estimated that contusion occurs in 30% to 75% of severe chest injuries with a mortality rate that varies greatly between 15% and 40%.

Patients with lung contusions must be followed up closely due to the high rate of post-accident ARDS (see Chapter 2 for further information on ARDS).

Interpreting Laboratory Results

Chest x-ray will show pneumothorax (air or collapsed lungs) and hemothorax (whiter color) over 20%.

CT scan is very sensitive for pulmonary contusion.

> **NURSING ALERT**
>
> *There is no single test or diagnostic procedure to confirm a pulmonary contusion, and often the clinical picture along with a high index of suspicion and close monitoring for signs/symptoms will help in diagnosis.*

Hallmark Signs and Symptoms

TABLE 6–6 Lung Injuries and Their Signs/Symptoms	
Lung Injury	**Signs/Symptoms**
Pulmonary contusion	May take up to 24–48 hours to develop
	Low SaO_2
	Circumoral and mucous membrane cyanosis
	Moist crackles in affected areas
Hemothorax	Dullness to percussion
	Decreased chest wall expansion in the affected lung
	Diminished breath sounds on the affected side
	Signs/symptoms of shock if a large hemothorax
Pneumothorax	Resonance on chest percussion
	Palpation of crepitus and rib fractures
	Tracheal shift from midline
	Diminished or absent breath sounds on the affected side
Tension pneumothorax	Dyspnea with acute respiratory distress
	Tachycardia
	Hypotension
	Tracheal deviation away from the affected side
	Diminished or absent breath sounds opposite the injured side
	Sudden chest pain that radiates to shoulders
	Traumatic cardiac arrest with pulseless electrical activity (PEA)

Treatment

Oxygen must be administered.

Chest tube compression in event of pneumothorax and hemothorax.

Emergency needle thoracostomy when time is of extreme essence.

Heimlich valve insertion if chest tube compression is unavailable.

Possible surgery if chest tube output does not decrease in a hemothorax.

Nursing Diagnoses for Lung Injuries	Expected Outcomes
Ineffective airway clearance due to pulmonary edema, blood, or exudate	The patient will maintain a patent airway
Ineffective gas exchange due to decrease in baseline	The patient will have alveolar oxygenation from increased SaO_2 and ABGs

Nursing Interventions in the Care of Patients With Lung Injuries

Assess the patient's vital signs as often as needed *to look for increase in pulse, respirations, and BP that signify impending respiratory failure.*

Suction the patient as needed *to maintain a patent airway.*

Administer supplemental oxygen *to help in alveolar oxygenation exchange.*

Monitor the arterial blood gases and SaO_2 *to detect changes from baseline status and worsening of respiratory acidosis, signifying respiratory failure.*

Set up and monitor chest tubes *to help restore negative pressure reexpanding lung tissue* (see Chapter 2).

Assist with insertion of Heimlich valve, which is *a stopgap measure until a chest tube is inserted. A Heimlich valve is a one-way valve that allows positive pressure to escape from the lungs and prevents air from entering back in.*

Administer fluids (blood and IVF replacement) cautiously *as it can result in increasing pulmonary edema.*

Administer pain medications via IV epidural or PCA *to control pain and allow ease of coughing and deep breathing without decreasing respiratory effort.*

Monitor closely for complications of pneumonia and acute respiratory distress syndrome *as 50% to 60% of patients develop this 24 to 48 hours after injury.*

NURSING ALERT

Massive left hemothorax is more common than a right hemothorax. Frequently associated with aortic rupture, a left hemothorax can lead to profound hemorrhage. If the chest tube output is greater than 200 mL/hr, the nurse should clamp the tube and notify the trauma surgeon, so exploratory thoracotomy can be performed.

Circulation

Hemorrhagic Shock

What Went Wrong?

Hemorrhagic shock is the most common shock in trauma patients. It is a type of hypovolemic shock that occurs when blood is lost in such large amounts that the organs and tissues cannot be supplied with oxygen or nutrients to sustain life. In traumatic injuries from penetrating and/or blunt trauma emanating from the MOI, forces rupture or tear organ structures, which causes the decreased blood volume. Compensatory mechanisms go into play to maintain blood volume to the brain and heart.

Catecholamines are released, causing the heart rate to speed up and breathing to increase to maintain cardiac output and oxygenated hemoglobin. Compensation in the early stages can maintain cardiac output, but if the cause is not corrected and enough blood is lost, decomposition occurs where the BP cannot be maintained and vital organ circulation is lost.

Prognosis

Prognosis is good if early treatment is initiated in the prehospital stage.

Interpreting Test Results

Serial hemoglobin and hematocrit to determine if blood replacement is needed

Respiratory acidosis from retaining pCO_2

Metabolic acidosis from decreased excretion of HCO_3 and lactic acidosis

Decreased glomerular filtration rate from decrease in kidney blood flow

Hypoglycemia

BUN and creatinine to determine if renal function has been compromised due to low blood flow

Hallmark Signs and Symptoms (Early)

- Tachycardia (one of the first signs)
- Hypotension
- Thready pulse
- Restlessness
- Decreased urinary output

Hallmark Signs and Symptoms (Late)

- Lethargy leading to coma
- MAP less than 60 mm Hg
- Decreasing hypotension
- Decreasing CO
- Doppler pulses

Treatment

Classification of hemorrhagic shock is important to identify and the treatment is matched with the signs/symptoms of shock the patient exhibits. Table 6–7 shows the classes of shock and treatment.

TABLE 6–7 Classifications of Hemorrhagic Shock and Treatment

Class of Shock	Estimated Blood Loss	Signs/Symptoms	Treatment
Class I	15% (750 mL)	Tachycardia may be only symptom May be slightly anxious	Crystalloid infusions
Class II	15%–30% (750–1,500 mL)	Tachycardia Decreased pulse pressure Anxiety Mildly decreased urinary output	Crystalloid resuscitation
Class III (uncompensated shock)	30%–40% (1,500–2,000 mL)	Heart rate >120 Change in mental status Drop in systolic BP 20 mm Hg drop in MAP	Crystalloid, colloid fluid resuscitation and blood replacement
Class IV	>40% (>2,000 mL)	Heart rate >140 Tachypnea Marked changes in mental status MAP <60 Pale, cool, clammy skin Sluggish capillary refill	Crystalloid, blood replacement Oxygenation with any means to increase the PO_2 to normal levels Pressor therapy

Nursing Diagnoses for Hemorrhagic Shock	Expected Outcomes
Fluid volume deficit	The heart rate will be below 100
	The BP will be above 100 systolic
	The patient's weight will be baseline
	The urinary output will be 30 cc/hr continuously
Tissue perfusion, decreased	All peripheral pulses will be intact
Decreased cardiac output	The heart rate will be below 100
	The BP will be above 100 systolic
	The MAP will be above 80 mm Hg
	The urinary output will be 30 cc/hr continuously

Nursing Interventions

Perform ongoing assessments of hemodynamic parameters prioritized by the ABC method including VS, SaO$_2$, MAP, and ABGs *to determine circulatory status.*

Elevate lower extremities *to enhance blood return to the heart and decrease peripheral venous pooling.*

Obtain estimated blood losses from first responders prn *to anticipate the level of shock and appropriate treatment.*

Administer oxygen *to prevent hypoxia.*

Administer and monitor the effects of fluid volume replacement therapy *to bring the amount of fluid in the intravascular space up quickly to prevent hypoxemia and resultant organ failure (see Table 6–3 and section on FVR for additional nursing care).*

Administer vasopressors like dopamine once IVF has been given *to raise the BP and prevent multiple organ system failure (MOSF).*

Apply external pressure to the bleeding site or prepare the patient for surgery *if bleeding cannot be controlled.*

Administer supplemental oxygen *to load up the hemoglobin molecules with oxygen in order to deliver more to the tissues.*

Monitor urinary output, weight, and BUN and creatinine *to determine if renal damage has occurred due to hypoperfusion.*

Assess neurological status *to determine if cerebral damage has occurred due to hypoperfusion.*

> **NURSING ALERT**
>
> *A patient who is cool, clammy to the touch, and tachycardic should be considered to be in shock unless proven otherwise. The critical care nurse needs to recognize these signs/symptoms and act as quickly as possible to identify and help correct shock.*

Spinal Cord Injury (SCI)

What Went Wrong?

Although head trauma is considered to be the most common type of traumatic injury, spinal cord injuries follow as a close second. MVCs are the number one cause of SCI. SCI is classified according to the level of injury and the amount of disruption to normal spinal cord function. Interventions are initiated with the goal of preserving any remaining neurological function. Descriptions of spinal cord injuries sustained depending primarily on the way in which the injury occurred or the mechanism of injury. These mechanical forces disrupt neurologic tissue and its vascular supply to the spinal cord. The spinal cord will become edematous and ischemic as it is deprived of adequate blood perfusion, nutrients, and oxygenation. The spinal cord can also become necrotic as a consequence of these secondary events. Neuronal conduction is no longer possible.

MOI for SPI are included in Table 6–8.

SCIs are either complete or incomplete. A complete SCI causes a total loss of sensory and motor function below the level of injury, despite the cause of the injury. The spinal cord is completely severed and the result is quadriplegia. An incomplete SCI results in a mixed loss of voluntary motor activity and sensation that occurs below the level of the injury. Any remaining function below the level of injury classifies the injury as incomplete. Common syndromes of incomplete injuries include Brown-Séquard, anterior cord, posterior cord, and central cord syndrome.

Brown-Séquard syndrome – Damage is located on one side of the spinal cord. There is a loss of voluntary motor control on the same side as the injury, but sensations such as pain and temperature continue to exist. On the opposite side of the body motor strength exists, but there is a loss of pain and temperature sensations. Clinically, the limb with the best motor strength has the poorest sensations, while the limb with the best sensations has the weakest motor strength.

Anterior cord syndrome – The anterior aspect of the spinal cord is damaged with paralysis evident below the level of injury. There is also a loss of pain, touch, and temperature. A sense of light pressure, position, and vibrations

TABLE 6–8 Mechanisms of Injury (MOIs) in Spinal Cord Injuries (SCIs)		
SCI	**Description**	**Common MOI**
Hyperflexion	Often seen in C5–6 level as most mobile area of spine. Compression of cord due to bony fragments or dislocation of vertebral bodies. Rupture or tearing of posterior muscles/ligaments creates spinal column instability	Seen in head on MVC
Hyperextension (whiplash injury)	Stretching and distortion. Results in contusion and ischemia of cord without significant bony involvement	Caused by rear–end collisions or diving accidents due to backward and downward motion of the head
Rotation	Severe turning of the neck or body. Results in tearing of the posterior ligaments and displacement or rotation of the spinal column	Occurs along with a flexion or extension injury
Axial loading	Vertical force along the spinal cord creates a vertical compression injury. Fractures of the vertebral body send bony fragments into the spinal canal or directly into the spinal cord	Commonly caused by a fall from a height where the person lands on his or her feet or buttocks such as falling from a tree or a roof
Penetrating injuries	Any objects that can penetrate the spinal cord can automatically sever the cord, causing permanent and irreversible damage	Blast or gunshot injuries

remain. This type of syndrome is most often caused by flexion injuries or an acute herniation of an intervertebral disk.

Posterior cord syndrome – Results from a hyperextension injury at the cervical level and is fairly rare. The senses of position, light touch, and vibrations are lost below the level of the injury. However, motor function, pain, and temperature remain intact.

Central cord syndrome – A combined cervical hyperextension/flexion injury. Motor and sensory deficits are more pronounced in the upper extremities than in the lower extremities. Bowel and bladder function can be impaired. This type of injury most typically occurs from contusion, compression, or hemorrhage of the gray matter of the spinal cord.

Autonomic Nervous Syndromes That Occur with SCI

Autonomic nervous syndromes can occur during SCI or the recovery phase. Common syndromes include spinal and neurogenic shock, orthostatic hypotension, and autonomic dysreflexia.

Spinal shock – A condition that occurs immediately after a traumatic spinal cord injury. Flaccid paralysis and a complete loss of all normal reflex activity below the level of injury is evident, including the loss of motor, reflex, sensory, and autonomic function. Bowel and bladder retention also occur. This condition can last for several weeks after injury, and its severity is determined by the level of injury. Spinal shock ends when spastic paralysis replaces flaccid paralysis.

Neurogenic shock – Known as a second shock state that can occur after spinal cord injury above the T6 level. Sympathetic nerve fibers are disrupted and the parasympathetic system becomes dominant, resulting in vasodilatation and a decreased heart rate. Blood pressure will also be decreased as a result of decreased venous return. The classic signs of neurogenic shock are hypotension, hypothermia, and bradycardia.

Orthostatic hypotension – This type of syndrome might occur after a spinal cord injury because the patient cannot compensate for position changes. Messages from the medulla are unable to reach the blood vessels, instructing them to vasoconstrict, and the result is an extreme hypotension as the patient's position changes from lying to sitting or standing.

Autonomic dysreflexia – Also known as autonomic hyperreflexia, this is a life-threatening complication of a spinal cord injury. It is caused by a massive nervous sympathetic response to stimuli such as a full urinary bladder, fecal impactions, kinked urinary catheter tubing, or excessive pressure on lower extremities, feet, and toes. Symptoms are bradycardia, hypertension, facial flushing, and extreme headache caused by vasoconstriction. The hypertension can be greater than 200 mm Hg systolic, with a diastolic reading of 130 mm Hg or greater. Immediate recognition of this problem along with immediate intervention is critical to the patient's survival. Recognize the cause; sit the patient up; and loosen tight clothing. Blood-pressure-reducing medications are needed to vasodilate the vessels if the symptoms continue and remain uncorrected, for example, nitroglycerin, nifedipine, and hydralazine.

Prognosis

The type of disability associated with SCI varies according to the location, amount of injury, and severity of the injured section of the cord. Many regain some functions during 1 week to 6 months after the injury. But the likelihood of full recovery diminishes after 6 months. Generally, serious, long-term rehabilitation is needed.

Interpreting Test Results

X-rays of C-spine

CT will be negative for injury

Hallmark Signs and Symptoms

Pain

Paresthesias

Paralysis

Palor above the level of the cord injury

Difficulty breathing if C4 or above

NURSING ALERT

A patient with a C5 or above SCI may have difficulty breathing. Monitor these patients closely and if respiratory distress occurs, prepare to support ventilatory efforts with BiPAP, intubation, or MV.

Treatment

Decompression of the spinal cord through realignment can be done medically or surgically depending on the types and extent of identified injuries. Medical management of SCI involves immobilization of the fracture site and realignment of any dislocation. Closed reduction of a cervical fracture can be done by using skeletal traction, which is indicated if the fracture is unstable or subluxated. Crutchfield tongs and halo vests are examples of skeletal traction devices for cervical injuries. They comprise two four-point tongs inserted into the skull through shallow burr holes under local anesthesia and connected to traction weights. The halo traction brace allows the patient to ambulate and participate in self-care. Thoracic and lumbar injuries can be treated by using fiberglass or plastic vests, canvas corsets, or a Jewett brace. These devices are fitted to the patient to provide support and stabilization of the spine. The recommended treatment for sacral and coccygeal injuries is bed rest.

Surgical management of SCI results in a more normal alignment of the ligaments and bone of the spinal column to provide spinal column stability and prevent a complete neurologic deficit or paralysis. Spinal surgery involves laminectomy, spinal fusion, or rods inserted into the spinal column.

Laminectomy – The spinal cord is decompressed by removing bony fragments or herniated disk material from the spinal canal.

Spinal fusion – Two to six vertebral disks are fused together to provide stability and to prevent motion. The fusion is achieved by using bone parts or bone chips taken from the iliac crest, or by using wire to achieve fusion, or by using acrylic glue.

Rods – Larger areas of the spinal column are stabilized and realigned by using rods attached to the posterior aspects of the spinal column by means of screws and glue. Rod procedures are most often done to stabilize the thoracolumbar area.

Nursing Diagnosis for SCI	Expected Outcomes
Ineffective breathing pattern related to transection of the spinal cord or edema above the level of C4	The patient will have normal rate, rhythm, and depth of respirations
	The patient will have baseline SaO_2, ABGs
	The patient will be able to cough and deep breathe

Nursing Interventions

Maintain head and neck alignment until spinal x-rays are completed and rule out a spinal injury or the spine is stabilized using an external fixation device like cervical traction or tongs.

Assess the patient's neurologic status including Glasgow Coma Scale, deep tendon reflexes, and spinal cord assessment *levels to determine if status is stabilizing and edema is subsiding.*

Monitor the patient for respiratory status with vital signs, SaO_2, ABGs, and respiratory mechanics *to check for early signs of respiratory depression.*

Observe for changes in cardiac status including BP and hemodynamic status *to identify neurogenic shock, which can be caused by hypotension.*

Prepare for administration of IVF *if hypotension occurs.*

Prepare to administer vasopressors *if IVF does not improve the patient's BP.*

Administer corticosteroids like methylprednisolone immediately and for the first 24 hours post SCI *to decrease inflammation and resultant edema.*

Assist with the application and care of cervical traction *to keep the alignment of the spine and to decrease muscle spasms.*

Prepare the patient for surgery *if internal stabilization is needed.*

Monitor the patients I & O *to detect fluid imbalances.*

Insert an indwelling catheter if SCI is in the cervical area *to monitor fluid status.*

Anticipate the insertion of a nasogastric tube *to prevent paralytic ileus if bowel sounds are absent.*

Monitor the patient for DVT and PE (see Chapter 3 for more information).

Provide emotional support for the patient and family. *Rehabilitation is a long and costly process that requires efforts of a multiple disciplinary team to keep the patient and family intact mentally, socially, and spiritually.*

Cardiac Tamponade

See Chapter 3 (Care of the Patient with Critical Cardiac and Vascular Needs).

Burns

What Went Wrong?

Burn injuries occur when energy is transferred to the skin from unwanted heat, chemical, radiation, or electrical current exposure. Exposure destroys layers of skin leading to tissue destruction and the stimulation of the inflammatory response. Burns are classified according to cause, location, body surface area burned, and depth. Location refers to where the burn occurs in the body. Burns of the head, face and respiratory tree, and genitalia are classified as more severe because they can compromise ventilation and/or can lead to infection. Inhalation of carbon monoxide competes with oxygen on the hemoglobin molecule, leading to hypoxemia. Inhaling superheated material can cause damage to the fragile lining of the respiratory system, leading to swelling and possibly early airway closure. Sloughing of necrotic tissue can lead to infection as the protective mechanisms of the skin are denuded.

Circumferential burns that encompass the entire distance around the extremity swell and lead to dysfunction and/or diminished blood supply. In the case of circumferential burns of the chest, swelling may lead to the inability of the chest muscle to expand during inhalation.

Severity according to body surface area (BSA) is calculated using the Rule of Nines. See Figure 6–3.

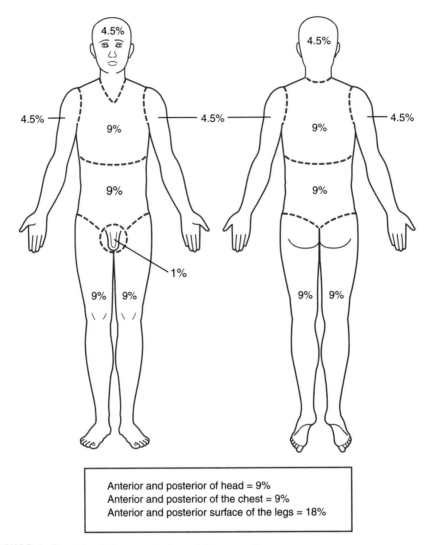

FIGURE 6–3 • Rule of Nines to calculate adult burn surface area.

Table 6–8 shows the causes of burn injury. The depth of the burn will be covered under Hallmark Signs and Symptoms in this section.

TABLE 6–9 Causes of Burn Injury		
Type	**Cause**	**Example**
Thermal burn (most common type)	Exposure to heat or flame	Scald from hot liquids/steam
		Fire and flame injury from residential fires

TABLE 6–9 Causes of Burn Injury (*Continued*)		
Type	**Cause**	**Example**
Electrical burn	Alternating current in households	Inserting objects in electrical outlets
	High–voltage exposures in work–related injuries	Lightning injury
Chemical burn	Exposure to strong alkali or acids	Common household cleaning agents (drain cleaners, ammonia)
Radiation burn	Sun exposure	Sunburn
	Work–related exposures	Nuclear power plant
		Medical or industrial accident

NURSING ALERT

Electrical burns have an increased mortality rate due to the susceptibility of the heart to ventricular fibrillation. Also, the current of energy sweeps through the body creating a path of cellular damage/necrosis with a small entrance and larger exit wound. Care of electrical burns requires continuous ECG monitoring.

Prognosis

Most burns are minor and can be treated at home. There are 500,000 burn injuries that occur annually that present to the ECU. Forty-six percent are thermal burns. There are 3,500 deaths due to burns annually; 75% occur at the accident scene. Deep thermal burns of 20% and burns of the respiratory system and genitalia require admission to burn units. Severe burns are life threatening; if the patient lives the burns result in amputations, surgical debridement with grafting, and long-term rehabilitation. Fourth-degree burns carry a high mortality rate.

Interpreting Test Results

SaO_2 and ABGs can show the extent of respiratory involvement in burns.

Carboxyhemoglobin level can show if the patient has carbon monoxide poisoning.

Creatine kinase and myoglobin levels may be high, indicating muscle damage.

Laryngoscopy or bronchoscopy determine the presence of carbonaceous material and the state of oral mucosa in inhalation burns.

Hematocrit and hemoglobin assist with fluid status.

Clotting factors may be elevated and PT increased.

Potassium levels will be high post-burn as it is liberated from damaged cells.

BUN and creatinine determine if renal failure is occurring.

Glucose temporarily elevated due to stress response.

WBCs can show if infection is developing.

Hallmark Signs and Symptoms

Nasal singeing and cherry red mucous membranes can indicate carbon monoxide inhalation injury.

Skin can be assessed using the depth of skin involvement at the burn surface area. Burn depths are known as superficial (first degree), partial-thickness (second degree), full-thickness (third degree), and fourth-degree burns (see Table 6–10).

TABLE 6–10 Depth of Burns		
Classification of Burn and Examples	**Layer of Skin Involved**	**Description/Healing**
Superficial burns: Scald Slight Sunburn	Epidermis or outer layer of skin	Pink to red in color and will be slightly edematous Heal within 3 to 6 days Painful, rarely require hospitalization
Partial–thickness burns: Severe scald Immersion thermal burn	Epidermis and the dermal layer of skin	Bright red; edematous with blister formation occurring within minutes of exposure Hair follicles and sebaceous and sweat glands remain intact Healing occurs within 3 weeks without scarring
Full–thickness burn: Severe chemical exposure	Encompasses all layers of the skin	Ranges from pale to bright red Capillary refill is compromised; blood vessels may appear black and thrombosed Little or no pain due to loss of pain receptors Hair growth will be absent due to loss of hair follicles Require skin grafting for full recovery
Fourth–degree burn: Severe electrical burn	Extends into the subcutaneous tissues, muscle, and bone	Black or charred, necrotic tissue Removal of necrotic tissue is required High mortality rate

Treatment

Remove any source of retained heat or chemicals (like clothing).

Maintain airway patency.

Administer oxygen.

Estimate the amount of fluid loss.

Fluid volume replacement if BSA greater than 15% or critical areas (genitalia).

Possible skin grafting.

Treat for infection.

How to Do It–Fluid Replacement Calculation

Estimation of fluid loss during burn injury using the Parkland formula: 2–4 mL × weight in kg × total body surface area burned

The first half of fluid is given in the first 8 hours and the rest is given over the next 16 hours. Time begins at the time of the event/injury, NOT the time the patient arrived at the unit.

Example:
The patient weights 110 lb and has a 50% burned area. The physician orders 4 mL of LR per kg.

Calculate the weight in kg: 110 divided by 2.2 lb/kg = 50 kg

Calculate the amount of fluid: 50 kg × 4 = 200 mL

Multiply by TBSA% burned: 200 × 50 = 10,000

The patient will receive 5,000 mL in the first 8 hours and the next 5,000 mL in the next 16 hours.

NURSING ALERT

Calculation of fluid to prevent hypovolemic shock due to large fluid loss is essential in the burn patient. Always time fluid replacement from the time of injury, NOT the time of admission to the ECU!

Nursing Diagnoses for Burns	Expected Outcomes
Impaired gas exchange due to thermal injury to airway and fluid translocation from intravascular space	The patient's VS will be stable The SaO$_2$ and ABGs will be baseline
Fluid volume deficit due to excessive loss of fluid from the intravascular space	The patient will have baseline BP The patient will have stable weight The intake will equal the output

Nursing Interventions (Early)

Assess the ABCs, especially respiratory status, of the patient *looking for signs/symptoms of carbon monoxide poisoning or inhalation of superheated air (nasal, eyelash, naris singeing; soot or sputum in mouth; stridor and hacking, productive cough).*

Prepare the patient for possible hyperbaric oxygenation therapy if carbon monoxide poisoning. *Hyperbaric oxygenation uses pressure to break the bonds to the hemoglobin molecule.*

Prepare for early intubation and ventilation *if airways swell.*

Administer oxygen *to prevent hypoxemia.*

Monitor temperature for signs of hyperthermia or hypothermia. *Hyperthermia can indicate infection; hypothermia can indicate large heat loss from burned area.*

Assess the cause, location, size, and depth of burn *to determine prognosis and treatment regimen.*

Administer large amounts of *fluid, calculated based on the burn area, to prevent burn shock.*

Monitor labs for H&H, serum sodium, and potassium. *H&H can show if anemia is resulting from bleeding from burned area. Serum sodium and potassium loss from the intravascular space may need to be supplemented.*

Perform neurologic and circulatory checks to determine level of consciousness and circulatory compromise in extremities.

Administer analgesics (like morphine) to control pain from injured areas.

Monitor intake and output *to determine fluid balance status.*

Perform weight check *to get a baseline for fluid retention or loss.*

Monitor urinary output via indwelling urinary catheter *to determine if fluid replacement is adequate. Output should be at least 30 to 50 mL/hr.*

Apply cool NSS dressings *to burns that are less than 10% to protect the areas from injury/infection.*

Apply dry, sterile dressings *to larger burns to prevent infection and hypothermia.*

Prepare to perform escharotomy (longitudinal surgical incisions) *to relieve pressure from burn swelling) if respiratory or circulatory compromise.*

Nursing Interventions (Late)

Assess degree of range of motion instituting ROM *to prevent further deformities.*

Monitor for signs of sepsis and infection *due to loss of protective skin layers.*

Administer topical or intravenous antibiotics *to prevent and treat infection.*

Provide emotional support, *as long-term therapy may be necessary and deformity can lead to issues with self-esteem.*

Prepare for dermal replacement *if new cells are not growing and the patient has third- or fourth-degree burns.*

NURSING ALERT

Carbonaceous (sooty) sputum, hoarseness, or facial burns and stridor are ominous signs. Prepare for early intubation due to airways swelling.

Abdominal Injuries

What Went Wrong?

Abdominal injuries are caused when a patient is launched forward over an object in high-speed accidents. Injuries may be blunt or penetrating and involve the stomach, liver, spleen, small and large bowel, bladder, and kidneys. Abdominal injuries can create life-threatening airway issues if abdominal contents enter the thoracic cavity compressing lungs and mediastinum. Massive herniation can compress lungs and decrease venous return and therefore CO. Blunt injury to the liver and spleen can lead to hemorrhagic shock. Penetrating injuries to abdominal viscera of the bowel can lead to peritonitis. Blunt trauma to the bladder and kidneys can lead to infection and renal failure.

Prognosis

These injuries may be difficult to diagnose and are usually found on secondary survey. Many of these injuries require hemodynamic stabilization or immediate surgical repair if signs and symptoms of shock continue during FVR.

Interpreting Test Results

Chest x-ray showing elevated hemidiaphragm on affected side and tip of nasogastric tube (NGT) above the diaphragm.

Focused assessment with sonography for trauma (FAST), which is a noninvasive test that examines the abdominal quadrants before a diagnostic peritoneal lavage (DPL).

DPL.

NGT shows blood if abdominal injury.

UA shows blood if kidney injury.

> ### NURSING ALERT
>
> *A DPL that is positive for frank blood or lavage fluid of greater than 100,000/mL indicates the presence of intraperitoneal hemorrhage.*

Hallmark Signs and Symptoms

Signs of respiratory distress if ruptured diaphragm.

Signs of hemorrhagic shock if spleen and liver are damaged.

Auscultation of bowel sounds in the chest if ruptured diaphragm.

Diminished breath sounds on affected side.

Diminished or absent bowel sounds if injury to small, large bowel.

Shoulder pain and SOB if ruptured diaphragm.

Elevated temperature and abdominal tenderness if peritonitis.

Blood at the tip of the urethra can indicate urethral trauma.

Nursing Diagnoses	Expected Outcomes
See nursing diagnoses for shock and ABCs	

Nursing Interventions

Assess the ABCs *to treat life-threatening emergencies on first priority basis.*

Hemodynamic monitoring with a central line *if shock is suspected.*

Observe for signs/symptoms of peritonitis including abdominal guarding, pain, tenderness, rigidity, discoloration around the umbilicus (Cullen's sign), decreased bowel sounds, tachycardia, and fever.

Assist with FAST and possible DPL to determine if blood has entered the peritoneum due to trauma.

Insert and monitor NGT drainage *to determine ruptured stomach or lower abdominal trauma.*

Monitor indwelling urinary catheter *to determine if injury to kidneys.*

NURSING ALERT

A patient with an acute abdomen with peritonitis can present with abdominal guarding, pain, rigidity, and Cullen's sign. Prepare for emergency exploratory abdominal surgery to determine the cause.

CASE STUDY 1

Roy Scott is on his way to your hospital with hypovolemic shock secondary to blood loss from an MVC. Roy has the following vital signs: pulse – 120, respirations – 28, and BP – 100/60. His GCS is 14; he is awake and oriented. An estimated Estimated Blood Loss (EBL) at the scene of 1 L was determined from a deep laceration in his right forearm. The prehospital care providers are instructed to start infusing Roy with LR via two large-bore peripheral IVs until he can be transported to the ECU. What is the preferred solution to start in this instance? Using the 3:1 rule, how much solution should this patient receive on his way to your Trauma I facility? How would you measure successful fluid resuscitation? What are the possible complications a nurse should monitor this patient for?

CASE STUDY 2

Prioritize nursing diagnoses for this patient with a traumatic injury.

E.B., age 21, was admitted to the ECU after sustaining a contact sports injury while playing college football as a quarterback in the final game of the school year. According to the EMS, the MOI was a hyperflexion injury from being tackled by six other players. E.B. was unconscious at the scene; his head and neck were stabilized immediately; C-spine collar was applied in the field and E.B. was transported to the hospital via helicopter.

In the emergency room E.B. begins to groggily regain consciousness and cannot recall the previous circumstances leading to his arrival at the hospital. He asks, "How many minutes are left in the game?" His vital signs are as follows: T – 99.0, P – 108, R – 24, BP – 138/62. C-spine x-rays reveal he has a partial high cervical fracture of C-5. CAT scan, blood work, EEG, and urinalysis were all within normal limits. He is able to slowly respond to all commands. E.B. is diagnosed as having a "moderate concussion, C-5 partial fracture, and a dislocated left shoulder."

REVIEW QUESTIONS

1. A patient arrives in the Emergency Care Unit unconscious with a suspected head and neck injury. Before x-rays are obtained, the best way to stabilize the head and neck while performing CPR is

   A. Head tilt chin lift.

   B. Modified jaw thrust.

   C. Hyperextension of the neck for placement of an endotracheal tube.

   D. No special precautions are needed in the above instance.

2. A mechanism of spinal cord injury that often results in a "whiplash" injury, occurs from

   A. Hyperflexion—compression of the cord due to vertebral column dislocation

   B. Rotation—tearing of posterior ligaments

   C. Axial loading—a vertical compression injury

   D. Hyperextension—stretched and distorted spinal cord without bony involvement

3. The nurse is assessing a patient newly admitted to the ECU with a complete spinal cord transection. The head-neck x-ray confirms that the level of the transection is above C3. The nurse's priority nursing observation should be

   A. Observation for full recovery without any neurological deficits

   B. Monitoring paraplegia with bowel and bladder control in question

   C. Monitoring for quadriplegia requiring ventilatory assistance

   D. Monitoring for hemiplegia requiring nasal oxygen only

4. The cortical evoked potential responsible for the sensory stimulation of hearing is

   A. VEP

   B. SSEP

   C. BAER

   D. CEP

5. A patient is admitted after an MVC where he was thrown through the windshield of his truck. Physical examination and facial x-ray reveals a horizontal fracture where the entire maxillary arch moves separately from the upper facial skeleton. The above describes the

   A. Le Fort I

   B. Le Fort II

   C. Le Fort III

   D. Le Fort IV

6. The nurse suspects a patient is experiencing neurogenic shock. The classic clinical symptoms of neurogenic shock include
   A. Facial flushing, headache, and hypertension
   B. Flaccid paralysis, pyrexia, and hypertension
   C. Spastic paralysis, tachycardia, and hyperthermia
   D. Hypotension, bradycardia, and hypothermia

7. A critical care trauma specialist is giving a lecture describing a perforating wound injury. Which of the following descriptions is most suggestive of a perforating wound injury?
   A. The body surface directly impacts and comes in contact with the offending object.
   B. Internal organ structures are seriously damaged with an object that enters but does not exit the body.
   C. Objects enter and exit the body causing severe internal trauma.
   D. There is evidence of a whiplash contusion injury.

8. A nurse is caring for a patient with third-degree full-thickness burns. While assessing the area, the nurse would anticipate which of the following in the traumatized area?
   A. Absence of pain, loss of hair, and thrombosed blood vessels
   B. Pain, hair growth, and blister formation
   C. Paresthesias, pallor, and capillary refill to be normal
   D. Loss of bone and muscle, charred appearance, and pain

9. A critical care trauma nurse is orienting a nursing student to the nursing care of trauma patients. The student asks why a nasogastric tube is contraindicated in patients with facial fractures. Which of the following would be the best response by this critical care nurse?
   A. "A nasogastric tube can lead to asphyxiation by obstructing the airway."
   B. "A nasogastric tube can cause hemorrhage if the sinuses are penetrated on insertion."
   C. "Passing the nasogastric tube into the cranium is possible with facial fractures."
   D. "Insertion of a nasogastric tube introduces bacteria into a traumatized area, which can lead to meningitis."

10. The nurse is assessing a patient with an incomplete spinal cord injury (SCI) often caused by a herniated intervertebral disk. This type of SCI is classified as a/an
    A. Anterior cord syndrome
    B. Central cord syndrome
    C. Brown-Séquard syndrome
    D. Posterior cord syndrome

ANSWERS

CASE STUDY 1

Roy should be started on LR with a total fluid replacement aimed at around 3 L (1,000 mL loss × 3 mL of fluid replaced = 3,000). Successful fluid resuscitation would be indicated by stabilization of vitals by a drop in pulse to less than 100, a drop in respirations to 18, and a BP between 110 and 120. His urinary output would also be light yellow with 30 cc/hr. Complications the nurse should monitor for include pulmonary edema from third spacing, hypothermia from rapid infusion of a room-temperature solution, and coagulopathies due to rapid dilution of the blood.

CASE STUDY 2

After an x-ray, E.B.'s shoulder is manipulated back into alignment and placed in a sling for comfort and support. He is admitted to a Critical Care Unit for observation of his moderate concussion and for continued neurological assessment of spinal cord damages resulting from a partial C5 fracture.

Possible Nursing Diagnostic Statements

Risk for ineffective airway clearance due to loss of gag reflex

Risk for ineffective breathing patterns due to spinal cord injury and swelling

Risk for impaired spontaneous ventilation due to swelling in the area of the spinal cord that controls respiration

Risk for decreased cardiac output due to lack of innervation to the spinal cord (spinal shock)

Altered Level of Consciousness related to a contact sports head injury

CORRECT ANSWERS AND RATIONALES

1. B. The head tilt chin lift would compromise the spine, leading to possible worsening of a spinal cord injury. The modified jaw thrust allows opening of the airway without added compression on the spinal cord. Endotracheal tubes can be placed without hyperextension of the neck.
2. D. There can be significant stretching and distortion of the spinal cord due to a downward and backward motion of the head, caused by rear-end collisions or diving accidents. Typically, a whiplash injury results from this type of trauma, with minimal to no bony disturbances.
3. C. A spinal cord injury above the level of C5 causes diaphragmatic and vagal nerve paralysis. Without the innervation to stimulate breathing, the patient will need to be placed on a ventilator.

4. C. BAER means brainstem auditory evoked potential. A sound stimulus is used to determine levels of hearing. A: VEP uses light sources to detect vision. B: SSEP (somatosensory evoked potential) assesses neurological responses below the level of a spinal cord injury by electrically stimulating the arm or leg. D: CEP means cortical evoked potential, which is the name for the entire diagnostic sensory process.

5. A: LeFort I are horizontal fractures in which the entire maxillary arch moves separately from the upper facial skeleton. B: Le Fort II involves an extension of Le Fort I, which includes the orbit, ethmoid, and nasal bones. C describes a serious craniofacial disruption with CSF leaks. D: There is no Le Fort IV category.

6. D. the classic clinical symptoms of neurogenic shock. A describes the symptoms of autonomic dysreflexia. B: Flaccid paralysis often describes the beginning of spinal shock. C: Spastic paralysis often describes the end of spinal shock.

7. C. With a perforating injury, items will enter and exit the body. A is an example of blunt force trauma. B: A penetrating injury where the item enters but does not exit the body. D: A whiplash injury is an example of a hyperextension injury.

8. A. A full-thickness burn is characterized by loss of pain receptors leading to no pain, loss of hair follicles, and thrombosed vessels.

9. C. The danger of passing the tube into the cranium is the most acute dilemma, which can lead to secondary dangers of edema, bleeding, CSF leaks, and eventual acute infection, all of which are life threatening and are to be avoided.

10. A. Anterior cord syndrome is most often caused by an acute herniated disk or damage from a flexion injury. B: A central cord syndrome is a combined hyperextension/flexion cervical injury. C: Brown-Séquard syndrome is where damage is located on one side of the spinal cord (incomplete). D: A posterior cord syndrome is a rare hyperextension injury found at the cervical site.

chapter 7

Care of the Patient With Endocrine Disorders

At the end of this chapter, the student will be able to:

1. Explain the essential anatomy and physiology of the endocrine system.

2. Describe the purposes and actions of specific secreted hormones.

3. Utilize appropriate clinical assessment skills while caring for the patient with endocrine disorders.

4. Discuss the therapeutic nursing management of endocrine disorders.

5. Describe tests/diagnostic tools used to identify endocrine disorders.

6. Recognize the implications of life-threatening endocrine emergencies.

KEY WORDS

Acromegaly
ACTH – adrenocorticotrophic
Addison's disease
ADH – antidiuretic
Adrenal glands – suprarenals
Aldosterone
AVP – arginine vasopressin
Cretinism
Cushing's syndrome
DI – diabetes insipidus
DKA – diabetic ketoacidosis
DM – diabetes mellitus

Dwarfism
ECF – extracellular fluid
Euthyroid
Graves' disease
HHNS – hyperglycemic hyperosmolar
            nonketotic syndrome
Hirsutism
Hypothalamus
Myxedema
Parathyroid
Prognathism

Introduction

During one's youth, hormone production can be perceived as "over active," "raging," or "running rampant." Sadly, as a person ages, organs atrophy, metabolism decreases, and hormone secretion diminishes and becomes underactive.

The endocrine system consists of various organs that function to maintain homeostasis within the body by releasing significant hormones throughout the bloodstream. The process of maintaining hormonal balance is intricate and delicate. An imbalance of hormones can provoke numerous and devastating individual health care problems. Hormones are chemical substances that either stimulate or prevent specific functions from occurring. These chemical substances have either a protein/amino acid structure or a steroid structure that is synthesized from cholesterol. An organ-specific hormone is something like prolactin, particular only to the mammary gland, while insulin, particular to the pancreas, affects almost all cellular functions of the body. Hormones tend to be released when the circulating level of that hormone is low, known as positive feedback. If the circulating hormone level is too high, the release of that hormone stops until a lower level is achieved, known as negative feedback. This process is performed to regulate blood hormone levels and to prevent an overproduction of hormones.

❶ Major Organs of the Endocrine System to Be Addressed (Figure 7–1)

Pituitary (hypophysis)

Thyroid

Parathyroid

Pancreas

Adrenals (suprarenals)

Structure and Function of the Pituitary Gland

Also known as the hypophysis, the pituitary gland is considered to be the "master gland" because it influences most bodily functions. It controls growth and metabolism and is found in a hollow depression at the base of the skull in the

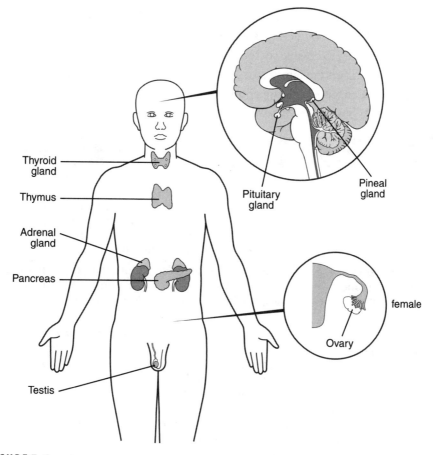

FIGURE 7–1 • Glands of the endocrine system.

sphenoid bone at the site of the "sella turcica." The pituitary gland is very vascular and well protected in this area. It is highly inaccessible and hard to reach for purposes of repair. The pituitary gland acts in partnership with the hypothalamus, which actually controls the release and inhibition of its hormones. The hypothalamus is located above the pituitary gland and is connected to the posterior pituitary gland by the "pituitary stem" or "infundibular stalk," also located at the base of the brain.

Areas of the pituitary gland are listed in Table 7–1.

The use of certain medications can create ADH imbalances. The release of ADH can be decreased by the use of medications such as Dilantin, chlorpromazine, and reserpine. Medications such as barbiturates, anesthetics, vincristine, and glucocorticoids will stimulate and increase the release of ADH. Other factors that affect ADH levels are pain, stress, surgery, alcohol, and malignant diseases.

What Went Wrong?

Pituitary malfunctions can lead to significant patient problems. An overproduction of growth hormone (GH) is almost always caused by a tumor or benign pituitary adenoma. Excessive secretions of GH (somatotropin) in children prior to puberty can result in giantism to an excess of 8 ft tall in height. Longitudinal bone growth occurs because the epiphyseal plate has not fully matured, making continued long bone growth possible.

❷ TABLE 7–1 Areas of the Pituitary Gland	
Anterior lobe or adenohypophysis—the largest portion of the pituitary gland	Hormones produced are ACTH—or the adrenocorticotrophic hormones, TSH—thyroid-stimulating hormones, FSH—follicle-stimulating hormones, LH—luteinizing hormones, growth hormone—somatotropin, and prolactin, which stimulates breast milk production during lactation.
Pars intermedia or the intermediate lobe	Located in the center of the pituitary gland between the anterior and posterior portions, it gradually merges with the posterior lobe in adulthood. Its function is unclear.
Posterior lobe or neurohypophysis	An extension of the hypothalamus, which collects, stores, and releases hormones produced by the hypothalamus. The two major hormones manufactured in the hypothalamus and stored in the posterior pituitary lobe are oxytocin (Pitocin) and ADH—antidiuretic hormone (arginine vasopressin or AVP). ADH is directly responsible for regulating bodily fluid balance by controlling sodium levels of extracellular fluid or ECF.

In adults post puberty, an excessive secretion of GH produces acromegaly. The adult bones are unable to grow longer as in the case of children whose long bones continue to grow. Adult bones increase not in length, but in width and thickness. Acromegaly usually begins gradually in the 3rd or 4th decades of life.

Hallmark Signs and Symptoms

Initial noticeable enlargement of the hand and fingers occurs with "clubbing" of the fingertips. The skin becomes thick, leathery, and oily. Speech difficulties become apparent as the tongue enlarges, the voice deepens, and vocal cords hypertrophy. Additional symptoms of acromegaly may range from mild joint pain to severe, debilitating arthritis. Sleep apnea can occur due to upper airway narrowing. Muscle weakness and neuropathy may also result. Marked prognathism or projection of the mandible forward can occur and interfere with the individual's ability to chew.

Cardiovascular involvement may develop associated with congestive heart failure (CHF), angina pectoris, and hypertension. Atherosclerosis may become apparent due to increased circulating fatty acids in the bloodstream. Women may develop menstrual disturbances. If the cause of acromegaly is a pituitary tumor, increased pressure within the brain can create visual problems and headaches. Excessive secretion of GH can lead to symptoms of hyperglycemia and eventual diabetes mellitus.

❸ Patient Assessment

The nurse should assess the patient for signs and symptoms of abnormal growth of bones and excessive soft tissue on the face and forehead and a thickening of facial features around the eyes, nose, and mouth. An enlargement of the mandible will cause the jaw to protrude forward. Question the patient about increases in shoe, hat, ring, and glove size and any noticeable changes in the patient's physical appearance. Such changes are usually gradual over the years, so a photographic comparison would be helpful.

Interpreting Test Results

The normal GH level in the adult, fasting and at rest, is 2 to 5 ng/mL. In some adults the results might be so low that the hormone remains undetected. Giving L-Dopa may stimulate GH to increase to measurable levels. Since blood GH levels fluctuate so much, the most reliable test for acromegaly is the oral glucose load challenge test, given to demonstrate that excessive release of GH cannot be suppressed. Under normal conditions, GH concentration levels *decrease* during an oral glucose tolerance test but *increase* with acromegaly because the cells become more resistant to insulin. The body strives unsuccessfully to handle increases in glucose and to metabolize carbohydrates. It has been noted that GH levels tend to increase during sleep, but the reasons are unknown. Severe malnutrition also creates a prolonged elevation of GH.

An MRI will determine the extension of a pituitary tumor into surrounding tissue, while a CAT scan with contrast dye will help to localize a pituitary tumor.

A complete ophthalmologic examination is also indicated due to potential increased pressure occurring over the optic nerves.

Treatment

Someone with a pituitary tumor may undergo radiation or surgery to remove the tumor. The surgical term is hypophysectomy and is accomplished using the transsphenoidal approach. An incision is made in the inner aspect of the upper lip and gingiva and the sella turcica is entered through the floor of the nose and sphenoid sinuses.

Radiation is indicated when surgery fails to produce successful results. It has also been used to reduce the size of a tumor prior to surgery. Gamma surgery or stereotactic radiosurgery can be used to treat small, inaccessible pituitary tumors. Radiation is delivered to a single site from multiple angles. It occludes the blood vessels feeding the tumor, which starves the tumor.

Drug Therapy to Decrease GH Levels

Table 7–2 contains three groups of drugs used to treat acromegaly.

TABLE 7–2 Drugs Used to Treat Acromegaly		
Category	**Drug Names**	**Dosages and Effects**
Somatostatin analogs	Octreotide or Sandostatin and two newer, long-acting drugs: Depot, Sandostatin LAR, and lanreotide SR (Ipstyl)	Given SQ, 3 times weekly to reduce GH levels Given IM every 2–4 weeks
Dopamine agonists	Cabergoline (Dostinex) has replaced Parlodel (bromocriptine)	Suppresses GH secretion, is more effective, and has fewer side effects
GH receptor antagonist	Pegvisomant (Somavert)	An alternative to the above dopamine agonists or somatostatin analogs. It blocks hormone action when there is continued hypersecretion of GH. It is best used for those who have received radiation therapy to control the disease process.

Prognosis

Since all soft tissues and organs of the body are enlarged and affected by excesses in the production and release of GH, marked improvement of symptoms can be achieved with careful monitoring of pituitary hormone serum levels, and adequate pharmacologic and medical management.

❹ Nursing Diagnosis for Pituitary Tumors	Expected Outcomes
Impaired nutrition less than body requirements related to increased GH hormone levels and difficulty chewing and swallowing	Patient will demonstrate an improved nutritional status within 1–2 weeks Patient's level of dysphagia will gradually improve GH levels will return to within normal limits (2–5 ng/mL)

Nursing Interventions

Weigh patient daily *to assess weight gain or loss.*

Provide a soft diet in small portions and *easy to swallow, enjoyable snacks for easier chewing.*

Maintain accurate intake and output *to ensure adequate hydration.*

Offer prn muscle relaxants if prescribed *to reduce discomfort of dysphagia.*

Assess for signs of aspiration such as choking, coughing, tearing, or cyanosis when ingesting food or fluids.

Allow the patient sufficient time *to eat and chew slowly without being rushed.*

Teach jaw movement exercises *to enhance mandibular movement.*

Suction patient if danger of aspiration is pronounced.

Maintain emergency tracheostomy equipment on standby.

Provide prescribed medications to lower GH levels and monitor laboratory results, for example, Sandostatin, Depot, Dostinex.

Recounting a True Story

In 1933, a young woman clutched her diploma with pride. She had just graduated after completing a rigorous 3-year nursing program and was ready to cure illness and conquer the world. In addition to all of the challenges facing new nurses in those days, she had one additional challenge—Giantism. She was well over 7 ft tall and despite what might be viewed as a considerable setback, this nurse was well adjusted to her condition, performed admirably, and never acknowledged any significant limitations in her abilities to function as a nurse. Throughout the years she traveled the world, cared for many people, and even managed to obtain a bona fide Florence Nightingale Lamp from England, return it to the United States, and present it to her School of Nursing. This woman faced her condition with dignity and will always be respected and admired for her many years of active, dedicated contributions to the profession of nursing despite all odds.

Hypopituitarism

What Went Wrong?

Hypopituitarism is caused by a lack of GH due to hypofunction of the pituitary gland. In children, a deficiency of GH causes dwarfism or an abnormally small stature as well as physical, mental, and sexual underdevelopment.

Sheehan's syndrome is a type of hypopituitarism that can develop after a complicated delivery with excessive bleeding and hypovolemic shock. Destruction of the pituitary gland occurs after circulatory collapse from uterine hemorrhaging.

Interpreting Test Results

In children the normal serum growth hormone level is 0 to 20 ng/mL. In cases of suspected dwarfism, the GH level is less than 10 ng/mL.

Prognosis

Treatment consists of lifelong hormone replacement therapy using certain medications such as Genotropin or Humatrope.

❹ Nursing Diagnosis for Hypopituitarism	Expected Outcomes
Knowledge deficit related to hormone replacement therapy	Family will be aware of need for lifelong GH replacement therapy in the child
	Family will understand actions and side effects of the medications provided

Nursing Interventions

Provide detailed instructions about specific medications.

Emphasize the need for lifelong follow-up care and medical interventions.

Assess status of child's mental and physical development.

Syndrome of Inappropriate Antidiuretic Hormone (SIADH)

What Went Wrong?

An *overproduction* or excess of ADH occurs due to a continuous release of ADH into the bloodstream, resulting in a condition known as syndrome of inappropriate antidiuretic hormone or SIADH. SIADH occurs most often in older adults and can be caused by a malignancy such as small cell lung cancer that releases ADH. It can also be caused by the use of antidepressant and psychotropic medications.

Hallmark Signs and Symptoms

This condition is characterized by fluid retention, increased body weight, and hyponatremia. Kidney tubules are stimulated to retain fluid through the excessive release of ADH, resulting in severe overhydration and an increase in body fluid volume. Sodium levels decrease (less than 120 mEq/mL) caused by an increase in urinary sodium excretion, and dilutional hyponatremia occurs. In an effort to equalize osmotic pressure, a fluid shift takes place from the extracellular to the intracellular spaces. It is important to mention that aldosterone is normally released by the adrenal glands to retain sodium but is suppressed by the condition of SIADH. The lack of ADH and aldosterone suppression causes water to be retained, urine output to decrease, and excessive amounts of sodium to be lost in the urine. Although there is a weight gain because of an expanded fluid volume, edema is absent due to the loss and lack of sufficient sodium. Hyponatremia causes muscle cramps and weakness. In addition to low concentrated urinary output and weight gain, dangerously low sodium levels can produce seizures, abdominal cramps, vomiting, muscle twitching, cerebral edema, lethargy, anorexia, confusion, headaches, and coma.

❸ Patient Assessment

The nurse should assess for a low, concentrated urinary output of less than 30 mL/hr with a high specific gravity greater than 1.030 (normal value 1.005–1.030), increased body weight indicating fluid retention, and a decrease in sodium levels. Identify any of the above-mentioned symptoms accompanying dangerously low sodium levels. It is also important to obtain a baseline patient weight and compare with daily weights, determine fluid intake and output and vital signs, assess skin turgor for dehydration or edema, and obtain a list of current patient medications. Goals of care include reduction of fluid intake and sodium replacement therapy. Accurate measurement of intake and output is required. Fluid intake is restricted to equal urine output until sodium levels return to normal. Determine the patient's status of elimination as constipation can occur when fluids are restricted. To correct hemodilution caused by severe sodium loss and fluid retention at the site of the kidney tubules, sodium can be replaced via 3% intravenous hypertonic saline solution infused at a slow rate of 0.1 mg/kg per minute on an infusion pump to prevent rapid volume overload and pulmonary edema.

Interpreting Test Results

Laboratory tests combined with the patient's clinical profile are the best indicators of the amount of ADH released into the bloodstream. The serum ADH test measures the amount of ADH present in a frozen sample of blood.

The normal result is 1 to 5 pg/mL. A more accurate direct measurement of ADH is possible through a sensitive radioimmunoassay serum ADH test. BUN, albumin, creatinine, hemoglobin, hematocrit, and electrolyte values may also be affected and should be evaluated.

Laboratory value changes associated with SIADH are shown in Table 7–3.

A water load test might be done to confirm a diagnosis of SIADH by creating a quasi-state of water intoxication. The patient is overhydrated with water after a period of fasting. Urine output and serum osmolality are monitored. Serum osmolality levels will decrease, and despite the excessive water load, an inability to excrete dilute urine will be evident. Overhydration is difficult for the patient and is generally never performed if the patient's condition is critical.

Prognosis

Individuals at risk for SIADH who are identified and cared for early in their illness can expect a full recovery.

❸ and ❺ Nursing Diagnosis for SIADH	Expected Outcomes
Fluid volume deficit related to dilutional hyponatremia and dehydration	Sodium levels will return to normal status Status of dehydration will improve

TABLE 7–3 Laboratory Value Changes Associated With SIADH

Test	Normal Values	Change
Serum ADH	1–5 pg/mL	Elevated
Serum osmolality	285–300 mOsm/kg	<250 mOsm/kg
Serum sodium	135–145 mEq/mL	<120 mEq/L
Urine osmolality	300–1400 mOsm/kg	Increased
Urine specific gravity	1.005–1.030	>1.030
Intake and output	Fluid intake will remain unchanged.	Urine output will be below normal.

Nursing Interventions

Obtain daily weights *to determine fluid retention or fluid loss.*

Assess urine and blood laboratory values and act upon changes.

Assess skin turgor and signs of tenting.

Monitor fluid intake and urine output; output should exceed intake.

Diabetes Insipidus (DI)

What Went Wrong?

Diabetes insipidus is caused by an *underproduction* of ADH. It occurs when there is a deficit or hypofunctioning of ADH, leading to water diuresis and dehydration. With an absence of ADH, the kidneys cannot reabsorb water or control fluid output. The body is then deprived of necessary fluid hydration and the kidney tubules cannot conserve enough water to reduce sodium levels. Hypernatremia and increases in serum osmolality occur, which stimulate the thirst receptors as the individual attempts to replace lost bodily fluids and prevent dehydration and severe hypernatremia. There are three types of diabetes insipidus:

1. Neurogenic or central DI – An interruption in the synthesis and release of ADH. ADH levels can be low. Causes include

   Primary – Abnormalities within the posterior pituitary gland, hypothalamus, or the infundibular stalk prevent the release of ADH. The cause can be sporadic or idiopathic in nature, which means the cause is either unknown or it has an abrupt onset.

   Secondary – Occurs from trauma or a pathologic condition such as benign or malignant tumors, neurosurgery, radiation, and infections of the posterior pituitary gland. Frequently found in patients in critical care units with head injuries or fluid loss from intracranial surgery.

2. Nephrogenic DI (NDI) – Enough ADH is available, but there is a decreased response to circulating ADH by the kidney. The problem can be drug induced by long-term use of lithium carbonate, which reduces kidney tubule responsiveness to ADH. The ADH level remains normal, the signs of diabetes insipidus are apparent, serum osmolality is elevated, and urine output is increased.

3. Dispogenic DI or psychogenic DI – A rare form of overhydration or water intoxication associated with excessive fluid intake of 5 or more liters per day. The individual generally favors iced or cold beverages. The ADH level remains normal but pure water is lost from the kidney leading to hypernatremia.

Hallmark Signs and Symptoms

The patient may experience generalized weakness, dehydration, increased thirst (polydipsia), a very low specific gravity of less than 1.005, increased sodium levels of greater than 145 mEq/mL and polyuria of greater than 300 mL/hr of very dilute (tasteless or insipid) urine. A huge cycle of polyuria and polydipsia continues, which creates significant disruptions in a person's schedules and quality of life. Hypotension, tachycardia, and shock can reveal signs of cardiovascular impairment. Also observe for signs of CNS involvement such as mental dullness, irritability, and coma. Additional problems that can occur include constipation from fluid loss or diarrhea from intestinal hyperactivity associated with vasopressin drug therapy.

❸ Patient Assessment

Obtain a medication history that could help to identify ADH imbalances. Drugs that *increase* ADH release are barbiturates, anesthetics, vincristine, and glucocorticoids. Those that *decrease* ADH are Dilantin, reserpine, and chlorpromazine. A social history is also necessary to identify the patient's compulsive or unsatisfied water drinking and unexplained weight loss. Continuously assess the patient's hydration status through accurate measurement of intake and output, daily weights, and determination of skin turgor and buccal membranes, as severe dehydration and hypovolemia can result from polyuria and polydipsia.

Fluid and electrolytes are routinely drawn and evaluated. ADH levels, serum osmolality, urine osmolality, and serum sodium levels are obtained and compared.

Interpreting Test Results

Laboratory value changes associated with DI are shown in Table 7–4.

Also of diagnostic value is the *Water Deprivation* or *Dehydration Test*. The patient is deprived of fluids for 24 hours. Urine and serum osmolality is measured during this time. In patients with DI, their urine will be minimally concentrated after forced dehydration and their serum osmolality will rise above 300 mOsm. Sodium levels will increase above 145 mEq/mL. Individuals with DI show no decrease in urine volume in response to strict water restriction, whereas healthy people respond with a rapid decline in urine volume when water intake is withheld.

The priority of care is to restore and maintain circulating fluid volume and osmolality and prevent circulatory collapse through ADH replacement. For those patients who can drink, they are given fluids orally and hourly in amounts to match their fluid loss and output. Intravenous hypotonic solutions of 0.45% NSS can be given to correct hypernatremia. A low sodium diet might be beneficial to the patient with DI, along with fluid restriction of 500 to 1,000 mL per day.

⑤ TABLE 7–4 Laboratory Value Changes Associated With DI

Test	Normal Values	Change
ADH	1.5 pg/mL	Decreased in central DI
		May be normal with nephrogenic or psychogenic DI
Serum osmolality	285–300 mOsm/kg	>300 mOsm/kg
Serum sodium	135–145 mEq/mL	>145 mEq/mL
Urine osmolality	300–400 mOsm/kg	<300 mOsm/kg
Specific gravity	1.005–1.030	<1.005
Urine output	1.5 L/24 hr	30–40 L/24 hr
Fluid intake	1.5 L/24 hr	50 L or more in 24 hours

ADH Replacement Hormone Therapy

This can be achieved by giving ADH preparations to replace the ADH, while enabling the kidney to conserve water. Examples are

DDAVP, or desmopressin acetate	Given subcutaneously or intranasally and has mild to infrequent side effects
Exogenous ADH such as vasopressin or Pitressin	Given sq, causes a temporary increase in urine osmolality. There is an appropriate response to ADH as the kidney conserves water, and urine output decreases while restoring ECF.

Prognosis

Chronic DI will not shorten ones life span. Lifelong medications are required to control the signs, symptoms and complications of this disorder.

Nursing Diagnosis for Diabetes Insipidus	Expected Outcomes
Impending hypovolemia related to severe dehydration and hypotension	Hydration levels will be within normal limits
	Patient will be normotensive

Nursing Interventions

Monitor fluid balance of intake and output

Assess daily weights

Measure electrolytes, BUN and Urine specific gravity

Teach the importance of taking prescribed medications and not discontinuing them abruptly

Provide meticulous skin and oral care

Assess for signs of dehydration

Assess vital signs for return to normal status

Wear Medical Alert bracelet to identify illness

❶ Structure and Function of the Thyroid Gland

The thyroid gland is considered to be the largest endocrine gland. Located at the front of the neck, it resembles a bow-tie and has two lateral lobes connected by a band of narrow thyroid tissue known as the thyroid isthmus. The thyroid gland is highly vascular. Its basic cells of function are known as follicles, filled with the protein thyroglobulin. A person with a normal functioning thyroid gland is said to be *euthyroid*. Thyrotropin, or TRH, is secreted by the hypothalamus. It activates the release of the thyroid-stimulating hormone (TSH), which is produced and secreted by the anterior pituitary gland. The thyroid gland secretes three hormones that affect all active metabolic processes of the body. These hormones are T3 – triiodothyronine, T4 – L-thyroxine, and calcitonin. Functions of these hormones include

1. Increasing the effects of epinephrine to activate heat production and lower serum cholesterol levels.

2. Enhancing the normal development of the central nervous system and stimulating the growth and normal metabolism of all body cells.

3. Calcitonin lowers serum blood calcium levels and increases calcium absorption by the bone.

An adequate intake of iodine by ingesting table salt is necessary for the continued production of these hormones. The iodine is absorbed and concentrated in the thyroid follicles. Iodine becomes iodide and, aided by thyroxine (an amino acid), binds to thyroglobulin to become T3 and T4. T3 is five times as potent and more metabolically active than T4, but most of the thyroid output is in the form of T4.

Conditions Affecting Thyroid Function

An enlarged thyroid or thyromegaly is referred to as a goiter. It is visible and palpable on the anterior neck and can be noted on inspection if the thyroid gland is excessively enlarged.

Cretinism is a congenital condition caused by a deficient amount of thyroid hormones, which produces growth failure, possible mental retardation, lowered basal metabolism, dystrophy of the bones and soft tissues, and myxedema. The required treatment is lifelong thyroid hormonal therapy. The symptoms of cretinism may not be apparent at birth because the newborn may still be carrying some maternal thyroid hormone.

Hypothyroidism (Myxedema)

What Went Wrong?
Iodine-deficient diets can cause hypothyroidism, especially in parts of the world where iodine availability is lacking, for example, Hashimoto's thyroiditis. Antibodies are produced that destroy substances needed to produce T3 and T4, creating a decreased metabolism throughout all body systems.

Hallmark Signs and Symptoms
These include fatigue, weight gain, intolerance to cold temperatures, lethargy, mental sluggishness, constipation, slowed and slurred speech, hoarse voice, a thickened tongue, anorexia, anemia, somnolence, dry and flaky skin, coarse hair, dry and brittle nails, and boggy, nonpitting edema seen around the eyes, hands, and feet. EKG changes are additional causes for concern. Hormone replacement therapy to reverse this disorder include

Synthroid – levothyroxine

Lugol's solution – small doses of iodine

Potassium iodide solution

Prognosis
The symptoms of Myxedema will subside and normal metabolic activity restored with continued adequate hormone replacement therapy.

Myxedema Coma

This is a medical emergency that progresses gradually or rapidly into coma or death as the symptoms of hypothyroidism continue unrelieved.

What Went Wrong?
Myxedema coma can be precipitated by infections, trauma, surgery, exposure to cold temperatures, and taking medications such as narcotics, barbiturates, and tranquilizers.

Hallmark Signs and Symptoms
Subnormal body temperatures below 80°F, as the patient with myxedema coma cannot shiver to produce body heat; hypotension; bradycardia; and hypoventilation.

Intravenous thyroid hormone replacement and critical care management is necessary for patient survival.

Prognosis

Intravenous thyroid hormone replacement and critical care management is necessary for patient survival. The mortality rate is 20–25% even with vigorous treatment and early intervention.

Hyperthyroidism (Graves' Disease, Thyrotoxicosis)

What Went Wrong?

An excessive amount of thyroid hormone is produced and released beyond the needs of the body. There is an increased metabolism level that can be caused by tumors, inflammation, or autoimmune disorders of the thyroid gland.

Hallmark Signs and Symptoms

These include exophthalmus or large, bulging eyes; goiter; weight loss; extreme irritability; nervousness; restlessness; and insomnia. The goal of care is to prevent the oversecretion and adverse effects of thyroid hormones. Surgical intervention such as a subtotal thyroidectomy, treatment with radioactive iodine, and antithyroid medications are considered.

Examples of antithyroid medications are provided in Table 7–5.

TABLE 7–5 Examples of Antithyroid Medications

Medication	Purpose
PTU (propylthiouracil)	Blocks the conversion of T4 to T3
Tapazole (methimazole)	Slower acting but more potent than PTU
SSKI (saturated solution of potassium and Lugol's solution)	Rapid-acting and short-term duration preparations of iodine used to control hyperthyroidism by reducing thyroid hormone release into the circulation
Lithium carbonate	Given to individuals who cannot take iodine preparations due to allergies
	Prevents the release of thyroid hormone
Decadron (dexamethasone)	A glucocorticoid medication that can be given 2 mg q 6 hours intravenously
	It suppresses thyroid hormone release
Propranolol (Inderal) and atenolol (Tenormin)	B-adrenergic blockers to provide symptomatic relief of hyperthyroidism

Thyroid Storm/Thyrotoxic Crisis

What Went Wrong?

Untreated or uncontrolled hyperthyroidism can precipitate a severe and rapidly worsening condition of a hypermetabolic, overactive thyroid state. It is a life-threatening and critical complication with an acute, sudden onset. Causes could be infection, trauma, or surgery in patients with preexisting hyperthyroidism. Emergency management must be provided quickly and aggressively.

Hallmark Signs and Symptoms

These include heart failure; severe tachycardia and tachypnea; intolerance to heat; excessive diaphoresis; hot, flushed skin; extreme pyrexia with body temperatures of 105.3°F; abdominal pain; nausea; vomiting; diarrhea; agitation; restlessness; seizures; delirium; and coma. Immediate therapy includes fever reduction with cooling blankets and acetaminophen. Assess body temperatures q 15 minutes until temperatures reach a safe level; institute appropriate intravenous fluid replacement to counter the effects of hyperthermia and fluid losses from vomiting and diarrhea. Reduce circulating thyroid hormone levels with the appropriate drug therapy. Verapamil, a calcium channel blocker, is effective in controlling tachycardia and esmolol, a short-acting beta-blocker used for short-term, rapid control of atrial fibrillation, are medications that might be ordered.

Prognosis

Current methods of diagnosing and treating hyperthyroidism have significantly reduced the incidence of Thyroid Storm, making it relatively uncommon.

❺ Interpreting Test Results

Specific laboratory tests are completed to diagnose and monitor progression of thyroid disease. As nurses, it is important to remember that certain medications can interfere with thyroid test results, such as heparin, dopamine, and corticosteroids.

The free thyroxine test (free T4) and TSH (released by the anterior pituitary gland) are the two main laboratory tests recommended for testing by the American Thyroid Association.

NURSING ALERT

The following three points should be emphasized: (1) High doses of corticosteroids and dopamine infusions can suppress TSH levels. (2) Thyroid hormones increase cholesterol metabolism. Therefore, people with hyperthyroidism tend to have low serum cholesterol levels, while those with hypothyroidism tend to have high serum cholesterol levels. (3) Test results can be inconclusive in the critically ill patient as the stress of illness interferes with normal hormonal production and regulation.

TSH (thyroid-stimulating hormone) – Determines if a problem is caused by the thyroid gland itself or is due to a secondary problem of the anterior pituitary gland. No fasting is required for this test. Normal values are 2 to 5.4 mU/mL. TSH levels will be very high in cases of hypothyroidism, in an effort to stimulate the failing thyroid gland, and very low in cases of hyperthyroidism, in an effort to reduce thyroid hormone output.

Total T4/L-thyroxine serum concentration – Measures both the free T4 and TBG (thyroxine-binding hemoglobin). Normal value for adults is 4 to 12 ug/dL. Infants, children, pregnant women and those taking oral contraceptives have higher results such as 15 to 16.5 ug/dL. Fasting is recommended for this test. Results will be elevated with hyperthyroidism and liver disease and decreased with hypothyroidism. It should be noted if the patient is already taking a thyroid preparation. Propranolol and Dilantin can also interfere with accuracy of test results.

T3 (triiodothyronine serum concentration) – This measurement is needed when a person has a normal T4 but presents with clinical symptoms of thyrotoxicosis. T3 value will be elevated with thyrotoxicosis while other test results remain within normal limits. Fasting prior to testing is recommended. Normal adult value is 110 to 230 ng/dL.

Thyroid scan and RAI (radioactive iodine uptake) – A thyroid scan in conjunction with an RAI is done to identify and diagnose hypo- and hyperthyroidism, nodules, cancer of the thyroid, and ectopic thyroid tissue. An RAI test measures the rate of iodine uptake by the thyroid gland after giving iodine 123 intravenously, by capsule, or by solution. Gamma rays are measured as they are released from the breakdown of the tracer in the thyroid gland. Radioactivity of the thyroid gland, neck, and mediastinum is visualized. A normal result will show even distribution of the radioactive iodine in the thyroid gland. Images visualized as *cold* nodules will aid in confirming cancer of the thyroid gland.

Ultrasound – A noninvasive study that utilizes high-frequency sound waves to produce an image of the thyroid gland. Cysts, masses, and enlargement of the thyroid gland can be detected.

Fine-needle biopsy – The diagnostic tool of choice to evaluate a thyroid mass or detect a malignancy of a thyroid nodule. Cytology of biopsied material will be positive for cancer cells even if thyroid tests were previously normal.

❸ Patient Assessment

The astute nurse will be able to distinguish the physical differences between hypo- and hyperthyroidism by obtaining a detailed health history and thorough physical assessment. A health history should reveal prior or current use of a thyroid hormone and other medications that can compromise thyroid function. Sufficient or insufficient dietary intake of iodine, intolerance to extreme changes in environmental temperatures, visual problems, goiter or anterior neck enlargement, and family history of thyroid disease should also be explored. Determine through questioning if the patient has had any changes in sleeping, elimination, or eating patterns such as insomnia versus excessive sleeping, weight gain or loss with increases or decreases in appetite, vomiting, diarrhea, or constipation. Is the patient feeling overly anxious and restless or simply tired, fatigued, and sluggish? Are there complaints of muscle weakness, tremors, heart palpitations, or outbursts of crying and bad temper? Do they suffer from extreme sweating and fever or has their skin, fingernails, and hair become dry, brittle, and scaly?

Upon inspection the nurse will observe that a normal-sized thyroid gland is not visibly obvious as a goiter or a bulge in front of the neck. Ask the patient to swallow to see if upward movement of the thyroid gland is apparent. Observe nutritional body mass, skin condition, emotional status, and signs of exophthalmus or bulging eyes. Evaluate diagnostic test results to determine increases or decreases in T4 and T3 serum levels. Evaluate glucose results as hyperglycemia can occur from an increase in nutrients minus a sufficient release of insulin.

Assess vital signs through palpation and auscultation. Attention is given to extreme highs or lows in body temperature and cardiac status such as tachy-dysrhythmias and PVCs.

Palpate the thyroid gland using the anterior or posterior approach according to varying recommendations. There are two schools of thought on how to palpate the thyroid gland.

How to Do It–Examining the Thyroid Gland

1. The examiner stands behind the patient with the patient in a sitting position.

2. Avoiding hyperextension of the neck, the examiner places his or her hands on either side of both lobes of the gland and isthmus and palpates for size, shape, symmetry, and the presence of tenderness.

3. Another source describes examining the gland with the examiner standing in front of the patient and asking the patient to swallow and then observing the upward motion of the thyroid.

4. The thyroid gland is then palpated with the index and middle fingers of both hands placed below the cricoid cartilage on both sides of the trachea.

5. Palpation may be unsuccessful if the patient has a short, heavy neck.

6. An enlarged thyroid found on palpation should be auscultated for systolic bruits, a positive sign of hyperthyroidism. Accelerated blood flow through thyroid arteries produces low, soft vibrations that can be heard by placing the bell of the stethoscope over one of the lateral lobes.

7. The patient should hold his or her breath while the nurse listens to prevent tracheal sounds from interfering with the bruits.

8. A bruit can be distinguished from a venous hum as the nurse uses his or her finger to lightly occlude the jugular vein on the side that the nurse is assessing while continuing to listen. Interestingly, the venous hum will disappear during venous compression, but a bruit will not. By definition, a venous hum is produced by jugular blood flow.

Additional Nursing Considerations

1. Obtain daily weights *to record changes in body mass.*

2. Provide adequate hydration *to counter the effects of fluid loss from nausea and diarrhea and hyperthermia if these complications are evident.*

3. Utilize warming or cooling blankets *to stabilize either hypo- or hyperthermia.*

4. The patient post thyroid surgery may develop risks due to hemorrhage or laryngeal nerve injury. Particular attention must be paid to airway compromises that can occur.

5. Signs of impending thyroid storm need *to be assessed and addressed.*

6. If the parathyroid gland has been excised or injured, signs of tetany could also occur.

7. Prescribed medications must be administered such as acetaminophen for pyrexia and thyroid or antithyroid medications according to the prevailing condition.

8. Continue to evaluate laboratory outcomes for thyroid gland status, blood glucose levels, and fluid and electrolyte imbalances.

9. Cardiac monitoring and EKG must be ongoing to identify cardiac dysrhythmias such as atrial fibrillation, sinus tachycardia, sinus bradycardia, and heart block.

⑥ Nursing Diagnosis for Thyroid Storm	Expected Outcomes
Disturbed metabolic state related to hyperthermia and loss of body temperature regulation	Body temperature will return to normal reading of 98.6°F Patient's metabolic rate will reveal a return to euthyroid status

Nursing Interventions

Hourly monitoring of body temperature *to determine return to normal range.*

Assess fluid status *by monitoring hourly intake and output.*

Assess hydration level by examining skin turgor, mucous membranes, and extremes of diaphoresis.

Determine patient's level of tolerance to variations in environmental temperatures, for example, too hot, throwing off clothes, demanding window opening.

Provide comfort measures to patient by offering more room ventilation, fan and window opening, cold fluids, and lighter clothing.

Administer acetaminophen prn *to reduce hyperpyrexia.*

Provide cooling blanket *to bring body temperature back to normal.*

Assess daily weights *to evaluate changes in body mass and nutritional status.*

Administer antithyroid medications as prescribed.

Evaluate diagnostic laboratory results for thyroid, glucose, and electrolyte status.

Teach coping strategies *in an effort to calm and decrease patient's emotional irritability.*

❶ Parathyroid Gland

The parathyroid gland consists of four small, oval-shaped glands arranged in pairs and located close to and behind the thyroid gland. The parathyroid gland is responsible for the production and release of parathormone (PTH). Functions of PTH are as follows:

1. Works in partnership with vitamin D to stimulate calcium and phosphorous absorption from the intestinal mucosa.

2. Promotes bone strength and movement of calcium from the bone. Ninety-nine percent of calcium is found in the bones and 1% is found in the bloodstream. Normal calcium value is 9.0 to 11.0 mg/dL or 4.5 to 5.5 mEq/L.

3. Promotes increased excretion of phosphorous in the urine as PTH also acts on the renal system. Phosphorous is measured as phosphate in the urine. Normal serum phosphate values are the direct opposite of calcium values: 2.8 to 4.5 mg/dL or 0.90 to 1.45 mmol/L.

4. Maintains neuromuscular activity.

5. Promotes blood-clotting functions.

6. Enhances cell membrane permeability.

The normal PTH value is 10 to 60 pg/mL. A feedback mechanism exists between the PTH and calcium, in that PTH secretion will increase when serum calcium levels are low and will decrease when calcium levels are high.

Conditions of the Parathyroid Gland

The parathyroid gland is sometimes damaged during thyroid surgery because of its close proximity to the thyroid.

Hyperparathyroidism

This is a condition of excessive overproduction of PTH. The result is hypercalcemia or increased calcium levels.

What Went Wrong?

Hyperparathyroidism is characterized by large amounts of bone decalcification that could result in pathological fractures particularly of the spine. The development of renal stones containing calcium could be another complication.

Hallmark Signs and Symptoms

Deep bone pain and possible fractures caused by bone demineralization lead to additional symptoms such as flaccid muscles, anorexia, nausea, vomiting, lethargy, confusion, and headaches.

Prognosis

Surgical removal of the parathyroid gland may be necessary in more severe cases. Mild cases have good outcomes with medication therapy.

Hypoparathyroidism

What Went Wrong?

Caused by deficient production of PTH manifested by hypocalcemic levels less than 5 mg/dL.

Hallmark Signs and Symptoms

This condition presents with neurological disturbances such as tetany or muscular hypertonia, tremors, and spasmodic movements that develop when calcium levels are very low. Additional complaints include numbness, tingling, and cramps in the extremities.

Tetany can be identified by evaluating the patient for

1. Trousseau's sign – Carpopedal spasm occurs after occluding blood flow to the arm for 3 minutes with the use of an inflated blood pressure cuff. The resulting tonic spasm of the hand is a positive sign of hypoparathyroidism.

2. Chvostek's sign – Twitching of the eye or mouth is a positive sign of hypoparathyroidism as the nurse taps over the facial nerve in front of the parotid gland to elicit such a response.

Interpreting Test Results

Diagnostic studies such as plain x-rays, bone scans, MRI, and ultrasound can be used to examine the parathyroid gland and to evaluate bone changes that may have resulted from this condition. Laboratory analysis will provide continuous data regarding PTH, serum calcium, and serum phosphate levels.

❹ Prognosis

Restoring calcium, phosphorous and PTH levels to within normal limits and preventing complications provides a positive outlook to recovery.

Care and management consists of restoring calcium, phosphorous, and PTH levels to within normal limits and to prevent further development of complications.

❺ Nursing Diagnosis for Hypoparathyroidism	Expected Outcomes
Altered comfort level related to excessive facial and hand tremors and decreased blood calcium levels	Calcium levels will return to within normal parameters
	Episodes of facial and hand tremors will be resolved

Nursing Interventions

Assess daily calcium levels to determine return *to normal ranges of 9.0 to 11.0 mg/dL.*

Assess for continued signs of tetany by provoking Trosseau's or Chvostek's signs through facial tapping or blood pressure cuff inflation.

Administer prescribed calcium-containing medications.

Provide nutritional teaching *to include a calcium-rich diet.*

Assess for additional neurologic disturbances such as numbness, tingling, and cramping in the extremities.

Maintain adequate fluid hydration and accurate measurement of intake and output.

❶ Pancreas

The pancreas is a fish-shaped organ located beneath the duodenum and the spleen. It is composed of the following parts:

1. The *head* of the pancreas is attached to and lies in the C-shaped part of the duodenum.

2. The body or *main* part of the pancreas is hidden behind the stomach. It extends horizontally across the abdomen.

3. The *tail* of the pancreas is *thin* and narrow and is in contact with the spleen.

4. The main pancreatic duct crosses the entire length of the pancreas and is known as the duct of Wirsung.

5. Digestive juices are emptied into an opening at the entrance to the duodenum, known as the ampulla of Vater.

The pancreas has two major functions:

1. Exocrine – Releases pancreatic enzymes that aid in digestion. These enzymes are composed of water, sodium, bicarbonate, and potassium and have an alkaline pH.

2. Endocrine function – Consists of cell types known as the islets of Langerhans that produce specific hormones that empty into the portal vein of the liver and are distributed into the general circulation to reach other target cells. Examples are

Beta cells	Produce insulin
Alpha cells	Produce glucagon
Delta cells	Produce somatostatin
F cells	Secretes polypeptide

Each hormone has specific purposes.

Insulin – Glucose is the primary energy source of the body. Insulin is released to lower rising levels of glucose in the bloodstream by transporting glucose from the bloodstream into the cells to be used for energy or stored for later use. *Glycogen* is an excess of glucose, stored in the liver and muscle cells for use as body fuel when needed. Hyperglycemia will occur if there is an abnormal or insufficient amount of insulin hormone available to decrease high blood glucose levels. Insulin is the only hormone with the ability to directly lower blood glucose levels. Without insulin, cells are deprived of their energy source. The body is forced to break down and use stored fats and proteins as fuel instead of glucose. This process is known as glucogenesis, where ketoacids are converted into glucose.

Glucagon – Has the opposite role of insulin, in that it increases blood sugar levels to prevent hypoglycemia, especially when stimulated by factors such as starvation and exercise. Stored glucose will be broken down (glycogenolysis), and noncarbohydrate molecules will be converted into glucose (glucogenesis).

NURSING ALERT

In a healthy person, insulin is released to decrease high blood glucose levels. When blood glucose levels are low, glucagon is released to increase blood glucose levels.

Somatostatin – A hormone that prevents the release of both insulin and glucagon.

Pancreatic polypeptide – Has the effect of creating smooth muscle relaxation of the gallbladder.

❺ *Interpreting Test Results*

Fasting blood sugar (FBS) – Measures abnormal carbohydrate metabolism after the patient has been fasting for at least 8 hours (patient may have water). Normal value is 70 to 110 mg/dL. An FBS greater than 126 mg/dL on two separate occasions suggests the condition of diabetes mellitus.

Fingerstick glucose test – A convenient, rapid, and economical test that can be done at the bedside or by the patient. Quick, accurate results make it easier to keep track of managing diabetes and provide information for insulin coverage.

Glycosylated hemoglobin (HbA1c) – Normal value is 4% to 7%. A recommended test for follow-up care only, not for an initial diagnosis. This study offers information about the average amount of glucose remaining in the bloodstream for the 120-day lifespan of the red blood cells. Glucose adheres to red blood cells through the process of glycosylation, making it possible for the health care provider to identify if the patient has adhered to diabetic dietary protocols within the 120-day time span.

Postprandial blood sugar (PPBS) – Two hours post meal. A blood sample is drawn after the patient eats a conventional meal or is given a meal containing carbohydrates. Its purpose is to determine the body's response to increases in carbohydrate intake after a meal and how quickly blood sugar levels return to normal. Levels that remain higher than 200 mg/dL after 2 hours suggest diabetes mellitus.

NURSING ALERT

Two-hour postprandial results increase in value by 5 mg/dL for each decade of life. Results of a PPBS for a 60-year-old person will be 15 times higher than that of a 30-year-old person.

Oral glucose tolerance test (OGTT) – Not routinely used but is the gold standard for making the diagnosis of Type 2 diabetes mellitus.

How to Do It–Oral Glucose Tolerance Test (OGTT)

1. Conventional meals are eaten for several days prior to this test. Fasting the night before is recommended. Water intake is allowed.

2. At the beginning of the test an FBS blood sample is obtained and a urine sample collected and tested for glycosuria.

3. The patient is then given 75 to 100 g of flavored glucose dissolved in water. Blood samples are drawn at 1-, 2-, and 3-hour intervals to evaluate the length of time it takes for blood sugars to return to normal levels. Individuals with diabetes mellitus may take longer to return to baseline readings or never return to fasting levels.

Disorders of the Pancreas

Disorders of the Pancreas are characterized by major changes in blood glucose levels as well as in fluid and electrolyte disturbances. Without the necessary insulin, glucose remains in the bloodstream and cells are deprived of energy.

The risk for developing diabetes mellitus (DM) increases with age. It is a metabolic disorder characterized by hyperglycemia and defects in insulin secretion. There are two main types of Diabetes Mellitus: Type 1—Insulin-Dependent Diabetes Mellitus and Type 2—Noninsulin-Dependent Diabetes Mellitus.

Type 1—Insulin-Dependent Diabetes Mellitus, Previously Known as Juvenile Diabetes

What Went Wrong? A complete deficiency of insulin secretion occurs and is caused by destruction of the beta cells of the pancreas. The onset is rapid and acute, usually occurring during childhood or at puberty.

Hallmark Signs and Symptoms Classic symptoms include the 3 Ps: polyphagia (excessive hunger), polydipsia (excessive thirst), and polyuria (excessive urination). Weight loss can occur as the body seeks other sources of energy such as fats and protein. Lifelong insulin replacement therapy is required.

Type 2—Noninsulin-Dependent Diabetes Mellitus, Previously Known as Maturity-Onset Diabetes

What Went Wrong? An insufficient amount of insulin is available to prevent hyperglycemia. Many of those affected can control their illness through diet, exercise, and oral antihyperglycemic medications. Initially, insulin medications may not necessarily be required. Type 2 diabetes mellitus can develop due to obesity or illnesses such as infection, trauma, or a myocardial infarction. It can go undetected for many years and progress slowly. It is best treated with weight loss, exercise, and oral antidiabetic medications.

Hallmark Signs and Symptoms The patient might experience some of the same classic symptoms associated with Type 1 DM. Additional symptoms include fatigue, recurrent infections, prolonged wound healing, and visual changes.

❸ Physical Assessment of the Patient With Diabetes Mellitus A multisystem approach is advised when assessing the patient with diabetes mellitus because glucose dysfunction affects literally every major body system. Obtain a family history to determine if others are also afflicted with DM. Question dietary habits such as too much food or inactivity, specific medications they are taking, symptoms such as the 3 Ps, weight changes, fatigue, blurred vision, frequency of urination, nocturia, chronic vaginitis in women, unhealing wounds, and frequency of dental cavities. Determine status of fluid hydration, skin turgor, weight, vital signs, breathing patterns, neurological status, urine specific gravity, and electrolytes.

Individuals with DM require much education regarding diet and a plan of healthy eating, exercise, foot care, medication administration, obtaining blood sugar levels, wearing a Medical Alert I.D. bracelet, and signs and symptoms of hypo- and hyperglycemia. Signs of hypoglycemia can resemble alcohol intoxication or drunkenness. Hypoglycemia can be quickly reversed by drinking a fast-acting fruit juice or soft drink. Commercial glucose gels and tablets can be purchased and carried around in the event of a hypoglycemic reaction.

Drug Therapy Oral antidiabetic medications are listed in Table 7–6.

TABLE 7–6 Classes of Drugs to Improve Control of Type 2 DM		
Class	**Characteristics**	**Drug Names**
Sulfonylureas – first generation	Increase insulin production from the pancreas For these drugs to be effective, the patient must still have some of his or her own circulating insulin.	Orinase (tolbutamide), Dymelor (acetohexamide), Tolinase (tolazamide), and Diabinese (chlorpropamide)
Sulfonlyureas – second generation	Have fewer side effects and are more potent, but more costly than first-generation sulfonlyureas	Glucotrol, Glucotrol XL (glipizide), Micronase, DiaBeta, Glynase (glyburide), Amaryl (glimepiride)
Meglitinides	Produce a more rapid and shorter–acting release of insulin from the pancreas Teach the patient to take these oral meds 30 minutes before each meal or right at mealtime because they are so short acting	Prandin (repaglinide) and Starlix (nateglinide)
Biguanide	Reduces glucose production by the liver Can be used alone or in combination with insulin or other sulfonylureas	Glucophage (metformin) Glucovance is a combination of metformin with glyburide. Metformin combined with rosiglitazone produces Avandamet and metformin combined with glipizide produces Metaglip
a–Glucosidase inhibitors	Delay the absorption of glucose from the gastrointestinal tract	Acarbose (Precose) and Miglitol (Glyset)

TABLE 7–6 Classes of Drugs to Improve Control of Type 2 DM (*Continued*)

Class	Characteristics	Drug Names
Thiazolidinediones	Promotes effects of insulin at receptor sites, resulting in glycemic control without creating hypoglycemia	Actos (pioglitazone) and Avandia (rosiglitazone)
Dipeptidyl peptidase–4 (DPP–4) inhibitor	Increases and prolongs the action of incretin, a hormone that increases insulin release and decreases glycogen levels, resulting in improved glucose control	Sitagliptin (Januvia) and vildagliptin (Galvus)

Insulin Therapy

Drug	Route of Administration	Action
Regular Iletin Humulin R, Novolin R	IV or subcutaneously Only type of insulin suitable for IV use	Onset 1 hour, peak 2–4 hours, duration 5–8 hours
Lispro (Humalog) Aspart (Novolog)	Subcutaneously	Onset 10–15 minutes, peak 45–60 minutes, duration 1.5–3.5 hours
Lente (Humulin L, Novolin L), semilente insulin	Subcutaneously	Onset 1–3 hours, peak 8–12 hours, duration 18–24 hours
NPH (Humulin N, Novolin N)	Subcutaneously	Onset 3–4 hours, peak 6–12 hours, duration 18–28 hours
Ultralente (Humulin U) Glargine* (Lantus), determir (Levemir)	Subcutaneously	Onset 4–6 hours, peak 18–24 hours, duration 36 hours
Combination therapy (premixed) NPH/Regular 70/30, Ex: (Humulin 70/30, Novolin 70/30) NPH/Regular 50/50 (Humulin 50/50) NPH/Lispro 75/25 (Humalog Mix 75/25)	Subcutaneously	Onset, duration, and peak times vary

*Glargine is given at bedtime and has no peak action.

Insulin Therapy Insulin cannot be taken orally because it will be destroyed by gastric juices. When exercise, diet, and oral agents can no longer maintain satisfactory blood glucose levels, insulin must be administered. The patient is no longer producing his or her own insulin to meet the patient's metabolic needs. Insulin is also required for the management of Type 1 diabetes.

Pramlintide (Symlin) Acts as a synthetic analog of amylin, which is an endogenous pancreatic hormone that aides in the control and management of postprandial hyperglycemia. Used with mealtime insulin, not in place of insulin. Preferrable to inject into the thigh or abdomen because absorption rates vary if injected into the arm. Never inject near an insulin injection site. Can be used with metformin and sulfonlyureas.

Exenatide (Byetta) This drug has been approved for Type 2 diabetes uncontrolled by metformin or a sulfonylurea. Mimics the action of incretin to control blood glucose levels. Injected twice a day within 1 hour before breakfast and dinner. It is not a substitute for insulin in patients who require insulin to control their diabetes.

Liraglutide (Victoza) This drug was recently approved for management of Type 2 diabetes. It is given as a once-daily injection and is not recommended for initial therapy.

Sample Guidelines to Control Glucose Levels With Regular Insulin

151–200 mg/dL: 6 U of regular insulin

201–250 mg/dL: 8 U of regular insulin

251–300 mg/dL: 10 U of regular insulin

301–400 mg/dL: 12 U of regular insulin

NURSING ALERT

Most commercial insulin is available as U 100, which means that 1 mL contains 100 U of insulin. U 100 must be used with a U 100–marked syringe. U 50 syringes may be used for doses of 50 U or less.

Alternate Insulin Delivery Methods

An insulin pen is a compact needle and syringe preloaded with insulin carried by the user in the event of an emergency (e.g., Novo Pen Insulin).

Insulin pump continuously infuses insulin subcutaneously and promotes the potential for tighter glucose control. It is a small battery-operated device worn on the belt and connected by a small plastic tube to a catheter inserted into the subcutaneous tissue of the abdominal wall (e.g., InDuo).

Complications of Insulin Therapy

1. Allergic reactions – Local reactions to insulin administration could include inflammation, burning, itching, or redness around the injection site. Could improve with a low dose of antihistamine. Urticaria or hives can signal a more systemic reaction, with anaphylactic shock occurring from the use of animal insulin.

2. Lipodystrophy – Hypertrophy or atrophy of subcutaneous tissue if the same injection site is frequently used. Hypertrophy is a thickening of subcutaneous tissue that can result in poor insulin absorption.

3. Somogyi effect – There is an undetected decrease in glucose levels during the hours of sleep in response to too much insulin. Specific hormones are released that produce a rebound hyperglycemia noticed in the morning when glucose levels are measured. The danger exists when the insulin dose is increased. The patient might complain of headache, night sweats, or nightmares upon awakening. Patient glucose levels should be assessed between 2 and 4 AM to determine if hypoglycemia is present. If so, the insulin dosage affecting the early morning blood glucose is reduced.

4. Dawn phenomenon – Also characterized by hyperglycemia upon awakening due to the release of growth hormone (GH) and cortisol in the pre-dawn hours. Treatment consists of increasing insulin dosage or the timing of insulin administration. Blood glucose levels should be assessed at bedtime, nighttime (between 2 and 4 AM), and morning fasting blood sugar. If predawn levels are less than 60 mg/dL and signs of hypoglycemia are present, the insulin dosage should be reduced. If the 2 and 4 AM blood glucose is high, insulin dosage should be increased.

Hypoglycemia

Glucose levels drop below 50 to 70 mg/mL or lower from taking too much insulin, eating late or skipping meals, and excessive unplanned exercise. Symptoms of hypoglycemia can occur quickly. They include pallor, confusion, slurred speech, palpitation, tremor, diaphoresis, hunger, anxiety, numbness, and tingling in extremities. Patients can even have seizures and lose consciousness. It is recommended that patients carry snacks or candy when out and about for a quick glucose fix between meals.

Gestational Diabetes

May develop during pregnancy; however, mother's condition returns to normal post delivery. Trends show that 40% to 60% of these women will develop diabetes later in life.

Impaired Glucose Tolerance

This condition involves no signs or symptoms of diabetes except high glucose levels. These patients are referred to as borderline diabetic because their blood sugar levels are not high enough to classify or treat them as diabetics.

Complications of Diabetes Mellitus

Serious illnesses requiring critical care can develop. Neuropathy, retinopathy, nephropathy, peripheral and cardiovascular diseases, hypertension, and hyperlipidemia are some examples.

DKA (Diabetic Ketoacidosis) Diabetic ketoacidosis is an acute complication of diabetes mellitus.

What Went Wrong? DKA is a severe disorder state of fat, carbohydrate, and protein metabolism caused by extreme insulin deficiency that manifests as severe hyperglycemia, metabolic acidosis, and fluid and electrolyte imbalances. It is a life-threatening event, especially to the patient with Type 1 insulin-dependent diabetes mellitus.

With hyperglycemia, excessive glucose rapidly escapes into the urine (glycosuria) because the filtering capacity of the kidneys is decreased and glucose cannot be reabsorbed into the bloodstream. Excessive glycosuria and hyperglycemia leads to electrolyte and *volume depletion*, as the patient with unregulated diabetes mellitus cannot ingest enough sodium bicarbonate and water to compensate for fluid and electrolyte losses.

1. As DKA progresses, ketoacidosis occurs due to the accumulation of highly acidic substances in the bloodstream (ketonemia) and the urine (ketonuria) faster than they can be metabolized.

2. Ketoacids are excreted in the urine as Na, K^+, and ammonium salts.

3. Respirations are affected as the body attempts to compensate for a carbonic acid buildup. Breathing becomes deep and rapid (Kussmaul's respirations) in an effort to release the carbonic acid in the form of carbon dioxide. Acetone is exhaled, giving the breath a sweet, fruity odor. It is the body's attempt to maintain a normal pH during the throes of metabolic acidosis.

❸ *Hallmark Signs and Symptoms* In addition to the initial symptoms of diabetes mellitus, which are unexplained weight loss and the 3 Ps of polyphagia (excessive hunger), polydipsia (excessive thirst), and polyuria (excessive urination), the patient with DKA will also experience nausea, vomiting, extreme fatigue, headache, and dehydration. The patient can become stuporous and unconscious, slipping quickly into a coma. The nurse, on inspection, will also observe flushed, dry skin; sunken eyeballs; poor skin turgor taking more than 3 seconds to return; parched lips; tachycardia; hypotension; variations in body temperature; and continued air hunger or Kussmaul's respirations.

❺ *Interpreting Test Results* DKA is rapidly confirmed through urine ketone testing and fingerstick blood sugar analysis. Decreased arterial blood gas pH and low bicarbonate levels are also evident with DKA. BUN, specific gravity, hematocrit, and serum osmolality increase. Sodium and potassium levels decrease.

Emergency medical management is needed to reverse ketoacidosis. Insulin and intravenous solutions are given to reduce hyperglycemia and restore fluid volume and electrolyte balance. Gastric motility is affected with DKA and the patient might require a nasogastric tube to decompress the stomach and relieve the patient of gastric distention, abdominal pain, tenderness, vomiting, blood-positive gastric contents, and paralytic ileus.

A Foley catheter needs to be inserted for accurate measurement of intake and output to determine fluid volume status and renal functioning. Skin assessment for moisture or dryness determines fluid volume distribution throughout the body.

Oral care is provided to moisten dry mucous membranes. Monitor vital signs to assess cardiac responses to fluid replacement. Signs of circulatory fluid overload include moist lung sounds, dyspnea without exertion, and neck vein engorgement.

Prognosis

Mortality rates are less than 5% in cases of DKA if underlying causes are identified and prevented through appropriate patient education.

HHNS (Hyperosmolar Hyperglycemic Nonketotic Syndrome)

What Went Wrong? The primary difference in this syndrome is that the patient with diabetes still has enough circulating insulin to prevent DKA, but not enough to prevent severe hyperglycemia, osmotic diuresis, and severe dehydration. A deficit of insulin and an excess of glucagon exist. Extracellular fluid loss can be as great as 9 L.

Hyperglycemic values can exceed 2,000 mg/dL, while hyperosmolality values can be as high as 350 mOsm/kg. The mortality rate with this syndrome exceeds the mortality rate of DKA.

The patient develops lactic acidosis from poor tissue perfusion and not ketoacidosis. An increase in hepatic glucose production occurs, dehydration worsens, and confusion, lethargy, and seizures result due to CNS dysfunction. Hemoconcentration of the blood can cause major organ infarctions and thromboemboli.

Secondary causes of HHNS include other illnesses such as stroke, MI, pancreatitis, trauma, sepsis, burns, or pneumonia. Dietary supplements such as TPN (a prolonged intravenous hypertonic glucose infusion), excessive carbohydrate intake from tube feedings, or peritoneal and hemodialysis can also create this syndrome.

Most of the signs are the same as with DKA except for the absence of Kussmaul's respirations and it takes longer to develop as compared to DKA. Volume depletion is usually greater in HHNS than in DKA but fluids should be replaced gradually to prevent fluid overload. Patients should be placed on seizure precautions.

Prognosis
There is a mortality rate of 10–40% primarily because of delays in seeking medical help, underlying illnesses and vulnerability of the elderly patient.

❹ Nursing Diagnosis for DM	Expected Outcomes
Risk for infection related to hyperglycemia and an open, unhealed foot ulcer	Signs of infection will be resolved
	Wound foot ulcer will show signs of healing
	Glucose levels will be within normal limits

Nursing Interventions
Use fingerstick glucose testing to obtain and evaluate blood glucose levels daily.

Administer prescribed antidiabetic and antibiotic medications.

Provide sterile wound care daily to open foot ulcer.

Examine wound for signs of infection, for example, warmth, redness, swelling, pain, odor, and purulent drainage.

Teach the benefits of proper foot care, for example, wash feet daily with warm soap and water. Do not walk barefoot. Do not wear tight-fitting shoes. Cut toenails straight across. Examine for unusual discoloration and openings.

❶ Adrenal Glands

There are two glands, one each perched on top of each kidney and composed of an

1. Outer layer or cortex – Produces aldosterone (mineralcorticoids) that regulate sodium and potassium balance and cortisol (glucocorticoids) that regulates metabolism, increases in blood glucose levels, and CNS responses to stress. Also produced are the androgens, which contribute to male and female growth and development and to sexual activity in adult women.

Progesterone, estrogen, and testosterone are the androgens. Production of these sex hormones increase when there is hyperplasia of the adrenal glands, which is verifiable through a urine test—17-ketosteroid (17-KS).

2. Inner core or medulla – Secretes catecholamines such as epinephrine, norepinephrine, and dopamine.

❺ Interpreting Test Results

1. Cortisol (hydrocortisone) – Elevated in adrenal hyperfunction and decreased in adrenal hypofunction. An excess secretion of ACTH by the pituitary gland can indicate Cushing's syndrome. Other causes of an elevation can result from high stress, trauma, and surgery. Adrenal hypofunction can be caused by anterior pituitary hyposecretion, hepatitis, and cirrhosis. Cortisol secretion is higher from 6 to 8 AM and lower from 4 to 6 PM, so this is when blood samples are drawn for analysis. Normal morning values are 138 to 635 mmol/L, and 83 to 44 mmol/L are the normal afternoon values.

2. Cortisol (dexamethasone) suppression – The test of choice to diagnose Cushing's syndrome. A low dose of Decadron, similar to cortisol, is given at bedtime and blood samples are drawn the next day at 8 AM and 4 PM. ACTH is suppressed in a healthy person. However, those with adrenal hyperfunction will continue to produce ACTH with no variation of levels occurring in the AM and PM readings. Medications such as estrogen, Dilantin, and cortisol-related products are discontinued 24 to 38 hours prior to this test. Radioisotopes *should not* be given within 1 week of this test.

3. Cortisol stimulation – The preferred test to diagnose Addison's disease. The response of the adrenal gland to a synthetic ACTH preparation such as Cortrosyn (cosyntropin) is measured. Cortrosyn is given I.M. or I.V. The dose is usually 0.25 mg. A fasting 8 AM cortisol level is drawn prior to giving Cortrosyn and then blood samples are taken 30 and 60 minutes after it is administered. The standard cortisol level is 20 mcg/dL. A normal response to the Cortrosyn synthetic drug will be an increase 2-3 times over the baseline level. If the gland is dysfunctional, the level will decrease or be absent in people with adrenal insufficiency hypopituitarism. Long-term steroid therapy will affect the results. The test should not be done if the patient has an inflammation or infection.

4. Urine vanillymandelic acid and catecholamine levels – A metabolite of catecholamine, it is highly concentrated in the urine. It is a 24-hour urine test done when hypertension in an individual is suspected of being caused by pheochromocytoma. Elevated levels are noted in patients with hypothyroidism, DKA, neuroblastomas, and ganglioneuromas. Certain foods

that may have an effect on the test results, such as tea, coffee, vanilla, and fruit juice, might be restricted for 2 days before and on the day of testing. Certain drugs may also be discontinued for 4 to 7 days before testing. Normal adult values for urine vanillymandelic acid are 2 to 7 mg/24 hr and for catecholamine 270 fg/24 hr.

5. Urine 17-ketosteroids and 17-hydroxycorticosteroids – These are 24-hour urine collection tests done to determine adrenal function by measuring the urinary excretion of steroids.

6. Adrenal scan – Done to determine tumor areas or sites that produce or hypersecrete catecholamines. An IV radioisotope (131I) is injected and scans are done on days 2, 3, and 4.

7. CT scan and MRI – Done of the skull and adrenal glands to detect tumors or pathology of both the pituitary and adrenal glands.

8. Electrolyte studies – Indicate an elevated BUN, hyponatremia, hyperkalemia, decreased bicarbonate levels, hypoglycemia, anemia, lymphocytosis, and eosinophilia. Metabolic acidosis may occur because of dehydration.

Adrenal Gland Dysfunction

Addison's Disease This is a primary *hypofunction* of the adrenal cortex or a secondary cause of adrenocortical insufficiency of the pituitary gland. It is also known as hypoadrenalism or hypocorticism.

What Went Wrong? With a primary cause, adrenal gland destruction occurs from antibodies attacking the patient's own adrenal cortex. Tuberculosis (TB), AIDS, hemorrhage from anticoagulant therapy, fungal infections, sarcoidosis, and adrenalectomy are a few causes.

With a secondary cause, pituitary/hypothalamic involvement occurs as a complication of cortisol therapy, lung or breast cancer, infection, basilar skull fractures, surgery, chemotherapy, or radiation. A rare but life-threatening condition, symptoms are not visible until 90% of the adrenal cortex has been destroyed. Therefore, the onset of symptoms is slow and the illness is often advanced before it is diagnosed.

❸ *Hallmark Signs and Symptoms* Clinical symptoms include progressive weakness, fatigue, weight loss, and anorexia. Hyperpigmentation of the skin is evident over bone joints and in the palmar creases of the hands. Hypotension, hyponatremia, hyperkalemia, nausea, vomiting, and diarrhea can also occur.

Complications of Addison's Disease—Addisonian Crisis This is a life-threatening emergency caused by an abrupt decrease in circulating adrenocortical hormones triggered by stressors of trauma, post adrenal surgery or infections, sudden pituitary gland destruction, or the sudden withdrawal of corticoid steroid hormone replacement therapy. Circulatory collapse and hypotension can lead to shock and a general unresponsiveness to fluid replacement and vasopressin therapy. The most common form of treatment is to administer hydrocortisone because it contains glucocorticoids and mineralcorticoid properties. Intravenous fluid therapy is given to reverse hypotension and electrolyte imbalances.

Prognosis

The onset of symptoms tend to be slow and the illness well advanced before it is diagnosed.

Cushing's Syndrome

What Went Wrong? Excessive levels of corticosteroids contribute to a condition of adrenal hyperfunction caused by exogenous factors such as the prolonged use of a corticosteroid medication such as prednisone, used to treat an inflammatory illness or arthritis, and endogenous factors such as an ACTH-secreting pituitary tumor, adrenal tumors, or lung or pancreatic cancer.

Hallmark Signs and Symptoms Symptoms include changes in physical appearance such as weight gain from sodium and water retention, leading to hypertension; a full, rounded and reddened moon face; a buffalo hump or fat accumulation in the trunk, face, and cervical area; purplish striae on the abdomen, breast, or buttocks; hyperglycemia muscle wasting and weakness in the extremities; bone and back pain from possible osteoporosis or pathologic fractures; thin skin; poor wound healing due to the loss of collagen; and quick bruising. Additional symptoms include unwanted, excessive facial hair (hirsutism) and menstrual difficulties in women; gynecomastia and impotence in men; insomnia; anxiety; and mood swings of depression, irritability and euphoria. Symptoms of diabetes mellitus could also be apparent because glucocorticoid hormones oppose the action of insulin.

Treatment depends on the cause of the problem with the goal of normalizing hormone secretions by suppressing cortisol production. Certain medications are given, such as mitotane (Lysodren), metyrapone ketoconazole (Nizoral), and aminoglutethimide (Cytadren).

Prognosis

Cushing's syndrome might improve if the chronic use of steroid medications could be prescribed to be taken every other day or the high doses of these medications could be tapered down. A diet high in protein and potassium but low in calories, carbohydrates, and sodium is provided. Surgery is recommended if the cause of Cushing's syndrome is an adenoma.

Nursing Diagnosis	Expected Outcomes
Cushing's syndrome—disturbed physical appearance	Patient will show a gradual loss of body weight
	A generalized improvement of physical appearance will occur
	Muscle strength will be increased
	Patient will develop a more positive body image

Nursing Interventions

Provide a low calorie, high vitamin diet.

Monitor daily weights.

Limit water intake *to reduce sodium and water retention.*

Measure intake and output.

Assess for signs of edema.

Encourage self-care methods *to improve personal appearance, such as good grooming and attractive clothing.*

Teach and practice range of motion exercises to improve muscle strength and dexterity.

Hyperaldosteronism

What Went Wrong? The culprit is an oversecretion of the aldosterone hormone produced by the adrenal glands. The syndrome results from sodium retention and excretion of potassium by the kidneys.

Primary causes of this disorder include adrenal tumors or adrenal hyperplasia (Conn's syndrome).

Secondary causes of this disorder could be a nonadrenal reason such as renal stenosis, chronic renal disease, and renin-secreting tumors.

❸ *Hallmark Signs and Symptoms* Hypernatremia, hypertension, and headache are caused by sodium retention. An increased loss of potassium creates hypokalemia and the additional symptoms of muscle weakness, fatigue, glucose intolerance, and metabolic alkalosis, which could further lead to cramps, tetany, or cardiac arrhythmias.

❺ *Interpreting Test Results* Normal aldosterone value is 2 to 9 ng/dL. Levels greater than 10 ng/dL signify hyperaldosteronism. Levels higher than 50 ng/dL indicate an adenoma.

A surgical adrenalectomy is usually the recommended treatment of choice. Prior to surgery, the patient is placed on a low-sodium diet and potassium-sparing diuretics such as

Aldactone (spironolactone)

Inspra (eplerenone)

Midamor (amiloride)

Cytadren (aminoglutethimide)

Antihypertensive medications are also administered.

Pheochromocytoma

What Went Wrong?   This is a tumor of the adrenal medulla that produces an excessive release of catecholamines such as epinephrine and norepinephrine, resulting in severe hypertension. Consequences of undiagnosed and untreated pheochromocytoma include diabetes mellitus, cardiomegaly, uncontrolled hypertension, and death.

Hallmark Signs and Symptoms   Profuse diaphoresis, tachycardia, anxiety, palpitations, pallor, tremors, weakness, nausea, chest or abdominal pain, and a severe, pounding headache. These attacks can be brought on by opioids, antihypertensives, radiologic contrast dye, and tricyclic antidepressants and can last from a few minutes to several hours.

Interpreting Test Results   CAT scans and MRI will be used to localize a suspected tumor. A 24-hour urine test to determine excessive levels of catecholamines or their metabolites is conducted and will show elevated results in a person with pheochromocytoma.

Prognosis

This type of endocrine tumor is successfully treated through surgical intervention.

CASE STUDY

J.F.K., a 64-year-old male, is admitted to the critical care unit in Addisonian crisis. He is exhibiting signs of tachycardia and extreme dehydration. Laboratory results reveal the electrolyte imbalances of hyponatremia, hyperkalemia, and hypoglycemia.

QUESTIONS
1. Discuss the initial care protocols for this patient.
2. What are the causes of Addison's disease?
3. How much of the adrenal gland is destroyed before clinical signs and symptoms of Addison's disease become apparent?
4. Discuss expected laboratory findings.
5. Develop an correctly written nursing diagnosis for this individual.

REVIEW QUESTIONS

1. Which of the following discharge instructions would be appropriate for the nurse to provide to a patient following a thyroidectomy?   **Select all that apply.**

   A. Report signs and symptoms of hypoglycemia.

   B. Take thyroid replacement medication as ordered.

   C. Report changes to the doctor such as lethargy, intolerance to cold, dry skin.

   D. Avoid all over-the-counter (OTC) medication.

   E. Carry injectable Decadron at all times.

2. A patient is to receive 10 U of regular insulin for a blood glucose level of 365 mg/dL. The vial is labeled 100 U/mL. How many milliliters of insulin should the nurse administer?

   A. 1 mL

   B. 0.5 mL

   C. 0.1 mL

   D. 0.375 mL

3. Which of the following findings should the nurse expect to find when assessing a newly admitted patient diagnosed with diabetes insipidus? Select all that apply.

   A. Extreme polyuria

   B. Excessive thirst

   C. Elevated systolic blood pressure

   D. Low urine specific gravity

   E. Bradycardia

   F. Elevated serum potassium level

4. Which of the following patient findings should alert the nurse of inadequate thyroid replacement therapy? Select all that apply.

   A. Tachycardia

   B. Low body temperature

   C. Nervousness

   D. Bradycardia and constipation

   E. Dry mouth

5. A 50-year-old woman seeks medical attention for the following symptoms: ravenous appetite with a 20-lb weight loss within the past month. A diagnosis of Graves' disease is confirmed. What other signs and symptoms of Graves' disease would the nurse expect to find? Select all that apply.

   A. Rapid, bounding pulse

   B. Bradycardia and constipation

   C. Heat intolerance

   D. Tremors and nervousness

6. The nurse teaches a preoperative patient that the surgical approach of choice for an hypophysectomy is accomplished via
    A. Laparoscopy
    B. Burr holes
    C. Stereotactic
    D. Transphenoid approach

7. The nurse knows that the purpose of medication therapy in the patient with acromegaly is to
    A. Reduce GH levels of production and secretion.
    B. Increase GH levels of production and secretion.
    C. Regulate glucose intake.
    D. Replace gonadotropin hormones.

8. The nurse should provide what information when teaching the diabetic patient about hypoglycemia?   **Select all that apply.**
    A. Excessive alcohol consumption can create hypoglycemia.
    B Skipping meals could lead to hypoglycemia.
    C. Thirst and excessive urination are symptoms of hypoglycemia.
    D. Strenuous activity can precipitate hypoglycemia.
    E. Symptoms of hypoglycemia include shakiness, confusion, and headache.
    F. Hypoglycemia is a harmless condition.

9. Which of the following electrolytes would the nurse expect to be abnormal in the patient with a parathyroid hormone (PTH) deficiency?   **Select all that apply.**
    A. Sodium
    B. Potassium
    C. Calcium
    D. Glucose
    E. Phosphorous

10. After a recent head injury, a patient develops SIADH. Which findings indicate to the nurse that the treatment the patient is receiving for this condition is effective?   **Select all that apply.**
    A. Decrease in body weight
    B. Increased blood pressure and decreased pulse
    C. Moist wheezes
    D. Increase in urine output
    E. Decrease in urine osmolality

ANSWERS

CASE STUDY

1. Management of an Addisonian crisis includes monitoring serum cortisol levels and hormone replacement therapy by administering a glucocorticoid such as Solu-Cortef. Start an intravenous infusion of 5% dextrose and sodium as fluid volume replacement and to correct imbalances of hyponatremia and hypoglycemia. Do not anticipate giving potassium because the patient is hyperkalemic. Mr. J.F.K. may require as much as 5 L of fluid replacement in the first 12 to 24 hours of his admission due to extreme fluid volume deficits. Especially monitor accurate intake and output. Provide close cardiac monitoring as there is a potential for the development of dysrhythmias such as heart block, bradycardia, ventricular fibrillation, and sinus arrest.

2. Causes of Addison's disease include autoimmune infections such as AIDS, tuberculosis (TB), sarcoidosis, hemorrhage from trauma such as postpartum Sheehan's syndrome, cancer, radiation, developmental or congenital abnormality, barbiturate medications, and long-term steroid use.

3. Clinical signs and symptoms of Addison's disease appear after 90% of the adrenal gland is destroyed.

4. Expected laboratory findings would include pH less than 7.3, BUN greater than 20 mg/dL due to protein breakdown and hemoconcentration, Na^+ less than 150 mEq/L, K^+ greater than 6.5 mEq/L, glucose less than 50 mg/dL, and cortisol less than 10 mg/dL.

5.

❺ Nursing Diagnosis	Expected Outcomes
Knowledge deficit related to long-term use of corticosteroids	Patient will state the need for corticosteroid therapy as a lifelong process
	Patient will follow appropriate medication guidelines for proper administration
	Fluid volume deficits will be restored to normal levels
	Electrolyte imbalances will remain within normal limits

Nursing Interventions

Monitor and measure fluid volume status through accurate intake and output.

Obtain and review cortisol levels, BUN, and electrolytes.

Provide patient education by teaching actions and side effects of prescribed corticosteroid medications.

Obtain and wear a Medical Alert bracelet identifying the disease process and emergency care guidelines.

CORRECT ANSWERS AND RATIONALES

1. B and C. Thyroid replacement medication needs to be taken after a thyroidectomy. Physical symptoms of lethargy, dry skin, and intolerance to cold may signal the need for a higher dosage of medication. Some nonaspirin OTC meds are allowable for discomfort, such as acetaminophen.

2. C. Use the following equation to calculate the correct administration amount:
   $x = \text{unknown}/10\ U = 1\ mL/100\ U$
   Then cross-multiply $100 \times \text{units} = 10\ U \times 1\ mL = 10/100$.
   Divide both sides by 100 to solve for $x = 10/100$. Result = 0.1 mL.

3. A, B, and D. Diabetes insipidus has an abrupt onset of polyuria, polydipsia, dry skin and mucous membranes, tachycardia, and hypotension. Diagnostic studies reveal a low urine specific gravity and osmolality and an elevated serum sodium level. The serum potassium level will be decreased, not increased.

4. B and D. The body is in a hypometabolic state when a person is hypothyroid and has symptoms of subnormal body temperature, constipation, and bradycardia.

5. A, C, and D. Graves' disease is a state of hypermetabolic hyperthyroidism and has symptoms of a rapid, bounding pulse; tremors; nervousness; and heat intolerance.

6. D. With the transphenoidal approach, an incision is made in the inner aspect of the upper lip and gingiva. The sella turcica is entered through the floor of the nose and sphenoid sinuses.

7. A. Since an overproduction of GH causes acromegaly, the purpose of medication therapy is to reduce the GH levels of production and secretion.

8. A, B, D, and E. Alcohol consumption, missed meals, and strenuous activity can cause hypoglycemia. Signs of hypoglycemia include headache, confusion, shakiness, and circumoral tingling sensations. Hypoglycemia is not harmless. It can result in seizures and death of brain cells if untreated.

9. C and E. PTH regulates the calcium and phosphorous electrolytes. The other electrolytes are not controlled or affected by the parathyroid hormone.

10. A, C, D, and E. SIADH is an excessive release of ADH with symptoms of water retention, edema, oliguria, and weight gain. Successful treatment should result in a loss of weight, increased urine output, and a decrease in urine concentration or osmolality.

chapter 8

Care of the Patient With Critical Renal Needs

At the end of this chapter, the student will be able to:

1. Identify nursing assessment skills needed to care for the patient with critical renal needs.

2. Discuss common laboratory and diagnostic tools used to confirm renal failure.

3. Relate the use of commonly used medications to the care of the patient in renal failure.

4. Differentiate between the different types of dialysis relating the nursing care involved with each.

5. Describe differences between acute and chronic renal failure including causes, prognosis, treatment, and nursing care.

6. Recall the symptoms of uremia according to body systems.

7. Identify ECG/EKG changes with hyperkalemia and treatment involved in reducing the potassium level.

8. Given a case study, prioritize collaborative and nursing care of the patient requiring dialysis.

KEY WORDS

ADH – antidiuretic hormone
ARF – acute renal failure
Arteriovenous (AV) fistula
Arteriovenous (AV) graft
ATN – acute tubular necrosis
Bruit
CRRT – continuous renal replacement therapy
Disequilibrium syndrome
ESRD – end-stage renal disease
FENa – fractional excretion of sodium
Fluid rebound
GFR – glomerular filtration rate

Hemodialysis
High-ceiling diuretics
KUB – kidney ureter bladder x-ray
Kussmaul's respirations
PD – peritoneal dialysis
Peritonitis
RAAS – renin-angiotension-aldosterone system
Renal osteodystrophy
Steal syndrome
Thrill
Vascular access sites

Anatomy and Physiology of the Renal System

The kidneys are two pear-shaped organs that lie in the superior, posterior abdomen or retroperitoneal space. They are coated with a protective layer of fat, which also covers the adrenal glands sitting on top of the kidneys. The kidneys contain 2 to 3 million functional units called the nephrons (see Figure 8–1).

The microscopic nephron contains an afferent arteriole that brings arterial blood to the glomerulus. The glomerulus is a tough working network that is encapsulated by Bowman's capsule. The job of the glomerulus is to filter out waste products that are molecularly small. It is the glomerular filtration rate (GFR) that determines the quality of kidney functioning.

GFR is dependent on the glomerular filtration, the pressure in Bowman's capsule, and the plasma oncotic pressure (pressure of the plasma proteins). A mean arterial BP must be maintained between 80 and 100 mm Hg to sustain blood flow to the kidneys. Because they are large particles, blood and protein cells are too large to filter out; therefore, they stay in the intravascular space, not the filtrate. The filtrate in the glomerulus starts the production of urine.

Once the filtrate proceeds to the proximal convoluted tube, it collects more sodium and water. The next stop for the filtrate is the loop of Henle, which is thinner and reabsorbs additional water. The loop of Henle is where loop diuretics work enhancing excretion of water.

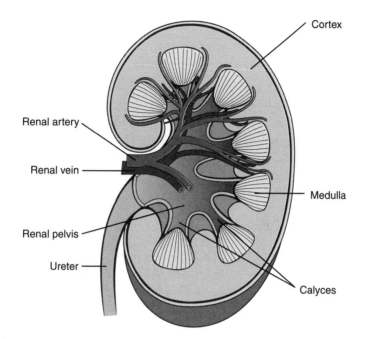

FIGURE 8–1 • Anatomy of the kidney.

Filtrate then travels to the distal convoluted tubule where sodium continues to be reabsorbed through active transport. Hydrogen, potassium, and uric acid are added to the urine by tubular secretion. Thiazide diuretics work in the distal tubule and H⁺ ions are also excreted for compensation during an acidosis.

Hormonal influences on the kidney depend on antidiuretic hormone (ADH) and the renin-angiotension-aldosterone system (RAAS). Hormonal control of the kidney is regulated by ADH secreted by the posterior pituitary gland. When there is an increase in serum osmolality, as with dehydration, the collecting tubes in the kidney increase their permeability to water, which concentrates the filtrate, ultimately causing the kidney to conserve water. Once the serum volume increases, the process stops.

The RAAS is stimulated when there is a decreased GFR as with sympathetic stimulation, as shown in the following box. In response to decreased blood flow, renin is secreted, which converts angiotension I in the liver to angiotension II in the pulmonary capillary beds. Angiotension II is a strong vasoconstrictor that increases SVR (systemic vascular resistance), increasing BP. This part of the system is short acting to increase fluid retention when the GFR drops.

Longer-term fluid retention is influenced by aldosterone, a mineralocorticoid excreted by the adrenal glands. An increased aldosterone leads to retention of water at the distal tubule, which again conserves sodium and water. The RAAS system does an excellent job in conserving water and sodium to increase intra-vascular volume when activated in hemorrhagic shock or dehydration. However, this system creates a vicious cycle of unwanted sodium and fluid retention when a poorly pumping heart is the culprit in dropping the GFR. Fluid and salt retention can quickly lead to heart failure and cardiogenic shock, especially in the patient with acute or chronic renal failure. Therefore, the RAAS is helpful in any type of shock except cardiogenic.

Renin-Angiotension-Aldosterone System

Decreased arterial BP
Decreased GFR
Increase in renin secretion
Increase in angiotension I
Increase in angiotension II
↓

Decrease in water and salt excretion   Increase in aldosterone
Concentration of urine excreted   Increase in water and salt reabsorption
(short term)   (Longer-term fluid retention)

Results in
↓
Increased intravascular volume
Increased GFR

The kidneys are essential organs impacting all body systems. The work of the kidneys is extensive, including

Excreting waste products and excess fluid in the urine

Maintaining water balance and controlling BP

Controlling electrolytes levels

Maintaining acid-base balance

Stimulating production of red blood cells through erythropoietin

Activating vitamin D synthesis

Secreting prostaglandins and growth hormones

Circulation to the kidneys is supplied by the renal artery, which branches from the abdominal aorta just above the mesenteric arteries. The kidneys receive one-quarter of the blood into the renal artery, which articulates with the afferent arteriole. Blood leaves the kidney through the renal veins, which return blood to the left side of the heart through the inferior vena cava.

> ### NURSING ALERT
>
> *Any surgery that involves decreasing blood supply to the kidney can potentially cause renal failure. Types of surgeries notorious for doing this are abdominal aortic aneurysm repair and open-heart surgeries.*

Assessment Skills

❶ Failing kidneys can affect all body systems, making a thorough history and physical of the patient important in determining the presence, extent, and complications of renal failure. The correct order of performing this assessment should proceed from inspection and auscultation to percussion and then palpation.

Patient History

A patient history should include height and weight patterns and past medical history for ureteral calculi, tumor, glomerulonephritis, cystic kidney disease, heart problems, diabetes, and hypertension. Patients at highest risk for renal failure are those with diabetes, hypertension, glomerulonephritis, and cystic kidney disease.

A nutritional assessment should obtain information about the patient's weight history and previous diets; food intake patterns; social economic status; and living arrangements. This information becomes important if the patient needs to be placed on special diets like protein sparing and potassium-sodium limiting to control edema and uremia. Inquire about weight gain and voiding patterns, which can develop if fluid is retained. Patients who develop uremia often describe having little appetite, nausea, and vomiting, which leads to impaired nutrition and fluid/electrolyte issues.

Ask the patient what medications he or she is taking and if they are nephrotoxic. Medications that can cause nephrotoxicity include aminoglycoside antibiotics, cephalosporins, sulfonamides, thiazide diuretics, and phenytoin.

Has the patient had recent tests where potentially nephrotoxic dye was injected like a cardiac catheterization or renal arteriogram? Dyes used in these tests are frequent causes of acute tubular necrosis (ATN) leading to kidney failure.

Ask patients if they have had changes in sexual habits like impotence or decreased sexual energy/drive, dysmenorrheal, or amenorrhea. Uremic poisoning can cause issues with sexual health.

Inspection

A close look at the patient can tell the astute critical care nurse a wealth of information. All body systems need to be inspected. Some of the following signs/symptoms can be seen in patients with renal disease.

Determine the patient's level of consciousness and reasoning. High levels of retained by-products of metabolism like urea and nitrogen can lead to changes in sleep patterns, fatigue, lethargy, headaches, blurred vision, confusion, and consciousness. They can also lead to symptoms of anxiety, depression, and psychosis.

Observe the patient for tremors or spasms. Hypocalcemia that can develop in renal failure can cause neuromuscular excitability, resulting in cells depolarizing unchecked. Placing an inflated BP cuff over an arm for 10 minutes can stimulate Trousseau's sign, which looks like carpopedal spasms, a clinical sign of tetany. The patient may also tell you that he or she has numbness and tingling (paresthesias) around the mouth or extremities. Tapping on the patient's facial nerve can also cause twitching of the facial muscles, which is known as Chvostek's sign. A calcium level should be checked as these muscular contractions can lead to seizure if not treated.

> ### NURSING ALERT
>
> *If the patient has a positive Chvostek's and Trousseau's sign, he or she is at risk for laryngospasm. Have intubation and cardiac arrest equipment available; notify the health care provider immediately.*

Look at the overall color of the patient's skin. A pale or sallow complexion can indicate renal-failure-induced anemia. Is the skin moist and intact? Frequently, patients with renal diseases will develop pruritus and have dry, itchy skin with areas of excoriation. Does the patient have periorbital, sacral, or pedal edema; is it pitting or nonpitting? Edema in the extremities can indicate fluid retention when failing kidneys stop excreting excess fluid.

Next, focus in on the patient's breathing; is the rate easy and unlabored? Compensation for metabolic acidosis can be seen by an increased rate and depth of breathing (Kussmaul's respirations). Kussmaul's respirations are caused by excessive building up of metabolic by-products leading to an increased respiratory rate to compensate with a respiratory alkalosis. The patient may also have a foul odor to his or her breath from urea exiting the body (uremic fetor). Ask the patient if he or she gets short of breath and if so, when it occurs—with rest or exercise? In renal difficulties, the lack of erythropoietin stimulation can lead to a reduction in red blood cell production, resulting in hypoxemia. Compensation for the lack of oxygen stimulates increased breathing.

Look at the patient's neck veins; are they flat or are the jugular veins enlarged when the patient is at high Fowler's position? Jugular venous distention (JVD) will result from the right side of the heart's inability to pump excess fluid from renal failure.

Next, focus on an abdominal assessment noting symmetry and contour; are there any scars, bruises, or abnormalities? Examine the abdomen, asking the patient if this is normal for him or her. Is it tense and shiny? This can indicate ascites, which can occur with fluid-retaining kidney conditions.

Look at the arms; if the patient has an arteriovenous (AV) graft for dialysis, you can see that the veins on the affected side are larger than those on the other arm. Make sure it is clearly communicated to the health care team that this arm should not be used for IVs, venipunctures, or BP. Doing these procedures can prevent clotting of these much-needed dialysis patient access lines or lifelines.

Auscultation

Take the patient's BP, noting the baseline or changes from normal. Is the patient hypertensive? Many patients with renal problems retain fluid, which increases intravascular volume raising the BP. Next, check the lungs for sounds of fluid by listening for crackles, gurgles, or wheezing. They can indicate that the patient has excessive retained fluid, too.

Auscultation is also used to determine if an AV fistula or graft for hemodialysis is functioning normally. It may be necessary to use a Doppler to detect a bruit or swishing sound in a new vascular access until spasm from the surgery diminishes.

NURSING ALERT

An AV fistula or graft patency is determined by auscultating a bruit and palpating a thrill over the access site. Absence of a bruit or thrill should be reported to the vascular surgeon/nephrologist immediately. The site may be thrombosed and can be reopened if discovered early. Otherwise the patient will need a temporary access site and a new permanent access site. Never use these sites for phlebotomy, IVs, or BPs. They can traumatize the access and set up clotting.

Normally the nurse will not auscultate any sounds over the kidneys. However, if the patient has renal artery stenosis a bruit may be heart over the left and right upper abdominal quadrants.

Percussion

Ask the patient to void before the percussion. Percussion of the kidneys may be done to check for enlargement from polycystic disease. Does the patient say he or she has pain or tenderness when you percuss this area? Reported discomfort can indicate infection or tumor. Percussion of the bladder should be done to determine fullness and pain.

Palpation

Palpate the patient for peripheral edema. In fluid volume overload, fluid translocates from the vascular system into the interstitial spaces. Check the patient for strength in the extremities. Weakness in the legs can signal that the patient is developing uremic neuropathy.

Palpate the patient's joints and move the patient's extremities through his or her range of motion. Does the movement cause bone or joint pain; does it illicit paresthesias or numbness in any of the extremities? Joint problems can result from vitamin D deficiency and demineralization of the bone from low calcium levels, leading to renal osteodystrophy. Uremic toxins can result in pain and paresthesias.

Usually the kidneys cannot be palpated as they lie deep within the abdomen and are protected by muscle. However, in thin patients they can sometimes be felt during deep inspiration. They should feel smooth and round without masses or lumps. The bladder can be palpated and should feel smooth, without masses or nodules.

In addition to performing a through and ongoing physical assessment, the nurse will also be involved in preparing the patient to undergo and screen diagnostic and laboratory tests.

Collaborative Diagnostic and Laboratory Tools

❷ The laboratory and diagnostic tools are monitored by the critical care nurse and it is essential to understand how they change if damage occurs to the kidneys.

Laboratory Tools

The following are a list of laboratory values that a nurse would need to monitor for a patient with kidney failure.

Blood urea nitrogen (BUN) – Serum level that increases with decreased blood flow to the kidney, which causes more urea to be absorbed and less to be excreted in the blood. Value will also rise in high protein diets and prerenal failure and is therefore not the best reflection of kidney damage. Normal value is 5 to 25 mg/dL.

Complete blood cell count (CBC) – Red blood cell (RBC) counts, hemoglobin, and hematocrit are all low in chronic renal failure due to lack of erythropoietin stimulation. RBCs are needed to help with oxygenation of the tissues. Normal values are RBC (4.2–5.9 million/mm³), hemoglobin (12–17 g/dL), hematocrit (36%–52%).

White blood cell counts (WBCs) – Needed to fight infection. Elevated with urinary tract infection (UTI), peritonitis, and transplanted kidney rejection. Normal value 5,000 to 10,000/mm³.

Creatinine clearance – Most accurate measure of GFR. Values below normal show 50% loss of nephron functioning. Normal value is 85 to 135 mL/min.

Fractional excretion of sodium (FENa) – Assesses how well kidneys concentrate urine and conserve sodium. Normal value is less than 1%.

Glomerular filtration rate (GFR) – Rate at which the urinary filtrate is formed. Usually 125 mL/min.

Serum calcium – Major components of bone and teeth. Found intravascularly playing strong roles in blood clotting, muscular contraction, and nerve impulse transmission. Usually low in patients in acute and chronic renal failure. Controlled by parathyroid and thyroid glands. Normal value 8.5 to 10.5 mg/dL.

Serum chloride – Major anion in the extracellular fluid. Important in acid-base balance, this level will increase when HCO_3 levels drop. Elevation suggests metabolic acidosis reflective of chronic renal failure. Normal value 96 to 115 mEq/L.

Serum osmolality – Reflects concentration of solutes in the serum. Normal value 275 to 295 mOsm/kg. Elevation in osmolality suggests dehydration while a drop suggests fluid overload.

Serum phosphorus – Found mostly in bone. Assists with ATP and acid-base balance. Moves the opposite of calcium in the serum so when calcium is low, phosphorus is high. Regulated by parathyroid-stimulating hormone. Usually high in renal failure. Normal value 2.5 to 4.5 mg/dL.

Serum potassium – Most common intracellular cation. Liberated with cell wall rupture. Also retained in renal failure, causing serious cardiac effects. Normal value 3.5 to 5.0 mEq/L.

Serum magnesium – Important in many enzymatic actions like carbohydrate and protein synthesis and contraction of muscle tissue. Magnesium and calcium are linked together; deficiency in one has a significant effect on the other as magnesium helps the absorption of calcium in the intestines. In decreased kidney function, greater amounts of magnesium are retained and therefore an increased blood level occurs. Normal value is 1.3 to 2.1 mEq/L.

Serum sodium – Most abundant cation in extracellular fluid. Usually where sodium goes, water goes. Influenced by ADH and aldosterone. Normal value is 135 to 145 mEq/L

Uric acid – In renal failure this rises as the kidney's are unable to excrete this by-product of purine metabolism. Normal value is 2.5 to 7.0 umol/L.

Urine osmolality – Tests concentration of solutes in the urine. Ability to concentrate urine is lost in renal failure. Normal value is 1.010 to 1.025.

Urine protein – The kidneys do not excrete protein as it is a large molecule and does not pass through the nephron. In renal diseases, proteinuria will result. Normal urine contains no protein.

Urinary RBCs – Since RBCs are large molecules, they do not normally pass into the urine. Presence is indicative of UTI, renal obstruction, inflammation, or trauma. Normal urine contains no RBCs.

Urinary WBC – Urinary infection and inflammation will result in an increase in WBC growth in the urine. Normal urine contains no more than four WBCs per high-powered field.

NURSING ALERT

Obtain a urine specimen prior to administering a diuretic. This will more accurately reflect the patient's urinary status.

Diagnostic Studies

ECG/EKG (electrocardiogram) – Shows the response of the heart to electrolyte imbalance by changes in waveforms and presence of rhythm disturbances.

KUB (kidney ureter bladder x-ray) – Shows position of kidney and presence of renal calculi or tumors. No contrast medium is used.

Renal biopsy – A small sample of the kidney is removed percutaneously to test for cellular type (tumor), damage (pyelonephritis), or rejection (renal transplantation). The nurse needs to perform frequent vital signs and monitor the site for bleeding and infection.

Renal angiography – Involves injection of contrast medium into the renal arterial tree to visualize kidney structures through fluoroscopy. Shows the presence of abnormal blood flow, renal artery stenosis, cysts or tumors, renal trauma, and abscesses or inflammation. Renal artery stenosis can lead to prerenal failure and hypertension, which can lead to heart failure. The nursing care pre and post care is similar to a cardiac catheterization (see Chapter 3 for nursing care).

Medications Commonly Used in Critical Care

❸ Medications that affect the renal system include a variety of complex types. These medications include diuretics, medications to control the unwanted effects of electrolytes that accumulate when the kidneys fail to function, and miscellaneous medications (see Table 8–1 to 8–3).

Table 8–1 will help the nurse identify representative medications from the diuretic group, their actions, their use, and precautions to take when evaluating the patient receiving these medications. These classes of diuretics work either at a different site in the nephron or by a different mechanism. It is not uncommon to have patients taking several different classes of diuretics to achieve a balanced fluid state.

TABLE 8–1 Diuretics

Class	Actions	Use	Precautions
Loop diuretics: Furosemide (Lasix) Torsemide (Demadex) Sometimes referred to as high–ceiling diuretics as they cause greater diuresis than other types	Work in the loop of Henle to prevent reabsorption of sodium and chloride resulting in sodium–rich diuresis	Fluid overload Heart failure Decreases pulmonary edema Peripheral edema (right–sided heart failure) Hypertension Renal disease	1. Check for drug allergy 2. Monitor the serum potassium and provide supplementation when values are near or less than normal 3. May not work with severe anuria from ARF 4. Monitor BP for drop related to fluid loss 5. May cause hyperglycemia with long-term use 6. Can cause reversible ototoxicity, which is exacerbated with concurrent use of aminoglycoside antibiotics 7. Carefully read any drug labels; furosemide and torsemide look alike and can be confused

TABLE 8–1 Diuretics (*Continued*)

Class	Actions	Use	Precautions
Thiazide diuretics: Hydrocholoro-thiazide (HCTZ) Chlorothiazide (Diuril)	Work in distal convoluted tubule to block action of chloride pump with sodium following passively More gentle in diuretic action than high-ceiling loop diuretics	Edema from heart failure, renal disease Hypertension	1. Sulfonamide drug, so look for allergies 2. Look for electrolyte imbalances, especially hypokalemia, hypocalcemia 3. Observe for GI upset 4. Monitor the BP and serum osmolality for hypovolemia 5. Can exacerbate digoxin toxicity due to changes in potassium levels
Potassium-sparing diuretics: Amiloride (Midamor) Spironolactone (Aldactone)	Primary site of action is the distal tubule and collecting duct Excrete sodium while retaining potassium	Edema from heart failure, renal disease Use for hypokalemia Adjunct for hypertension control	1. Monitor the potassium and hold if elevated 2. Signs of high K include lethargy, confusion, ataxia, muscular cramping, and rhythm disturbances 2. Avoid foods containing potassium
Osmotic diuretics: Mannitol (Osmitrol) Isosorbide (Ismotic)	Act in the glomerulus and tubule Create an osmotic effect pulling fluid from kidney	Edema from heart failure, renal disease Used to prevent oliguric phase of renal failure Some drug overdoses to clear toxic substances from the kidney tubules	1. Monitor the patient for osmotic-mediated drop in BP 2. Causes GI upset 3. Contraindicated in anuria from severe renal diseases 4. Monitor fluid and electrolyte levels

TABLE 8–1 Diuretics (*Continued*)

Class	Actions	Use	Precautions
Carbonic anhydrase inhibitors: Acetazolamide (Diamox)	Work in the proximal tubule Slow down movement of hydrogen ions leading to more sodium and bicarbonate loss	Diuresis in heart failure Adjunct to other diuretics when more intense diuresis is required	1. Contraindicated in patients with thiazide and sulfonamide allergies 2. Cause GI upset 3. Urinary frequency 4. Monitor the patient for metabolic acidosis as a result of bicarbonate loss 5. Monitor fluid and electrolyte status

NURSING ALERT

A fluid rebound effect can take place if patients limit their fluid intake while taking a prescribed diuretic. The body adjusts to fluid limitation by decreasing extracellular fluid and therefore decreasing GFR. Compensation for this by stimulating the RAAS can increase the retention of fluid. Patients need to be taught not to severely limit fluids while taking diuretics.

NURSING ALERT

Nursing education of the patient taking potassium-depleting diuretics should include dietary increases in potassium-rich foods. These include avocados, bananas, nuts, tomatoes, broccoli, cantaloupe, dried fruits, and oranges.

TABLE 8–2 Medications That Help Control Electrolytes

Name	Actions	Use	Precautions
Calcitriol (Rocaltrol) or Calcijex (IV vitamin D)	Vitamin D analogue Regulates absorption of calcium in the small intestine	Management of calcium level in CRF and hypoparathyroid-ism	1. Contraindicated with high serum calcium; substitute with Renagel 2. Do not give if patient is hyper-sensitive to drugs 3. Administer with meals 4. Mostly GI effects like nausea, vomiting, and dry mouth

TABLE 8–2 Medications That Help Control Electrolytes (*Continued*)

Name	Actions	Use	Precautions
Calcium gluconate (IV) Calcium acetate (PhosLo) (PO) Calcium carbonate (Os–cal) (PO)	In acute hypocalcemia, rapidly restores calcium levels quickly (IV) Also used in mild or severe hyperkalemia Oral forms regulate long–term management of high phosphate levels	Severe hypocalcemia with ECG and patient changes (tetany, changes in level of consciousness [IV]) Used in severe hyperkalemia with ECG changes and symptoms in patient (hypotension)	1. Give IV 2. Use with caution in patients on digoxin 3. Contraindicated in ventricular fibrillation 4. Do not give IM or subcutaneously 5. Monitor the calcium level frequently
Glucose and insulin	Drives potassium into the cell, thus decreasing hyperkalemia	Severe hyperkalemia and metabolic acidosis	1. Monitor serum potassium 2. Monitor glucose levels for hyperglycemia
Sevelamer HCL (Renagel) or Lanthanum carbonate (Fosrenol)	Calcium free phosphate binders Removes intestinal phosphate	Management of phosphate level in patients with high serum calcium and high phosphorus levels in ESRD	1. Monitor serum phosphate and calcium levels 2. Preferred over calcium–based binders 3. Do not give if low phosphate levels, fecal impaction, or bowel obstruction 4. Administer with food
Sodium bicarbonate ($NaHCO_3$)	Reverse metabolic acidosis in patients with ESRD	Severe metabolic acidosis Cardiac arrest after ABGs completed	1. Monitor the ABGs for correction 2. Do not administer if patient is in an alkalosis 3. Watch for IV drug incompatibility

TABLE 8–2 Medications That Help Control Electrolytes (*Continued*)

Name	Actions	Use	Precautions
Sodium poly-styrene sul-fonate (Kayexalate)	Reduces potassium levels by removing it via the GI tract	Lowers potassium levels in mild hyperkalemia	1. Given by mouth or enema 2. Given with sorbitol to prevent constipation 3. May need to be repeated every 4-6 hours 4. Use cautiously in patient with GI motility issues (surgery, bed rest, opiate use)

TABLE 8–3 Miscellaneous Medications Used With Patients in ARF and CRF

Medication	Actions	Use	Precautions
Folic acid (vitamin B9) (Folacin, Folvite)	Synthesis and maintenance of red blood cells (RBCs)	Used in the synthesis of RBCs in CRF-induced anemia	1. Monitor Hct and Hgb for effectiveness 2. Monitor site if given IV for warmth and flushing
Histamine-2 receptor blockers Cimetidine (Tagamet) Famotidine (Pepcid)	Blocks the release of hydrochloric acid in the stomach	To prevent stress ulcers and GI bleeding in ARF/CRF Treatment of gastric esophageal reflux disease (GERD)	1. Check for decreased dosage used in renal failure 2. Monitor for adverse reactions including dizziness, confusion, cardiac dysrhythmias, and hypotension

TABLE 8–3 Miscellaneous Medications Used With Patients in ARF and CRF (*Continued*)

Medication	Actions	Use	Precautions
Iron supple-mentation Ferrous sulfate (Feosol) Iron sucrose (Venofer) IV form	Increase needed for red blood cell stimulation	Anemia associated with CRF	1. Poorly absorbed if taken with phosphate binders, H2 blockers, and proton pump inhibitors 2. Causes constipation and black stools; patient teaching required to increase fiber/fluid to prevent constipation 3. Assess neurologic changes due to iron toxicity 4. Give IM injections Z track
Procrit (EPO)	Synthetic erythropoietin Increases quality of life as increases energy, appetite, and functional/role abilities	To promote red blood cell stimulation in the absence of erythropoietin in ESRD Prevents increased frequency of blood transfusions	1. Takes several weeks to take effect 2. Does not replace transfusions in emergency blood loss 3. Monitor the BP as hypertension can result
Proton pump inhibitors Pantoprazole (Protonix) Esomeprazole (Nexium)	Inhibits HCL release in the lumen of the stomach	To prevent stress ulcers and GI bleeding	1. Monitor for hypersensitivity to these drugs 2. Administer before meals 3. Monitor for GI upsets including nausea, vomiting, and diarrhea 4. Monitor for *Clostridium difficile*, which has been reported to be three times higher in patients on this group of drugs

TABLE 8–3 Miscellaneous Medications Used With Patients in ARF and CRF (Continued)			
Medication	**Actions**	**Use**	**Precautions**
Water–soluble vitamins like B, C	Needed for cellular growth and repair Important in RBC formation	CRF	1. Monitor the response to the drugs like alleviation of anemia 2. Must be given after dialysis or they are removed during dialysis treatment 3. Observe for hyper-sensitivity

Dialysis

❹ Dialysis is an artificial method to replace the functioning of the kidneys. During all types of dialysis, excess fluids, electrolytes, and toxins are removed from the blood by a filter. Dialysis can be used on a short-term basis, as in removing drugs and toxins from a patient who overdoses on medications, or it can be used for long-term therapy in patients with end-stage renal disease (ESRD). There are three types: hemodialysis (HD), peritoneal dialysis (PD), and continuous renal replacement therapy (CRRT). Table 8–4 shows a summary of the different types of dialysis.

TABLE 8–4 Differences in Types of Dialysis	
Type of Dialysis	**Differences**
Hemodialysis (HD)	1. Can be done via a special temporary central line inserted in an emergency 2. Can be inserted at the bedside by a physician 3. Long term requires a surgically implanted AV fistula or AV graft 4. Quick; fluid, medications, and electrolytes can be dialyzed quickly in several hours 5. Requires trained nursing staff to care for the machines and the patient 6. Notorious for dropping the BP profoundly, so cannot be used in patients who are hemodynamically unstable

TABLE 8–4 Differences in Types of Dialysis (*Continued*)	
Type of Dialysis	**Differences**
Peritoneal dialysis (PD)	1. Fast; can be done at the bedside but is usually done in a surgical suite 2. Fluids and electrolytes removed at a slower pace than HD 3. Catheter placed in the peritoneal cavity, which is used as a dialyzing membrane 4. Can cause respiratory distress when intraabdominal pressure pushes up on diaphragm 5. Contraindicated in patients with abdominal surgery or peritonitis 6. Can cause peritonitis from invasion of peritoneal cavity by contaminated catheter or dialysis fluid 7. Requires training but not as extensive as HD 8. Can be done at home overnight if cycling machine used 9. Is more economical and nearly as effective as HD 10. Observe for peritonitis
Continuous renal replacement therapy (CRRT)	1. Slower; venovenous CRRT can be used in patients who are hemodynamically unstable because fluid/electrolyte shifts are gradual 2. Extracorporeal; so an access site is needed 3. Can be combined with HD, so fluid can be replaced as well as solutes removed 4. Can be done at the bedside by the critical care nurse with additional training and educational support

Hemodialysis (HD)

Hemodialysis (HD) is frequently used in the critical care environment for acute situations like uremia, electrolyte, and fluid overload and some drug overdoses. Its most frequent use is for long-term therapy in chronic renal failure (CRF). Usually CRF is treated at home or in a community-based outpatient clinic; however, dialysis patients can be admitted to ICUs with other critical conditions like cardiac tamponade, heart failure, and severe anemia. Although the critical care nurse usually does not perform HD, he or she must monitor the patient, working in tandem with a specially trained HD nurse in coordinated care of the patient.

There are contraindications to HD. A patient who is hemodynamically unstable will not tolerate additional removal of blood from the body. The drop in BP while the blood is extracorporeal can lead to cardiogenic shock. A patient with a coagulopathy can hemorrhage when given heparin while the extracorporeal

Blood removed
for cleansing

Dialyzer

Clean blood returned
to the body

FIGURE 8–2 • Hemodialysis.

blood is running through the machine filters in HD. The patient needs either a patent internal or external access site (see Figure 8–2).

In HD, blood is removed from the body, pumped through a machine where toxins are removed by a filter, and returned to the patient. An internal or external vascular access is needed to remove and return blood. For short-term or emergency therapy, an external vascular access in the form of a dual-lumen central access line is inserted to access the arterial and venous systems. These are known as vascular access sites.

Internal jugular or femoral veins are usually catheterized in the case of ARF or when a previously placed internal access is not functioning. These can be inserted quickly at the bedside. The catheter's terminal end is in the central vein. Once inserted by the physician, blood can be removed and returned to the patient when caps on the lines are removed and connected to the appropriate HD line without sticking the patient. Caps are color-coded red for arterial and blue for venous. Once the dialysis treatment is finished, the central lines are capped, flushed with heparin, and clamps are closed to prevent accidental exsanguination. Follow your institutional guidelines for accessing these lines, but most physicians prefer that the external venous access is restricted to dialysis use only (see Figure 8–3).

Complications of external sites include infection, clotting and/or kinking of the central line catheter, and hemorrhage from the catheter if clamps are not closed and capped. Nursing care of this site includes

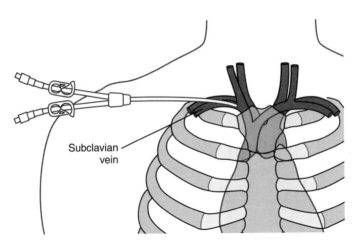

FIGURE 8–3 · Subclavian vascular access site.

Monitoring VS for elevated temperature, which can indicate infection

Checking and redressing the insertion site and monitoring for infection and kinking

Maintaining strict aseptic technique when accessing the site

A permanent type of internal vascular access site is needed if the patient is in CRF or requires long-term dialysis. The most frequently used internal accesses are the arteriovenous (AV) fistula and the AV graft. An AV fistula is the more common surgically inserted internal vascular access. The most frequently accessed site is the radial artery, although an artery and vein in the upper arm can be used as well. A fistula is created when an artery and a vein are surgically connected. This is done so that arterial pressure from the artery can strengthen the vein so that less trauma occurs from faster blood flow in HD. The strengthening process or maturing requires several weeks to months before a fistula can tolerate needles and the HD process. Attempting to access an underdeveloped AV fistula can cause arterial vascular spasm, reduced blood flow to the extremity, and damage it. This preferred method of vascular access has blood vessel durability and fewer complications than other types of internal access sites (see Figure 8–4).

An AV graft is used when a patient's veins are too weak or too small to tolerate a fistula. A graft is a synthetic tube that connects an artery to a vein. Grafts are generally placed in the forearm or the thigh, creating a telltale bulge that can be seen and palpated under the skin at the site.

Accessing both fistulas and grafts requires two large-bore needles for each HD treatment. Large bores are needed so that there is less trauma to the red blood cells (RBCs) as they are shunted back and forth from body to machine.

FIGURE 8–4 • AV Fistula and graft.

Once the treatment is finished, the needles are removed, pressure is applied until hemostasis has been achieved, and a dry, sterile dressing is placed over the site.

Checking the patient for complications at internal access sites is critical to maintain the patient's lifeline for HD. Complications include thrombosis, infection, ischemia, and hemorrhage. Nursing care includes:

Auscultating a bruit and palpating a thrill to determine site patency.

Checking the site for infection indicated by erythema, edema, and exudate.

Monitoring the patient's temperature for signs of infection.

Maintaining a clean, dry dressing to prevent infection.

Monitoring for changes in vascular status (temperature, sensation, color, and capillary refill). Steal syndrome can occur where arterial ischemia is noted at the affected extremity. Notify the surgeon if this occurs.

Monitoring the patient for hypotension, which can lead to site clotting.

Elevating the extremity to prevent edema.

Communicating to all health care members that no BPs, blood work, or IVs should be performed near the access sites, which can clot the site; usually this information is included on a special bracelet that the patient wears on the extremity or noting this at the patient's bedside.

Notifying the physician if clotting is suspected and if there is bleeding at the insertion site.

Teaching the patient and significant others how to check for graft patency and to speak up if someone tries to perform BPs, venipunctures, or laboratory work on that extremity. The most common reason for admission to the hospital for HD patients is clotting of the internal access site. Preservation of this graft is a high priority for the patient and nursing staff.

> **NURSING ALERT**
>
> *A bruit should be auscultated and thrill felt over the AV fistula or graft. If this is not observed, then the surgeon or nephrologists should be notified as soon as possible!*

> **NURSING ALERT**
>
> *A patient with an AV fistula or graft should have no BPs, venipunctures, or laboratory work in the extremity of the internal access site. Trauma to the site from these procedures has been known to clot the site.*

Prior to starting HD, there are critical assessments that need to be completed by the critical nurse. These assessments include:

History, including reasons for HD.

Taking VS and comparing them to baselines.

Reviewing current laboratory studies confirming the need for dialysis.

Predialysis weight, which is subtracted from the postdialysis weight to determine fluid removed.

Checking intake and output history confirming the need for dialysis.

Evaluating the function of the access site.

Describing the outcomes of the HD—is the treatment for fluid removal, electrolytes, or drugs?

Performing a neurological assessment to determine baseline.

Assessing the patient's knowledge of the procedure.

Hold any medications that could cause hypotension like beta-blockers and may be dialyzed out of the patient (see Table 8–5).

TABLE 8–5 Medications Frequently Held That Would Be Removed by HD
Acyclovir (Zovirax)
Ceftazidime (Fortaz)
Folic acid
Iron
Gentamycin (Garamycin)
Multiple vitamins (MVIs)
Salicylates
Tobramycin (Tobrex)
Vitamins B1, B6, B12, and C

Once the access site has been inserted and HD has begun, it requires teamwork between the critical care nurse and the HD nurse to care for the patient. During dialysis the nurse will be observing for possible complications related to HD. These include

Monitoring the patient for hypotension, which is caused by removal of blood from the body and can lead to shock and/or clotting of the access site.

Observing/documenting the cardiac rhythm, which can change if electrolyte disturbances, especially potassium, occur.

Monitoring the site and VS for external or internal bleeding. Signs/symptoms can include hypotension; tachycardia; tachypnea; cool, clammy skin; and changes in the level of consciousness. Heparin is used during the procedure, which could lead to bleeding.

Observing the patient during and after dialysis for disequilibrium syndrome, which can include headache and twitching, which can lead to seizures, nausea, and vomiting. This is caused by rapid shifts in fluid and electrolytes. The physician needs to be notified immediately.

Protecting all health care workers from blood-borne infection by using appropriate personal protective equipment while caring for the patient.

Teaching the patient and significant others about the equipment, procedure, access site care, and complications that could occur.

Peritoneal Dialysis (PD)

Peritoneal dialysis (PD) allows the removal of fluid and waste products with the use of the peritoneal cavity as the filter. The principles of diffusion and osmosis come into play in this type of dialysis. Diffusion allows substances of high concentration to move to lower concentration across a semipermeable membrane. In this case the semipermeable membrane is the gut, which removes urea and electrolytes.

Osmosis is the movement of fluid from areas of lower solute concentration to areas of higher concentration; the water goes to salt principle. So diffusion allows excess fluid to be drawn out by an osmotic gradient between the peritoneum and the dialyzing fluid.

PD can be used temporarily before an AV fistula or graft can be placed. It is easy to teach, which is why some patients prefer this method of dialysis. It is not as expensive and does not require the special training that restricts HD. The patient must have an intact abdominal cavity free from adhesions or surgery; however, it is slower than HD and therefore is not the treatment of choice in an emergency. Since it is slower, it poses fewer risks than HD. PD can be performed intermittently or constantly depending on the amount of fluid and electrolytes to be removed.

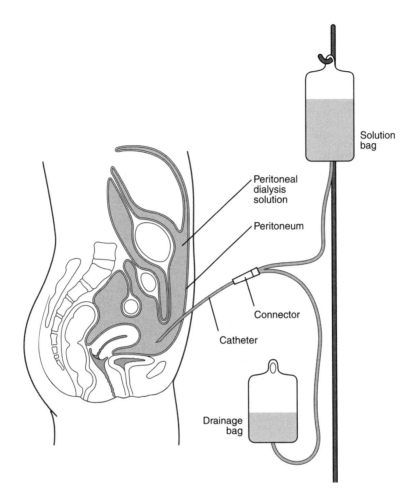

FIGURE 8–5 • Peritoneal dialysis.

In PD, a warmed dialyzing solution in what looks like a super-large intravenous bag is attached to a specially inserted abdominal catheter that is made of soft plastic. The PD catheter is surgically placed with use beginning immediately. There is no contraindication for immediate dialysis after placement like there is with HD, AV grafts and shunts. The intraperitoneal catheter exits usually above the umbilicus and can be flushed with heparin and capped in between PD treatments (see Figure 8–5).

Complications of the PD catheter can include

Bleeding from surgery or heparin used to keep it patent

Peritonitis leading to systemic infection and sepsis

Clotting of the catheter with fibrin and debris from dialysis

The warmed dialysate is infused through the PD catheter into the peritoneum dwelling in this space according to physician preference. The longer the fluid is intact with peritoneum in the abdomen, the more fluid and electrolytes it will remove. Next, the IV tubing is clamped and the dialysate is allowed to flow by gravity into a drainage bag, which, except for its size, looks like an indwelling urinary catheter drainage bag. The dialysate is ordered to be drained at a specific amount of time. Once measured and determined to be more than what was infused, the process begins again. An infusion, dwell time, and drain time is considered one cycle and time limits are placed by the nephrologist. A cumulative tally of fluid removed is kept.

Before starting PD, the nurse should perform the following:

Explain the procedure to the patient.

Perform baseline VS measurements.

Perform an abdominal assessment to check for peritonitis.

Take the patient's predialysis weight (wet weight; the patient has retained fluid).

Monitor electrolytes, BUN, creatinine, and WBC levels to observe for renal function and infection.

Instruct the patient to void to prevent inadvertent perforation.

Check the PD catheter dressing observing for infection, bleeding, and for the catheter to be intact without kinking.

Gather all equipment, which includes dialysate, IV pole, tubing to and from the catheter, and medications that can be added to the dialysate like antibiotics to protect from peritonitis and heparin to prevent clotting of the catheter. Bring appropriate personal protective equipment, which includes mask, gloves, eye shields, and gown.

Prep the peritoneal catheter according to protocol; this may include cleansing the catheter exit port with a disinfectant.

During the procedure, the patient will require close observation to prevent complications associated with PD. The nursing care of this patient requires the nurse to:

Monitor for respiratory distress, which could happen from increased intrathoracic pressure from increased intraabdominal pressure as fluid enters the peritoneal space.

Monitor the patient for changes in temperature, which can indicate peritonitis.

Closely watch dialysate infuse and drain. A kink or clotting of the catheter from exudate can cause slower infusing and draining times. It can also stop the drainage.

Record the output of the dialysis and relate it to the amount infused and the total amount + or − the patient during the treatment period.

Observe the dialysate for bloody drainage. During the first several cycles, the dialysate may have blood-tinged drainage that will clear with each passing cycle. If bleeding persists, notify the surgeon who placed the PD catheter.

Reposition the patient frequently. Patients are usually more comfortable in a high Fowler's position during initiation and indwelling because it assists with ease of breathing.

At the end of the PD treatment nursing care includes:

Capping the dialysis catheter using sterile technique

Repeat VS, abdominal, and neurological checks

Observing for signs of respiratory distress, which is associated with fluid retention (crackles, decreased SaO_2, air hunger, tachypnea, hypertension)

Weigh the patient analyzing the weight with the amount of fluid taken from the patient (dry weight: weight has been reduced with treatment)

Recording the number of cycles and total amount of fluid removed

Capping the dialysis catheter and redressing the site

Administering any medications that were held due to dialysis

Asking the patient if he or she has any questions about the procedure and how the patient tolerated it

Supporting the patient and listening to fears as this is a life-altering procedure

NURSING ALERT

Peritonitis is a serious complication of PD. Fever, abdominal cramping that increases, pain or swelling at the catheter insertion site, and cloudy dialysate can indicate peritonitis. Notify the physician, prepare to take a dialysate specimen, and anticipate that the physician will start the patient on antibiotics.

Continuous Renal Replacement (CRRT)

The last type of dialysis that can be seen in the critical care environment is continuous renal replacement therapy (CRRT). CRRT is similar to HD because it is an extracorporeal procedure and requires a temporary external access site.

Like PD, CRRT uses the principles of diffusion and osmosis to remove fluid and waste products from the patient's system. Unlike HD and PD, it is much slower and is administered over a longer period of time. Because body changes occur at a much slower rate, CRRT can be used if the patient is hemodynamically unstable, making it a clear choice in many shocky patients. It can be done over 24 hours until the patient is stabilized and can tolerate other forms of dialysis (see Figure 8–6).

Similar to HD, CRRT uses a temporary external central dual lumen catheter in the subclavian or femoral areas. Blood flows from this catheter into a hemofilter, which is composed of multiple hollow semipermeable fibers that allow smaller molecules to pass through and yet retain the patient blood and protein. These smaller molecules, such as potassium, urea, nitrogen, and fluid, are filtered and

FIGURE 8–6 • Continuous renal replacement therapy (CRRT).

removed from the body into a drainage bag. The bag is drained according to institutional protocols, not unlike PD, and a tally is kept of how much fluid the CRRT has removed from the patient.

There are several different types of CCRT that are distinguished by the solutes they remove and how and why they remove them. Table 8–6 describes the types of CRRT and how they differ.

TABLE 8–6 Types of CRRT		
Type of CRRT	**What It Is**	**What It Does**
Slow continuous ultrafiltration (SCUF)	Requires an arterial access Pressure from systolic BP propels blood into hemofilter Problem if patient becomes hypotensive Mean arterial pressure of >70 mm Hg required or clotting can occur	Removes fluid from the patient No solutes are removed; not used for severe azotemia No replacement fluids are administered Not used with low BP
Continuous veno-venous hemofiltration (CVVH)	Blood is taken from venous system Requires an extracorporeal pump to run blood from patient into system	Fluid removal Fluid replacement Solutes removed No dialysate used
Continuous veno-venous hemodialysis (CVVHD)	A combination of hemofiltration and slower form of HD An infusion pump drives dialysate No replacement fluid used	Removes solutes/fluid Safe for patient with hypotension and fluid overload No replacement solution is used
Continuous veno-venous hemodiafiltration (CVVHDF)	Fluid is removed Blood propelled through pump Large volumes of fluid removed and replaced, so total volume lost from patient is small Solute is removed Counter flow of dialysate removes solutes from blood Faster rate than other forms of CRRT	Removes solutes/fluid Fluid replacement Safe to use for low BP

Predialysis nursing care is similar to that for HD external access sites. During dialysis, the nurse is responsible for:

Monitoring the patient's vital signs and cardiac rhythm.

Checking for hypothermia from blood removal from the body.

Evaluating hemodynamic and perfusion status via a pulmonary artery catheter with readings including central venous pressure, pulmonary artery pressure, and pulmonary artery occlusion pressure.

Monitoring fluid volume status and laboratory values to confirm this.

Administering anticoagulants (heparin) if needed to prevent clotting of the hemofilter.

Assessing for signs of bleeding or clotting.

Checking the system for patency, alarms, flow rates.

Calculating hourly intake and outputs with replacement solutions as indicated by the type of CRRT.

Looking for indications of infection at the access site; dialysate should be clear and not cloudy.

Observe for signs of blood in the filtered fluid, which can indicate a leak in the hemofilter; this should be preceded by an alarm as bacterial invasion can contaminate the patient's blood.

Calculating weight gain or loss from pre- and post-dialysis weights.

Acute and Chronic Renal Failure

Acute Renal Failure

What Went Wrong?

❺ Acute renal failure (ARF) is the sudden, reversible loss of partial kidney function. ARF has three types: prerenal, intrarenal, and postrenal failure (see Table 8–7). Prerenal failure involves a decreased blood supply or perfusion to the kidney. The most common causes are decreased cardiac output, dehydration, renal artery stenosis, and shock. All of these have in common that blood supply is not getting to the kidney, which stimulates the RAAS to conserve sodium and water. This leads to an increased intravascular volume, which increases the BP and decreases urinary output.

Intrarenal failure is caused when something injures the kidney tubules or nephrons directly. The most common cause of intrarenal failure is acute tubular necrosis (ATN). ATN occurs when destruction of tubular epithelial cells results in increased intraluminal pressure, which greatly reduces GFR and renal function. Direct damage of the nephrons or cortex results in tubular swelling and then necrosis, thus the title ATN. Debris from swelling and necrosis leads to blocking blood and filtrate flow further leads to stasis of urine and more necrosis.

Other causes of intrarenal failure include acute glomerulonephritis, nephrotoxic drugs (contrast dye, aminoglycoside antibiotics) and ischemia.

Postrenal failure is basically obstructive in nature. Obstructions can occur anywhere in the kidney or the ducts and organs that drain to the urethra. Abnormalities like kidney stones or tumors can lead to backup of urine and stasis leading to dilation of the system, increased GFR, and increased edema from water and sodium reabsorption and infection.

No matter where the renal failure occurs, the end result of this insult will lead to retention of wastes, chiefly nitrogen and electrolytes, and metabolic acidosis, which can lead to organ failure.

NURSING ALERT

A large amount of radiographic dye is injected during arteriograms of many organs like the heart, brain, and kidney. ATN from intrarenal failure can start 48 hours after drug administration and peak in 3 days. If the patient is discharged earlier than these times, nursing teaching at discharge regarding signs/symptoms of ATN is imperative to preserve kidney functioning.

TABLE 8–7 Types of Acute Renal Failure (ARF)

Type of ARF	Location of Failure	Causes
Prerenal failure (60% of cases)	Reduced blood flow to kidneys	Decreased blood supply* from low cardiac output disorders like dysrhythmias, cardiogenic shock, heart failure and MI
		Hypovolemia from burns, diuretics, dehydration, hemorrhage, shock, sepsis, and trauma
		Severe vasoconstriction from DIC
		High doses of dopamine ACE inhibitors/ARBs in combination with diuretics
		Mechanical ventilation with PEEP

TABLE 8–7 Types of Acute Renal Failure (ARF) (Continued)		
Type of ARF	**Location of Failure**	**Causes**
Intrarenal failure (30%–40% of cases)	Damage to kidney tissue	Prerenal failure ATN* Acute glomerulonephritis Pyelonephritis Nephrotoxic substances like radiographic contrast dye, aminoglycoside antibiotics, heavy metals, analgesics, cancer chemotherapy like cisplatin Myoglobin release from massive trauma (rhabdomyolysis), sepsis or transfusion reactions
Postrenal failure (5%–10% of cases)	Obstruction of out-flow tracts from kidney to the bladder and urethra Backflow results in distention decreasing GFR	BPH or prostate cancer* Kidney stones or tumors Ureteral stones or tumors Blood clots Strictures of ureters and bladder neck

*Most common causes.

Three Distinctive Phases

In ARF, patients transit through three phases: oliguric, diuretic, and recovery. Oliguria is characterized by a drop in urinary output less than 400 mL in 24 hours. In this phase, the BUN and creatinine rise as a result of decreased blood flow to the kidneys. As the insidious RAAS kicks in, sodium and water are conserved leading to hypertension, edema, and weight gain.

The diuretic phase is signified by an increase in urinary output. Fluid output during this phase can be excessive leading to dehydration and electrolyte disturbances, especially loss of potassium and sodium. Twenty-five percent of deaths due to ARF occur in this phase.

The recovery phase is characterized by return of kidney functioning. Urinary output returns to normal between 1 and 2 L per day. The concentrating ability of the kidney is signified by return of the BUN and creatinine to normal levels.

Prognosis

ARF occurs in 20% to 30% of critical care patients. It can be corrected if the precipitating factor is identified early. Sources vary but ARF can lead to organ failure, and the more organs that fail the higher the mortality rate. Patients who develop renal failure in the ICU have higher mortality rates than patients admitted with previous renal failure. Mortality rates can vary from 30% to 90% and are higher in patients over 65 years old.

Interpreting Test Results

Decreased GFR

Increased BUN and creatinine

Worsening metabolic acidosis

Hyperkalemia

Decreased hemoglobin (Hgb) and hematocrit (Hct)

Azotemia

Uremia

Hallmark Signs and Symptoms

A marked decrease in urine output less than 30 cc/hr or less than 400 mL/day.

Tachycardia.

Hypertension.

Pulmonary and peripheral edema.

Lethargy leading to coma.

ABGs will show worsening metabolic acidosis (elevated HCO_3 and decreased pH).

Treatment

Find the underlying cause.

If prerenal and related to renal hypovolemia, increase fluid to the kidneys.

If intrarenal, antibiotics and fluids are used to flush toxins out of the system.

If postrenal, care involves removing obstructions to urine flow such as calculi removal or prostate surgery.

Nursing Diagnoses for ARF	Expected Outcomes
Fluid volume excess related to decreased renal blood flow (prerenal) or nephron damage (intrarenal) or urinary obstruction (postrenal)	The patient will have a urinary output of >30 cc/hr The patient's weight will be stable The patient's intake will equal output

Nursing Interventions

Monitor the patient's vital signs, especially the BP, *which can indicate fluid overload if it elevates above baseline.*

Monitor the patient's heart and lung sounds *for signs of failure like S3, pericardial friction rub, and crackles*

Assess the patient's SaO$_2$ and/or ABGs *to determine if pulmonary edema is a result of retained fluid.*

Monitor the urinary output to keep it above 30 cc/hr and 400 mL/day, *which is the minimal amount of renal output required to prevent ARF.*

Perform neurological checks looking *for signs of uremic toxicity signified by changes in the level of consciousness, tremors, numbness, and tingling and can lead to coma.*

Check the patient's ECG *for rhythm changes due to metabolic acidosis and signs of hyperkalemia (see section on hyperkalemia).*

Maintain daily weights, which is the most critical indicator of fluid status.

Maintain intake and output hourly *to detect fluid deficit or overload.*

Monitor the patient's electrolyte status with close attention to sodium, potassium, chloride, and magnesium levels, *which will change with phases of ARF.*

Closely observe patients who require PEEP during mechanical ventilation. *Evidence-based research shows that decreased venous return leads to low CO, which can cause prerenal failure in patients with normal renal functioning.*

Prepare to insert a pulmonary artery catheter *to measure the heart's ability to handle preload and afterload.*

Observe strict aseptic techniques *as the patient is at high risk for infection.*

Prepare to insert an indwelling urinary catheter *for strict measurement of output.*

Administer diuretics *to decrease hypertension and excrete excess fluid.*

Monitor Hgb and Hct and prepare to administer Procrit or red blood cells according to protocols *to increase oxygenation.*

Institute safety measures to prevent injury or falls *due to uremic changes in brain functioning.*

Teach and maintain renal diets, *which include low-potassium, low-sodium, high-calorie, and low-protein foods to prevent azotemia, hyperkalemia, and fluid overload.*

Prepare the patient and significant other for dialysis or CRRT if the patient fails to recover.

NURSING ALERT

Recent evidence-based research shows that the use of low-dose dopamine does not prevent/treat renal dysfunction. It may cause more harm by worsening splanchnic oxygen need, decreasing GI motility, increasing tachyarrhythmias, and decreasing pulmonary response to hypercarbia. Dopamine is beneficial for inotropic and vasoactive effects in heart failure and septic shock.

Chronic Renal Failure (CRF)

What Went Wrong?

❺ Chronic renal failure (CRF) is a progressively worsening, irreversible loss of kidney function. Although CRF is irreversible, it can be slowed by medications and diet. In CRF, the kidneys lose their ability to maintain homeostasis with fluid balance and waste accumulation leading to end-stage renal disease (ESRD) and the need for dialysis. CRF is identified by glomerular filtration rate (GFR) and is divided into three stages: reduced renal reserve, renal insufficiency, and end-stage renal disease (ESRD; see Table 8–8).

CRF can be caused by all the processes outlined for ARF; however, the patients with the highest risk of developing CRF are those with diabetes mellitus (DM). Around 30% of patients treated with dialysis have DM. The second largest group is patients with hypertension.

Prognosis

The prognosis for patients with CRF provides hope. There are almost a half million patients in the United States being treated for CRF. Well more than half are maintained on hemodialysis and the next largest number, around 28%, have received kidney transplants. Five percent are treated with PD. The cause of death in most CRF patients is cardiovascular disease.

❷ TABLE 8–8 Stages of CRF

Stages	GFR	Signs/Symptoms
Reduced renal reserve	40%–70% decrease in GFR	Asymptomatic; observe BUN, creatinine, and GFR
Renal insufficiency	75% decrease in GFR	BUN, creatinine elevated Anemia Electrolyte imbalances Nocturia; polyuria (with inability to concentrate urine)
End-stage renal disease (ESRD)	90% reduction in GFR	Oliguria <500 mL/day Uremic toxins (uremia) elevate, creating severe fluid and electrolyte imbalances in all body systems

Interpreting Test Results

CRF affects all body systems and therefore many laboratory tests are affected.

GFR of less than 10 to 20 mL/min (uremia will be evident)

Elevated BUN and creatinine

Hyperkalemia

Hypocalcemia

Hyperphosphatemia

Proteinuria

Elevated triglycerides

Metabolic acidosis

Low Hct and Hgb

Hallmark Signs and Symptoms

CRF leads to uremia, which affects all body systems; therefore, a broad range of symptoms may occur depending upon the level of CRF. Table 8–9 shows changes that can occur in a patient with CRF with uremia.

❻ TABLE 8–9 Signs and Symptoms of Uremia According to Body Systems	
Respiratory system	Kussmaul's respirations in response to metabolic acidosis
	Pleural effusion
	Pulmonary edema
	Pneumonitis
Cardiovascular system	Hypertension
	Dysrhythmias
	Uremic pericarditis (pericardial friction rub) leading to cardiac tamponade
	Heart failure as seen by crackles, gurgles, drop in SaO_2, respiratory acidosis; fluid seen on CXR
Neurologic system	Headaches
	Inability to sleep; irritability
	Change in level of consciousness leading to coma
	Asterixis (tremors of the hands)
	Peripheral neuropathy

⑥ TABLE 8–9 Signs and Symptoms of Uremia According to Body Systems *(Continued)*

Hematological system	Anemia with low H & H
	Increased bleeding
	Impaired white cell functioning with resultant infections
Gastrointestinal system	Nausea, vomiting
	Diarrhea
	Constipation
	Stomatitis
	Uremic fetor (characteristic odor to breath)
Skeletal system	Joint pain and swelling
	Bone pain and pathological fractures from low calcium levels
Integumentary system	Dry and itchy skin (pruritus)
	Edema from right–sided heart failure
	Pallor from anemia
Reproductive system	Decreased libido
	Males: impotence; gynecomastia, decreased sperm counts
	Females: decreased sexual drive; amenorrhea, dysmenorrhea

Treatment

Treatment for CRF involves preserving renal function and delaying dialysis. To accomplish this the following should be done:

Controlling diabetes through diet, weight management, and medications

Controlling hypertension through diet, weight management, and medications

Restricting protein to 50 g of high biologic value

Controlling hematologic changes with epoetin alfa

Decreasing cardiovascular disease with statins

Nursing Diagnoses for CRF	Expected Outcomes
Fluid volume, excess RT inability of kidneys to excrete urine	The patient will maintain fluid gain of <5 lb between dialysis treatments
Imbalanced nutrition less than body requirements due to lack of appetite, dietary limitations, and stomatitis	The patient will have a stable weight
	The patient will select a menu with high–biologic protein
	The patient will have a stable weight

Nursing Interventions

The care of the patient in CRF is very similar to that of the patient with ARF with the following additions:

Monitoring vital signs, especially temperature and BP, *for infection and hypertension.*

Assess for signs and symptoms of worsening uremia *to prevent complications like confusion, pericarditis, hyperkalemia, and bone changes.*

Limit fluid volume intake *to decrease amount of fluid removed by diuretics or dialysis. Usual amount is calculated to be 500 to 600 mL from previous 24-hour urine output.*

Calculate the amount of fluid the patient is receiving including orally and through medications and irrigations as *considerable amounts may add to fluid intake from these sources.*

Administer antihypertensive medications *to lessen the workload of the heart and prevent heart failure.*

Monitoring for sodium and water retention by checking laboratory values *to reduce the edema.*

Observe the patient for twitching, headache, change in the level of consciousness, or seizure activity, *which can be caused by neurologic changes due to uremia.*

Administer vitamin D and calcium *to prevent renal osteodystrophy (removal of calcium from the bone, causing them to become brittle and break) and lower phosphate levels.*

Observe for pericarditis, *which can lead to pericardial tamponade caused by uremic wastes and inadequate dialysis.*

Assess the potassium level for hyperkalemia, *which can elevate in the blood when the kidneys cannot excrete it.*

Check the Hct (less than 30%) and Hgb (less than 12 g/dL) levels *to observe for anemia secondary to the absence of erythropoietin usually formed in the kidney.*

Administer synthetic erythropoietin after dialysis *to increase formation of red blood cells and prevent anemia.*

Monitor for range of motion (ROM) and functional abilities *as low serum calcium and high phosphate levels cause removal and weakness of bone structure.*

Check all medications for magnesium-containing compounds. Patients with chronic renal failure cannot excrete magnesium. Giving magnesium-containing compounds like antacids can lead to magnesium toxicity.

Provide frequent oral hygiene *to decrease oral dryness and improve appetite and overall feeling of wellness.*

Monitor for weight changes *to determine if patient is adhering to dietary restrictions.*

Assess for symptoms that lead to decreased dietary intake *to determine if other interventions may help the patient, such as a dietary consult.*

Promote a diet consisting of limited high-biologic protein, *which includes eggs and dairy products, to help maintain positive nitrogen balance, decrease nitrogenous waste production, and promote growth and healing.*

Limit the amount of potassium and sodium in the diet and medications *to prevent hyperkalemia and fluid overload.*

Administer phosphate-binding resins and calcium *to keep the phosphate levels low and prevent calcium from being absorbed from bones.*

Monitor the patient for bleeding tendencies (Hct and Hgb; platelet count, PT, PTT), *which can be caused by platelet impairment.*

Avoid administering aspirin or nonsteroidal anti-inflammatory drugs (NSAIDs), *which can further alter platelet function.*

Administer vitamin supplements after dialysis *as water-soluble medications are removed by the dialysis process.*

Recounting a True Story

My husband worked with a gentleman who had CRF for many years. I knew his wife as she was the head of the OR at a local hospital. I played golf with Pete once and noticed how enlarged his AV graft arm was. He was still able to remain physically active; however, he needed my assistance to look for his golf ball as his vision was failing. He was particularly proud that he had maintained this graft for many years without complications, but his other body systems were not as fortunate.

He started requiring frequent blood transfusions as the Epogen he was taking no longer maintained his oxygen levels, and he had had several bouts of infections that took their toll.

One day my husband came home and told me Pete and his wife decided he had had "enough." He refused any more dialysis treatments. It was very hard on his wife and family, but with the support of physicians, family, counselors, and fellow church members, Pete had a peaceful death with family and friends in attendance. But it was the constant vigilance and support of the nursing staff that made the most difference to Pete's family.

Hyperkalemia Related to CRF

What Went Wrong?

❼ Hyperkalemia occurs when the potassium level is greater than 5.5 mEq/L. High potassium levels are one of the most severe complications of ARF and CRF. Hyperkalemia is caused by retention of potassium, metabolic acidosis, excessive intake of potassium-containing foods and medications, and cellular catabolism. The critical care nurse must be aware of cardiac changes with hyperkalemia and emergency treatment to lower blood levels quickly.

Prognosis

The prognosis is excellent for treating hyperkalemia, but early recognition is key.

Interpreting Laboratory/Diagnostic Results

Potassium level greater than 5.5 mEq/L.

ABGs show a metabolic acidosis.

Early ECG changes show tall, tented T waves, QRS widening.

Later changes show flattened P waves and PR interval prolongation.

Hallmark Signs and Symptoms

Muscle cramps and weakness

Abdominal pain accompanied by nausea, vomiting

Treatment

Restrict potassium-containing intake in foods, IV fluids, and medications.

Administer Kayexalate therapy.

Dialyze potassium from the body.

Administer glucose and insulin to drive potassium into the cells.

Administer $NaHCO_3$ and monitor ABGs.

Administer calcium salts.

Nursing Diagnosis for Hyperkalemia	Expected Outcomes
Decreased cardiac output due to electric conduction disturbances	The potassium level will remain between 3.5 and 5.2 mEq/L
	The patient will describe foods containing potassium and limit the amount in his or her menu

Nursing Interventions

Monitor the patient's VS to determine *if cardiac output is diminished by decreased pulse rate or if temperature elevation indicates an infection.*

Observe potassium fluctuations *to prevent and treat hyperkalemia early.*

Monitor the patient's ABGs for acidosis, *which is caused by the inability of the kidneys to excrete H$^+$ ions and can create hyperkalemia by K$^+$–H$^+$ exchange.*

Monitor the patient for ECG/EKG changes that include high-peaked T waves, then widening of QRS and large, rounded T wave, concluding with P wave flattening and prolongation of PR interval, which are symptoms of hypokalemia.

Administer diuretics or sodium polystyrene if the hyperkalemia is mild (less than 6 mEq/L) *to excrete potassium (diuretic) or bind the potassium into the gut with removal in fecal material.*

Administer sorbitol with sodium polystyrene sulfate and/or give a cleansing enema after administration *to prevent constipation.*

Administer calcium gluconate or chloride IV, *which is the first priority in severe, life-threatening hyperkalemia to stimulate cardiac contractions.*

Administer glucose-insulin IV *treatment for* severe hyperkalemia *to shift potassium into the cell.*

Administer sodium bicarbonate *only if severe acidosis (pH less than 7.2 and HCO$_3$ less than 12 mEq/L) to correct metabolic acidosis.*

Administer calcium gluconate or chloride IV, *which is the first priority in severe, life-threatening hyperkalemia.*

Teach the patient to avoid potassium-containing foods like green, leafy vegetables and salt supplements, limiting potassium intake to 2 g/day *to prevent recurrence between dialysis.*

NURSING ALERT

Cardiac dysrhythmias from hyperkalemia can be fatal. Patients in ARF and CRF need to have their serum potassium monitored, especially if the hyperkalemia is of new onset.

CASE STUDY

8 R.R. is a 32-year-old female with juvenile onset DM, HTN, and CRF who has been admitted to the intensive care unit for severe hyperkalemia and clotting of a right forearm AV fistula. R.R.'s CRF is a result of an aspirin overdose with the diagnosis of CRF less than 3 months ago.

RR has been extremely depressed according to her husband and not taking care of herself or going to her dialysis treatments for the past week. He is afraid she has "given up" and "wants to end it all."

You perform vital signs (TPR = 100.1°F-120-34, BP 80/40, SaO_2 90% on 4 L nasal cannula) and attach R.R. to the cardiac monitor. You call for a 12-lead ECG because you see changes indicative of hyperkalemia and premature ventricular contractions on the bedside cardiac monitor. You identify her abnormal laboratory values: Na 155, K 7.2, Ca 5, and phosphate 7; Hct and Hgb 8 g/dL and 25%. ABGs are pH 7.25, pO_2 100, pCO_2 30, HCO_3 15. She has an S3 and crackles at both bases with pitting edema bilaterally below the knees.

QUESTIONS

1. What essential assessment finding will alert you to a blocked AV fistula?
2. What symptoms confirm that this patient has hyperkalemia?
3. Why are her laboratory values so abnormal?
4. What treatment would you anticipate R.R. will be receiving?

   After stabilizing R.R.'s collaborative needs (laboratory levels and vital signs, especially the potassium level and hypotension) you have time to formulate other less life-threatening nursing diagnoses.

QUESTIONS

5. What nursing diagnostic statements take priority in this scenario?

   Once stabilized, R.R. says she just cannot stand the way she is living and is overwhelmed with the dialysis treatments, the complex medication regime, and dietary restrictions. You notify the nephrologist about this and contact former patients who volunteer to talk to patients about adjusting to dialysis. You also tell her that depression might be induced by uremic poisoning due to an infection she might have. A dietary consult might be beneficial in this case and you continue to monitor the patient while making plans to discuss the blocked AV fistula and a new site replacement with the surgeon.

   She stays on your unit with 1:1 surveillance until feeling much better; she gives permission to insert a central line for HD continuation until a new AV fistula can be placed.

REVIEW QUESTIONS

1. A patient with acute renal failure (ARF) can have adverse cardiac signs and symptoms. Check all of the cardiac symptoms below a nurse would see in a patient with ARF.

   A. Crackles

   B. Severe pruritus

   C. Uremic fetor

   D. Melena

   E. Pericardial friction rub

   F. Lethargy

2. A nurse is analyzing the following arterial blood gases in a patient with renal failure. Describe what is occurring in this arterial blood gas and how the kidneys and lungs are involved.

   $pH = 7.32, pCO_2 = 30, pO_2 = 150, HCO_3 = 18$

3. The nurse suspects that a patient with acute renal failure (ARF) has early hyper-kalemia. What 12-lead ECG changes would confirm this suspicion?

   A. Shortened PR and QT intervals

   B. Tall, peaked T waves

   C. A widened QRS measurement

   D. Disappearing P waves

4. True or False. Predialysis and postdialysis weights are critical nursing care procedures to perform in all three forms of dialysis.

5. A patient has ARF due to prerenal failure. Which of the following risk factors would the nurse assess in a patient with prerenal failure?

   A. Dehydration

   B. Fluid overload

   C. Kidney stones

   D. Nephrotoxic medications

6. A patient has an arteriovenous (AV) fistula created for hemodialysis. At the beginning of the shift, assessment of what vital information would be required by the nurse to ensure proper functioning of this access site?

   A. Enlarged arteries around the access area

   B. A bruit and a thrill

   C. A patient dialysis catheter exiting at the abdominal area

   D. Distal pulses in the extremity as well as color, motor function, and sensation

7. The ICU nurse is starting peritoneal dialysis (PD) in a patient who has end-stage renal disease (ESRD) and was admitted to the ICU for uremic pericarditis. The patient states, "My abdomen is red and swollen; this is not like what I usually experience." During the assessment, the nurse notes the following VS: TPR = 101.8°F-110-28, BP 150/90. The abdomen is large, shiny, and tense with erythema around the PD catheter site. This patient is most likely experiencing

   A. Dialysis disequilibrium

   B. Hypokalemia

   C. Catheter kinking due to fibrin

   D. Peritonitis

8. A patient with ESRD has a serum potassium level of 8 mEq/L with hypotension, short runs of ventricular fibrillation, and a widened QRS. The critical care nurse should anticipate which drug for administration to counteract this patient's lethal rhythm?

   A. Do nothing; this is a normal potassium level

   B. Give the patient sodium polystyrene

   C. Administer sodium bicarbonate

   D. Give calcium gluconate IV

9. The nurse is evaluating the admission information of a patient with CRF needing dialysis. Which of the following medications would the nurse question?

   A. Milk of Magnesia (MOM)

   B. Folic acid (folate)

   C. Cimetadine (Tagamet)

   D. Procrit (Epogen)

10. A patient with ESRD requiring HD is admitted to your unit with heart failure. During the HD you note new onset of twitching. The patient also states leg cramping has developed in both lower extremities. The hemodialysis nurse also notes these changes in status. After completing a head-to-toe assessment, you call the nephrologist who asks you what your evaluation of these symptoms might be. Considering the information above, this patient is most likely experiencing

   A. Pericarditis

   B. An infection

   C. Disequilibrium syndrome

   D. Hyperkalemia

ANSWERS

CASE STUDY

1. When you palpate the right forearm fistula site, you should feel a thrill (rushing of blood pulsating under your fingers) and auscultate a bruit (swishing noise), which will determine patency. Do not forget to use a Doppler if you do not hear anything.

2. Hyperkalemia is confirmed by tall, tented T waves; widening of the QRS; and flattening of the P wave. Confirmation is done by the laboratory value of 7.2 mEq/L.

3. Her findings are indicative of a patient in CRF who has not been dialyzed. She is retaining sodium, potassium, and phosphate, which are seen as the kidneys cannot excrete these and they cannot be dialyzed due to her clotting AV fistula. Since calcium is opposite of phosphate in CRF, her levels are low, causing this level to rise.

    ABGs indicate a metabolic acidosis because the pH is 7.25 with an HCO_3 level of less than 22. She is partially compensating for this as her low pCO_2 indicates she is blowing off her CO_2 (creating a respiratory alkalosis). But the acidosis is her primary problem as indicated by the pH, which will always tell you the primary acid-base disturbance. This is confirmed by her respiratory rate in the 30s; she probably has Kussmaul's respirations if she is breathing fast and deep.

    Her low Hgb and Hct tell you to ask the husband or patient if she has been taking her Procrit, folic acid, and iron to help compensate for the lack of kidney production of native erythropoietin.

4. The priority treatment is to give this patient calcium gluconate IV to help stimulate the heart to contract and prevent death by dysrhythmias (ventricular fibrillation or asystole). A solution of glucose and insulin should be given to help drive the potassium back into the cell. This can also reverse the hyperkalemia.

    She will need blood later due to her low Hct and Hbg. She cannot wait for Epogen to work.

5. Decreased cardiac output related to hyperkalemia as noted by ECG changes, hypotension, and dysrhythmias. Fluid volume excess related to lack of dialysis treatments as manifested by elevated serum sodium and peripheral edema.

CORRECT ANSWERS AND RATIONALES

1. A, E, and F. A patient in ARF can develop right- and left-sided heart failure. Failure to excrete excess fluid can result in crackles as fluid backs up into the lungs from the heart's inability to pump the extra fluid load. Pericarditis develops due to uremic poisons, which affect the heart and can lead to cardiac tamponade. Lethargy can be due to hypoxemia when the excess fluid interferes with O_2 and CO_2 exchange in the lungs and heart.

2. This patient is in an acidosis as the pH is less than 7.35. The acidosis is not caused by the respiratory system as the pCO_2 indicates a respiratory alkalosis as a secondary problem, not the primary one. The HCO_3 is less than 22 mEq/L, which shows that the kidneys are giving up base or retaining acid, leading to an acidosis. Since the pH will always tell the primary problem, linked with the HCO3, this is a metabolic acidosis. The nurse needs to look at the clinical situation to find the metabolic acidosis. In the renal patient, it is because the kidneys cannot maintain pH balance and acid is retained. The lungs are compensating by excreting CO_2. Since the pH is not normal, we have a partially compensated metabolic acidosis. It would be fully compensated if the pH were less than 7.40 but in the normal range.

3. B. High, peaked T waves are indicative of early hyperkalemia. The others are late signs of hyperkalemia.

4. True. All dialysis types look at how much weight via fluid loss (wet weight minus dry weight) occurs during each treatment. Weight gain or loss is the number one indicator of fluid balance, and it should be confirmed with the intake and output, serum sodium, and hematocrit.

5. A. Prerenal failure is due to decreased blood flow to the kidney, so dehydration lowers BP, therefore lowering GFR. Fluid overload is a symptom of ARF and CRF. Kidney stones (postrenal) and nephrotoxic medications (intrarenal) can cause other types of ARF.

6. B. A bruit is a swishing sound like a heart murmur but heard peripherally over the fistula site. A thrill is a vibration like a pulsating water hose felt over the insertion site. If these are not present, call the nephrologist right away!

7. D. Peritonitis is the most common complication of PD. The patient is febrile, tachycardic, and tachypneic—all signs of possible infection. The abdominal insertion site is red and the patient states that it is swollen—all confirming the possible problem.

8. D. Calcium gluconate IV is needed to stimulate the heart to contract and prevent sustained ventricular fibrillation or asystole. This is an abnormally high potassium level as it is greater than 5.1 mEq/L. Sodium bicarbonate is given to correct a metabolic acidosis, and there is no evidence that this patient has this in the information provided. Sodium polystyrene is given with sorbitol in situations of mild hypokalemia. The level ventricular fibrillation and symptoms in the patient indicate an emergency!

9. A. Patients with CRF cannot excrete magnesium-containing compounds; so MOM would be contraindicated in the care of this patient. The other medications are used to treat CRF.

10. C. New-onset twitching, positive Trousseau's and Chvostek's signs, and cramping can all indicate disequilibrium syndrome. There is no information to support a pericarditis (temperature or friction rub), infection (elevated temperature, pulse, or infected HD site), or hyperkalemia (high-peaked T waves).

chapter 9

Care of the Patient With Critical Hematologic Needs

LEARNING OBJECTIVES

At the end of this chapter, the student will be able to:

❶ List key components of the hematologic system and their functions.

❷ Describe the steps in the hemostasis process.

❸ Identify nursing assessment skills needed to care for the patient with critical hematologic needs.

❹ Discuss common laboratory and diagnostic tests to confirm hematologic problems.

❺ Explain the risks and benefits of commonly used medications in the care of the patient with hematologic needs.

❻ Incorporate the nursing process in the care of a patient with hematologic issues.

❼ Distinguish between sepsis, septic shock, SIRS, and MODS.

KEY WORDS

Agranulocytes
Albumin
ANC – absolute neutrophil count
Clotting cascade
Erythrocyte
Erythropoietin
Glossitis
Granulocytes
Hematopoiesis
Leukocytes
MODS – multiple organ dysfunction
      syndrome
Neutropenia

Petechiae
Plasma proteins
Platelets
Pluripotent stem cell
Sepsis
Septic shock
Shift-to-the-left
SIRS – systemic inflammatory response
      syndrome
Stem cells
RBCs – red blood cells
Reticulocyte
WBCs – white blood cells

Anatomy and Physiology of the Hematologic System

❶ Hematopoiesis is the production and maturation of blood cells in the body. Blood consists of plasma, red blood cells, white blood cells, platelets, and lymphocytes. Plasma is the largest component of blood and includes water along with the plasma proteins albumin, globulin, and fibrinogen. Albumen is important in maintaining fluid balance in the vascular space by acting like a magnet to hold on to water. Globulin is necessary for immune responses, and fibrinogen is important for clotting.

Red blood cells (RBCs) or erythrocytes are the most numerous type of cell in the blood. In their mature state, RBCs contain no nucleus so they cannot reproduce and must be constantly formed. They are flexible, biconcavelike, and move quickly through the vascular system. RBCs have a short life of only 120 days, degrading as they age with excess iron converted to bilirubin. Bilirubin is reused by the liver or excreted in the urine. If it cannot be excreted, bilirubin can be excreted in the skin, creating the yellow color seen in jaundice.

RBCs are 90% hemoglobin. Hemoglobin is made up of iron, which binds with globin which attaches to and carries the oxygen molecule. The primary role of RBCs is to carry oxygen-rich arterial blood to all cells and major organs. Pluripotent stem cells stimulated by erythropoietin create RBCs. Immature forms of RBCs are called reticulocytes. Reticulocytes are released when erythropoietin from the kidney is produced in response to stress from hypoxemia, anemia, and other disease states. Failure to produce mature RBCs creates anemia and possible hypoxemia.

White blood cells (WBCs) or leukocytes originate in the bone marrow and circulate through the body within the lymph system. All WBCs protect the body from infection, defend against cancer formation, and promote wound healing. Their normal values and actions can be reviewed in Table 9–2.

WBCs can be further classified according to their cell type, including granulocytes and agranulocytes. Granulocytes have cytoplasmic granules that stain a certain color. Granulocytes are further subdivided into neutrophils, eosinophils, and basophils. Segmented neutrophils make up the greatest number of WBCs circulating throughout the body in search of pathogens. Eosinophils and basophils are primarily stimulated in response to allergic reactions.

Agranulocytes are also further divided into monocytes and lymphocytes. When stimulated by foreign substances, monocytes transform into macrophages that remove debris from proteins and phagocytize bacteria. Lymphocytes are produced in bone marrow and produce T cells and B cells. T and B cells are the principle mediators of the immune system and are stimulated to produce antibodies and identify foreign, "non-self" organisms. Failure to produce mature WBCs leads to an immunocompromised patient, with septic shock as a possible consequence.

Platelets are granular fragments of once giant cells, which play a dominant role in controlling bleeding. When there is an internal or external injury to the endothelium, the platelets get "turned on" and start collecting at the injury site(s). A platelet plug is then formed to temporarily stop bleeding.

Fibrin then adheres to the plug, creating a stable clot that is eventually decomposed as the wounded area heals. The life of a platelet is from 7 to 10 days. Failure to produce platelets results in bleeding and possible hemorrhagic shock.

All of the blood cells are produced by the pluripotent stem cells. They are differentiated according to what the body needs most. A major concept is that these cells are not produced immediately and if one group of cells proliferates, it is at the expense of the others. Also, immature cells do not perform the function of mature cells. This is why in leukemia the overproduction of immature white cells does not lead to more protection from infection; it leads to neutropenia, which is the absence of infection-fighting cells. The immature cells do not fight against infection.

The body is constantly maintaining a delicate balance between clotting and bleeding. Hemostasis is the ability of the blood to clot when injury has occurred. The normal clotting mechanism is a complex process called the clotting cascade. Platelets carefully work to keep the endothelial wall intact. When there is an assault on the endothelial lining from inside the body (intrinsic) or from outside (extrinsic), pathways are initiated that start a cascade of events to produce hemostasis.

Injury to the vessel results in muscular spasm also releasing neural reflexes and humoral factors. Platelets start "clumping" together adhering to the site of injury and each other with spinylike projections. A plug of platelets forms, stimulating the clotting cascade.

Thromboplastin is released from damaged tissues, activating numerous steps until prothrombin activator is produced. The amount of prothrombin activator released is directly proportional to the amount of tissue damaged. Prothrombin activator changes prothrombin to thrombin, which in turn leads to fibrin formation. Fibrin is the gel that holds together the platelets and other blood components. The thrombus or blood clot usually stays on site but may break away and embolize.

Further strengthening of the clot occurs as fibroblasts invade the meshwork of the clot. Next, the clot retracts, pulling its edges together and further protecting the injury. Almost immediately, the body starts breaking apart the thrombus by a process of fibrinolysis. The end result is healing of the injury, smoothing of the endothelial lining, and reestablishment of blood flow.

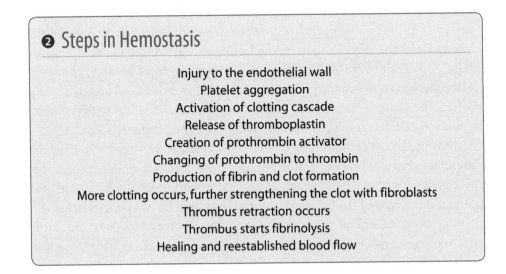

❷ Steps in Hemostasis

Injury to the endothelial wall
Platelet aggregation
Activation of clotting cascade
Release of thromboplastin
Creation of prothrombin activator
Changing of prothrombin to thrombin
Production of fibrin and clot formation
More clotting occurs, further strengthening the clot with fibroblasts
Thrombus retraction occurs
Thrombus starts fibrinolysis
Healing and reestablished blood flow

Assessment Skills

❸ Observation and care of the patient with hematologic disorders involve looking for signs and symptoms of bleeding, infection, or anemia.

History

The patient's age and cultural background are important as hematologic system functioning decreases with age, and some types of anemias are more frequent in cultural/ethnic groups. For example, sickle cell anemia is frequent in African-Americans.

Check to see if the patient is in pain. If so, perform a complete pain assessment. It is common for patients to say they have achy joints or pain upon movement if they are having a sickle cell crisis. (See OPQRST method in Chapter 3, Table 3–2.)

A functional history should be performed with special attention to any comments regarding fatigue, weakness, or inability to perform previous activities. The lack of RBCs and increase in WBCs can cause fatigue and an inability to perform life roles. Ask the patient if he or she has a history of headache, bleeding, or dyspnea. Does the patient have a loss of appetite?

What is the chief problem stated by the family or significant other? Many times hematological problems are chronic and much valuable information regarding care can be elicited. Does the patient have a past medical history (PMH) of anemia, leukemia, trauma, or clotting disorders such as PE and DVT?

What medications are taken regularly by the patient? Do they include anticoagulants, chemotherapeutic agents, or iron?

Do they describe any numbness and tingling in the extremities? If they can walk, do they have a sense of balance? Neurological signs of anemia can include these along with apathy and irritability.

NURSING ALERT

The patient's medications should be assessed as many can cause myelosuppression, which is a decrease in all three cell lines. Common medications that can cause myeosuppression include Dilantin (phenytoin), some antibiotics, and chemotherapeutic alkalyating agents. Medications like aspirin, clopidogrel (Plavix), and ibuprofen (Advil) can decrease platelet function.

Inspection

First, a generalized inspection of the skin is needed. An overall pale color can signify loss of hemoglobin. Jaundice of the skin and eyes can signify an inability of the liver to reuse bilirubin from older, spent RBCs. Does the patient have petechiae—small, pinpoint hemorrhages seen in platelet dysfunction? Are there bruises or hematoma formations? These would indicate bleeding into larger areas.

Check the patient's oral cavity. Is the tongue large, smooth, and beefy red? Is the mouth inflamed? Both of these conditions can be seen in iron-deficiency anemias. Is there easy bleeding of the mucous membranes? Are there white, patchy areas that can be invasion of the mucous membranes by thrush in a patient with low white cell counts?

Can you see an enlarged spleen or liver? Examine the lymph nodes for swelling; you will be palpating these areas next.

Palpation

Palpate the patient's peripheral pulses. Thrombus formation can cause diminished blood flow to the extremities, but a pulse should be present. Is there peripheral edema; is it pitting or nonpitting?

Lymph nodes can be palpated for signs of infection or an immune disorder. They are usually palpated from head to groin and include cervical, submandibular, axillary, and inguinal (see Figure 9–1). As you gently palpate these nodes note if they are hard, firm, soft, or freely moveable. Also note if they are painful or tender. Enlarged, hard, inflamed nodes could indicate infection or tumor.

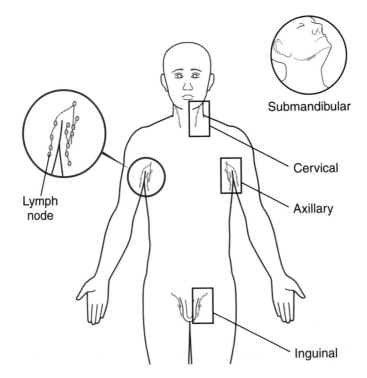

FIGURE 9–1 • Location of lymph nodes.

Percussion

Percussion of the liver and spleen can be done to determine enlargement. Normally the liver can be palpated under the right lower rib cage when the patient takes a deep breath. The spleen is located under the left costal margin and is only palpable when it is greatly enlarged.

Auscultation

Listen to the patient's heart sounds. Are they regular; do you hear any extra or skipped beats? Next, take the BP on both arms; a lower BP and hypotension can be caused by extreme blood loss. Listen to the abdomen for bowel sounds. Remember to do inspection and auscultation of the abdomen before percussion and palpation. Patients with high-pitched, loud bowel sounds can have an intestinal obstruction caused by lymphomas.

Collaborative Diagnostic and Laboratory Tools

Laboratory Tests

❹ The tests in Table 9–1 are frequently monitored in a patient with a hematologic problem.

TABLE 9–1 Analyzing Test Values for RBCs and Platelets		
Laboratory Tool	**Normal Value**	**Meaning of Abnormal Values**
RBC (erythrocyte count)	5 million × 10.6 cells/mm³	Decreased in anemias Increased in polycythemia vera
Hemoglobin	12–18 g/dL	Decreased in anemia Decreased with active bleeding Increased in polycythemia
Hematocrit	35%–50%	Decreased in anemia Decreased in fluid volume excess
Platelets	150,000–400,000/µL	A drop can indicate DIC, a reaction to heparin, extra-corporeal blood circulation, and disorders that decrease platelet formation

> **NURSING ALERT**
>
> *A drop in hemoglobin below 10 g/dL or a trend downward from baseline should be reported to the physician. A sudden drop can indicate bleeding, and a gradual drop can point to anemia.*

> **NURSING ALERT**
>
> *A decrease in platelets below 30,000 warns the nurse that bleeding, especially intracranial, can occur. Institute bleeding precautions and notify the physician ASAP!*

One of the most important tools to determine abnormalities of the hematologic system is the white blood cell count (WBC) with a differential. Table 9–2 reviews the components, values, and action of specific WBCs.

TABLE 9–2 WBC With Differential

WBC Component	Differential	Number*	Action
Neutrophils (also known as polymorphonuclear leukocytes—PNM) Largest number of WBCs Band neutrophils are types of immature WBCs that elevates in sepsis	60%–70%	3,000–7,000	Preserve normal defense against bacteria, fungi, and variety of non–self substances Increase in neutrophils can be caused by pathogenic invasion, stress, epinephrine, exercise, and steroid use Look for an elevation of the band neutrophils in sepsis >5%
Lymphocytes	25%–33%	1,000–4,000	Defend against infection Responsible for humoral and cellular immunity Produce B (humoral) and T cells (cellular)
Monocytes	3%–7%	100–800	Powerful macrophages They engulf foreign cells, necrotic tissue, and debris Also involved in immune response

TABLE 9–2 WBC With Differential (*Continued*)			
WBC Component	**Differential**	**Number***	**Action**
Eosinophils	1%–5%	50–400	Release enzymes that neutralize allergic responses
			Attach to parasites releasing enzymes that destroy them
			Increased in allergic reactions and parasitic infestations
Basophils	0–0.75%	25–100	Least numerous
			Granules contain heparin, histamine, and other inflammatory mediators
			Increase in production in allergic and hypersensitivity reactions
Total WBC count	100%	5,000–10,000	

*Reported in microliters of blood.

The Absolute Neutrophil Count (ANC)

The absolute neutrophil count (ANC) is an important value to determine whether the patient is immunocompromised due to a drop in neutrophils (neutropenia). Frequently laboratories report this number, but if they do not, the critical care nurse can calculate this value from the WBC with a differential. First, add up the total percentage of neutrophils. Then multiply this value by the total number of WBCs. An example of how to calculate this value follows. The normal value is greater than 1,000 cells/mm^3.

   Example: Segmented neutrophils = 30%

   Band neutrophils = 10%

   Total WBCs = 11,000 cells/mm^3

   30% + 10% = 40% = 0.40

   11,000 × 0.40 = 4,400 cells/mm^3 (ANC)

The patient in this example does not have an elevated ANC because the ANC count is greater than 1,000. Therefore, the patient is not neutropenic.

Coagulation Studies

Because the patient can develop bleeding disorders from hematologic problems, close monitoring and trending of coagulation studies is imperative. Table 9–3 summarizes important values the critical care nurse needs to know.

TABLE 9–3 Coagulation Studies

Test	What It Shows	Normal Values
Bleeding time	Infrequently done as it is highly insensitive Shows platelet interaction and capillary constriction	1–6 minutes
D–dimer	Positive in inflammatory responses where plasmin carries out fibrinolytic action on a clot that has formed	0 or <250 ng/mL
Erythrocyte sedimentation rate (ESR)	RBCs in anticoagulated blood fall faster in a specimen. Fall rate increases in presence of fibrin and other inflammatory problems	0–20 mm/hr
Fibrin degradation products (FPD)	Helps in confirming DIC When fibrinolysis occurs these products are liberated into blood	<10 mg/dL
Fibrinogen levels	Lack of fibrinogen in the bloodstream	200–400 mg/dL
International Normalized Ratio (INR)	Best standardized measurement, better than a PT	1
Prothrombin time (PT)	Shows extrinsic clotting factors Used to monitor Coumadin (warfarin) effectiveness—prolonged in this therapy 1.5 to 2.5 × normal value	12–15 seconds
Activated partial thromboplastin time (aPTT)	Shows intrinsic clotting factors Used to monitor therapeutic values of heparin drips for PE, MI, DIC—prolonged in this therapy 1.5 to 2.5 × normal value	30–45 seconds

Other Tests

There are other tests that can be used to help monitor patients with acute hemolytic anemia. These include tests for iron and its storage and are listed in Table 9–4.

❹ TABLE 9–4   Other Tests for the Presence of Iron

Test	What It Shows	Normal Values
Serum iron (Fe)	Decreases with serum iron concentration	75–150 µg/dL
Serum ferritin	Highly sensitive test for total body iron stores Decreased in iron–deficiency anemias	30–300 ng/mL
Serum transferring (total iron–binding capacity)	Production increased with low iron stores as this is transport protein	250–460 µg/dL

Diagnostic Tests

ECG/EKG – Electrocardiogram to check for MI, which can be caused in severe anemias.

CT scan – Can help locate source of sepsis.

Bone marrow aspiration/biopsy – Microscopic study of cells growing in bone marrow. This study is done by the physician with the nurse assisting. The physician inserts a coring needle for an aspiration and a special larger needle for an aspiration.

How to Do It–Assisting With a Bone Marrow Aspiration

1. Check that a consent form is signed.

2. Identify the patient with at least two qualifiers and perform time-out.

3. Monitor preprocedural coagulation studies to determine if the patient is subject to bleeding.

4. Assess the patient's knowledge of what to expect during the study and as far as the results of the study. It will take approximately 30 minutes.

5. Identify the medications the patient is taking. Aspirin, anticoagulants, and other medications can increase bleeding tendencies.

6. Check the IV site for patency for delivery of medications.

7. Administer any preprocedural medications like antianxiety and systemic opiates, if protocol. Request medications if not.

8. Perform baseline vital signs.

9. Prepare the patient, assisting him or her into a fetal position if the posterior iliac crest is used.

After the Procedure

1. Monitor/record VS and status of procedural site according to protocols, usually every 15 minutes for the first hour, then every hour for the next 4 to 8 hours.

2. Assess the patient's ability to swallow prior to allowing to eat if premedication was given to prevent aspiration.

3. Observe for delayed hypersensitivity reactions like urticaria, itching, tachycardia, and hypertension.

4. Report any excessive bleeding at the aspiration site.

5. Support the patient, recognizing that anxiety can result pending test results.

Medications Commonly Used in Critical Care That Affect the Hematologic System

❺ TABLE 9–5 Medications That Can Be Used in Hematologic Needs

Medication	Action	Uses	Precautions
Albumin 5% and 25%	Increases intravascular volume by creating an osmotic pull from plasma proteins	Shock	1. Watch for fluid overload and pulmonary edema 2. Only use clear yellow solutions; cloudiness or sediment can indicate infection 3. May leak back into interstitial fluid; monitor for dropping BP and serum albumin levels

⑤ TABLE 9–5 Medications That Can Be Used in Hematologic Needs (*Continued*)

Medication	Action	Uses	Precautions
Aminocaproic acid (Amicar)	Hemostatic agent helps control excessive bleeding Inhibits plasminogen activator substance and plasmin	Disseminated intravascular coagulopathy (DIC)	1. Avoid rapid infusion by regulating on IV pump 2. Rapid infusion can cause dysrhythmias, bradycardia, and hypotension 3. Change the administration site immediately if extravasation or thrombophlebitis occurs 4. Can cause renal failure; watch the BUN, creatinine, and urinary output 5. Report symptoms of myopathy like myalgia, fever, myoglobinuria 6. Discontinue if signs of DVT or PE develop
Anticoagulants	See Chapter 3 medications (see Table 3-9)		
Dobutamine (Dobutrex)	Increases cardiac contractility by stimulating beta-1 myocardial receptors Increases CO and decreases PAOP Increases conduction through AV node Decreases rhythm disturbances	Hypotension related to septic shock	1. Use infusion pump to titrate continuous infusion according to the HR and BP 2. Correct acidosis and hypovolemia prior to initiating 3. Check the VS frequently during initial therapy then every 15 minutes after stabilizing 4. If marked increase in HR, BP, or dysrhythmias, decrease the dose

❺ TABLE 9–5   Medications That Can Be Used in Hematologic Needs (*Continued*)

Medication	Action	Uses	Precautions
Intropin (dopamine)	Increases BP by systemic vasoconstriction	Used for hypovolemic shock	1. Fluid resuscitation should be implemented before dopamine 2. Check the VS frequently during initial therapy then every 15 minutes thereafter
Drotrecogin alpha (Xigris) Activated protein C	Severe sepsis with evidence of three or more SIRS criteria or evidence of MOSD	Combats thrombosis, inflammation, and fibrinolysis in septic shock Prevents secondary organ dysfunction	1. Check frequently for bleeding (epistaxis, hematemesis, hematuria, ecchymoses, and hematomas) 2. Monitor baseline Hgb and Hct, coagulation profiles, and urinalysis 3. May prolong aPTT, so not a reliable indicator of clotting abilities 4. Contraindicated in hypersensitivity to drug, active internal bleeding, hemorrhagic stroke (within 3 months), recent (3 months) intracranial or spinal surgery or trauma; use of epidural catheter; intracranial tumor or mass lesion 5. Further evidence of effectiveness is required before it becomes the standard of care

⑤ TABLE 9–5 Medications That Can Be Used in Hematologic Needs (*Continued*)

Medication	Action	Uses	Precautions
Epinephrine	Pure catecholamine that increases cardiac contractions and increases systemic vascular resistance	First–line drug used in cardiac arrest due to shock May also be used in hypotensive episodes due to septic shock	1. Continuous cardiac monitoring is needed to see HR increases 2. Given as IV push in an arrest. Infusion may be prepared via pump 3. Assess VS frequently during initiation and during infusion 4. Destroyed in alkaline solutions like bicarbonate, so use separate line for infusion 5. Check label as comes in varying solutions
Epoetin alfa (Epogen)	RBC stimulator	Used in chronic renal failure to prevent anemia Used for chemotherapy–induced anemia	1. Contraindicated in patients with HTN 2. Mostly central nervous system adverse effects: headache, fatigue, and dizziness 3. If dose does not give the response (elevation in RBCs, Hct) discontinue the drug. The patient may have RBC aplasia from the medication neutralizing antibodies

⑤ TABLE 9–5 Medications That Can Be Used in Hematologic Needs (*Continued*)

Medication	Action	Uses	Precautions
Norepineph-rine bitartrate (Levophed)	Increases BP in shock as a direct-acting sympathomimetic identical to epinephrine Vasoconstriction and positive ino-tropic agent	Restores BP in hypotensive states such as shock, MI, blood transfusion, and drug reactions Can be used in cardiac arrest	1. Given as IV push 2. Baseline and ongoing HR, BP, and cardiac monitoring 3. Titrated according to BP 4. Can cause stroke; monitor neurologic status 5. Headache, vomiting, palpitations, chest pain, photophobia, and blurred vision are signs of overdose 6. Contraindicated in mesenteric or peripheral vascular thrombosis, hypertension, and hyperthyroidism

Blood Products Used for Hematologic Problems

There are a variety of blood products that can be used in the patient with a hematologic problem. The workhorse still remains packed RBCs (see information in Chapter 6 for packed RBC replacement and nursing care, Table 6–4).

Medical Conditions That Require Critical Care

The Immunocompromised Patient (a Review)

What Went Wrong?

Immunocompromised patients lose their ability to fight off infections. They can develop infections from opportunistic organisms that we normally fight off like fungi, molds, and other bacteria. Common risk factors include young age or older aged and chronic disease such as diabetes mellitus, leukemia, anemia, and other cancers.

Any time the skin is invaded by surgery or instrumentative procedures, our first line of defense is lost. Close observation of these sites is important. An indwelling urinary catheter and central lines can increase the risk of infection. Medications can suppress the blood cells.

Prognosis

Unfortunately, prognosis is poor for patients with immunocompromised status. Many patients with anemias, leukemias, and lymphomas are particularly prone to developing infections. Even simple infections can become deadly as patients have limited ability to fight off even molds, fungi, and other organisms that usually lie dormant in other people. Infection control measures must be meticulously observed.

Interpreting Laboratory/Diagnostic Tests

Decreased ANC below 1,000 cells/mm^3

WBC less than or greater than normal (may be an increase in immature cells)

Treatment

Close surveillance of VS and laboratory/diagnostic studies

Monitoring and early treatment with antibiotics if infection starts

Strict neutropenic precautions observed

❻ Nursing Diagnosis for Risk for Infection	Expected Outcomes
Risk for infection due to a compromised immune system	The patient will have a stable temperature The patient's ANC will be >1,500 The patient will have negative cultures

Nursing Interventions

Wash hands according to CDC protocols (before and after patient contacts; before and after wound redresses and suctioning, etc). *Number one nursing intervention to prevent infection.*

Admit patient to a private room with positive pressure or laminar flow *to protect him or her from pathogens from other patients.*

Assess all invasive lines for edema and erythema. Remove and culture lines if signs of infection occur. *Invasive lines are a direct pathway into the blood, which can lead to sepsis.*

Monitor staff and visitors for infections; you may have to teach donning of personal protective equipment (PPE). *To prevent the patient from infections in others.*

Avoid use of enemas, suppositories, and rectal temps, *which can increase the likelihood of bleeding and infection.*

Provide only cooked food. *Raw food, especially fruits, can contain molds or fungi that can invade the patient's bloodstream.*

Change sources of stagnant water frequently deleting the use of fresh flowers and plants at the bedside. *Standing water such as tubing from ventilators and IV bags can grow bacteria.*

Recounting a True Story

Nursing involves using evidence-based research in order to improve patient care and safety. Back in the day, students were taught the SASH method of maintaining a peripheral IV site: Saline, Administer medication, Saline, and lastly Heparin. This was a quick way to remember the order of how a piggyback or IV push medication was delivered to prevent clotting the IV line. Clots in a capped IV line would necessitate a restart. This procedure was called "flushing a heparin lock."

Research findings in the new millennium found that heparin was not needed to keep peripheral lines open. Also, heparin-induced thrombocytopenia was found to be caused by a second exposure to heparin and was signified by a severe drop in platelets after repeated use of heparin.

It was easy to stop administering heparin as we know that unnecessary drugs and procedures can increase the chance of sepsis. This also added nursing time to do other things; most new procedures increase nursing time so "dropping the SASH" caught on quickly. Now if we could only drop the term "heparin lock" from our vocabulary all would be less confusing in teaching new nurses.

---

❼ Septic Shock

What Went Wrong?

Septic shock is hypotension due to an overwhelming pathogenic infection. This type of shock results in a decreased blood flow and an increase in blood clotting. The decreased blood flow leads to tissue hypoxia and inadequate cellular functioning. The infection-producing organism releases vasoactive substances when the cell wall is phagocytosed, releasing cytokines that increase inflammation. So it is the death of the causative organism releasing endotoxins that causes septic shock. Vasoactive substances like histamine, tumor necrosis factor, and interleukins increase vasodilatation by increasing capillary permeability. Overall this decreases systemic vascular resistance (SVR), which is seen in a dropped BP and CO.

Results of Septic Shock

Decrease blood flow
↓
Increase cellular hypoxia
↓
Anaerobic metabolism
↓
Increase in irreversible cell damage

To compensate for a decreased circulation in septic shock, the sympathetic nervous system increases the release of native catecholamines like epinephrine. Epinephrine increases the heart rate and vasoconstricts the blood vessels to try to maintain circulation to core organs like the heart and brain. Blood is shunted to the heart and brain controlling vital functions and is decreased to the kidneys. The kidneys sense a decrease in renal blood flow and stimulate the renin-angiotension-aldosterone system (RAAS) to conserve much-needed sodium and water and maintain intravascular volume.

Those at risk for septic shock include patients with:

Genitourinary (GU), biliary, or intestinal diseases

Immunosuppressant therapy or AIDS

Indwelling catheters left for extended periods of time (central lines, urinary catheters)

Use of long-term antibiotics and steroids

Recent infection or surgery

In recent years, terminology regarding septic shock has tended to become more confusing. The terminology used in septic shock and their definitions are listed in Table 9–6.

Visit these web sites for more information on septic shock: http://sites.google.com/site/nursing211fall09/wk-9-spinal-cord-injury-burn-injury-septic-shock/211a-group-5, http://www.xigris.com/Pages/sepsis-continuum-animation.aspx (last accessed July 28, 2010).

❼ TABLE 9–6   Terminology Used in Septic Shock Classification

Infection (SIRS—sudden acute inflammatory response syndrome)	Elevated temperature >100.4°F or <96.8°F
	Tachycardia
	Tachypnea
	Elevated white cell counts
Sepsis	Infection resulting from pathogens like bacteria, fungi
Severe sepsis	Sepsis resulting in failure of one or more organs
Multiple organ dysfunction syndrome (MODS)	Occurs when two or more organs are dysfunctional and cannot maintain homeostasis without some type of medical intervention. For example:
Secondary MODS is due to infection	Cardiovascular – dysrhythmias, tachycardia, hypotension
	Respiratory – tachypnea, hypoxemia, respiratory acidosis; ARDS
	Renal – prerenal failure, decreased urinary output
	Hematologic – coagulopathy

Prognosis

The mortality rate of septic shock is the highest of all the different types of shock and varies greatly from 28% to 50%.

Interpreting Laboratory/Diagnostic Results

Positive blood cultures.

Elevated WBCs with a shift-to-the left.

Chest x-ray positive for pulmonary congestion leading to ARDS.

ABGs indicate metabolic and respiratory acidosis with hypoxemia.

BUN, creatinine are elevated.

GFR reduced.

Coagulation profile indicates increased bleeding times (PT, PTT, etc.) as well as fibrin split products. Platelets are decreased.

Blood glucose elevated early; later decreased.

Hepatic and pancreatic levels are elevated.

CT scan may show source of sepsis.

> **NURSING ALERT**
>
> *Seventy percent of all septic shock is caused by* Escherichia coli, Klebsiella pneumo-niae, Seratia, Enterobacter, *and* Pseudomonas. *Culturing the patient's secretions and wound sites are important before starting on antibiotics.*

Hallmark Signs and Symptoms
Warm Shock

Increased temperature above 38°C (100.4°F) and below 36°C (96.8°F) from endotoxin release

Tachycardia

Full and bounding pulses

High cardiac output and decreased SVR

Change in the level of consciousness (LOC)

Tachypnea and hypopnea

Decreased urinary output less than 30 mL/hr

Cold Shock

Decreased temperature below 36°C (96.8°F)

Hypotension

Increased SVR, decreased CO; decreased PAOP

Worsening of LOC

Crackles and gurgles

Mottling of extremities

Cyanosis

Decreased or absent urinary output

> **NURSING ALERT**
>
> *All may not be well if the patient is warm. In the early stage of septic shock, the pa-tient maybe hyperthermic.*

Treatment

Identify patients at risk, which includes immunocompromised patients and those with antibiotic resistance.

Identify the causative organism and remove any potential infection source (IVs, debridement of wound).

Institute the ABCs of assessment and care.

Support cardiovascular functioning with fluids, medication, and hemodynamic monitoring.

Give oxygen.

Combat infection by administering antibiotics after body fluid cultures.

Dialysis to decrease high electrolytes like potassium and phosphorus and to replace kidney functioning.

❻ Nursing Diagnoses for Septic Shock	Expected Outcomes
Tissue perfusion, alteration in (peripheral) due to invasion by foreign organisms	The patient will be normothermic The cultures will be negative The BP, CO, and SVR will be normal Urinary output will be >30 mL/hr
Hyperthermia due to release of endotoxins from pathogenic cell walls	The patient will be normothermic

Nursing Interventions

Assess the patient's VS for recovery from shock *indicated by baseline temperature, pulse, respirations, and return of BP above 100 systolic.*

Prepare to insert a pulmonary artery pressure *to more accurately measure preload, afterload, contractility, cardiac output, and system vascular resistance.*

Monitor the patient's peripheral perfusion by assessing urinary output greater than 30 mL/hr, skin color normal tone, all peripheral pulses intact.

Culture all possible infectious sources (blood, urine, wounds, etc.) before starting antibiotics *to determine the causative organism.*

Remove and reinsert all invasive lines *to eliminate the possible causative organism.*

Monitor the patient for bleeding, *which can be caused by coagulopathy.*

Administer antibiotics *to eliminate causative organism.*

Institute mechanical ventilation in patient *who becomes severely hypoxic.*

Start continuous renal replacement therapy, which can be used to combat effects of metabolic acidosis and electrolyte imbalances.

Administer IV fluids, albumin, and blood products *to increase intravascular volume.*

Administer Levophed *to vasoconstrict blood vessels elevating the BP.*

Initiate drotrecogin alfa (Xigris) therapy for patients with severe sepsis and MOSD.

Use strict aseptic technique when performing invasive procedures *to decrease introduction of pathogens.*

Introduce nutritional support early *to help with repair and replacement of injured cells.*

Institute deep vein thrombosis prophylaxis, which includes turning, antithrombic stockings, sequential inflation stockings, and low molecular weight heparin to prevent blood clots and pulmonary emboli.

Provide emotional support to patient and significant others *as this is a highly fatal situation.*

Disseminated Intravascular Coagulopathy (DIC)

What Went Wrong?

DIC is a complex, serious disorder of the vascular system where massive clotting factors are stimulated and used up. Since the body cannot manufacture platelets immediately according to need, the patient starts to bleed. So this syndrome of events is a paradox. Either the intrinsic and/or extrinsic clotting cascade is activated, leading to massive clotting throughout the body. Causes of DIC include those listed in Table 9–7.

TABLE 9–7 Extrinsic and Intrinsic Causes of DIC		
	Method of Injury	**Types**
Extrinsic causes	Injury of the inner lining of the endothelium exposing the surface to circulating clotting factors	Abruptio placenta
		Fetal demise
		Pre-eclampsia and eclampsia
		Trauma from burns, crushing injury
		Malignant disease like leukemia
Intrinsic causes	Clotting is activated by substances like free radicals, chemical irritants, and inflammatory mediators like necrosis factor and cytokines	Bacterial, fungal, and viral infections, especially gram-negative sepsis
		Acute hemolytic blood reaction
		Trauma from internal injuries can result in this as well

Regardless of cause, the end result is the same: massive use of clotting activation and clotting factors cannot be replaced quickly enough by the liver and bone marrow. This ultimately leads to bleeding and possible hemorrhagic shock.

Tissue hypoxia also results as clots formed in smaller capillaries and blood vessels prevent delivery of nutrients to the cells and organs.

DIC can be recognized by three basic abnormalities that occur:

1. Massive clotting resulting in organ damage from tissue hypoxia

2. Accelerated production of natural anticoagulants

3. Splitting apart of existing clots

Prognosis

DIC carries a high mortality rate, especially in the elderly and in patients with coexisting medical problems.

Interpreting Laboratory/Diagnostic Results

The following is an accounting of the levels of coagulation studies in DIC.

Decreased Levels	Increased Levels
Platelets counts	FDP
Fibrinogen levels	PT and PTT
Factor V	D–dimer
Factor VIII	BUN
Hct and Hgb	Creatinine

Diagnostic Studies

There is no diagnostic study that confirms DIC. These studies look for possible complications due to clotting then hemorrhage.

ECG – Can show changes indicative of MI (Q waves, ST elevation, T wave inversion) if circulation to heart is decreased

Stools – May be positive for occult blood

CT scan – Can show evidence of stroke if there is cerebral hemorrhage

Hallmark Signs and Symptoms

Signs and symptoms affect many body systems and reflect tissue hypoxia and bleeding, which occur with DIC. These include those found by systems in Table 9–8. No one sign or symptom can tell the critical care nurse that DIC is

TABLE 9–8 Signs and Symptoms of DIC by Body Systems

Body System	Signs/Symptoms
Central nervous system	Changes in the level of consciousness
	Changes in behavior or mentation
	Confusion
	Seizures
	Symptoms of stroke; paresthesias, paralysis
Cardiovascular	Tachycardia
	Chest pain
	Hypotension
	Symptoms of MI
	Pain in extremities
	Decreased peripheral pulse
	Gangrene in fingers, toes, nose, and ears (prolonged hypoxemia)
	Bleeding around IV and central line sites
Respiratory	Shortness of breath
	Tachypnea
	Symptoms of PE
	Bleeding around ETT if intubated
Genitourinary	Oliguria or anuria
	Hematuria
	Bleeding around uretheral indwelling catheter
	Vaginal bleeding
Gastrointestinal	Bloody stool
	Hematemesis
	Abdominal cramping or pain
Integumentary	Pale skin
	Petechiae and ecchymosis
Musculoskeletal	Back pain or tenderness
Other	Bleeding from any traumatized or surgical sites

taking place, so a close look at the patient's risk factors and watching laboratories and body systems can help identify DIC early.

Treatment

There is no single acceptable treatment for DIC. Few studies confirm the best treatment.

Find and treat the underlying cause.

Continuous IV heparin is used in severe cases of DIC.

Administration of antifibrinolytic agents like aminocaproic acid (Amicar).

Drotrecogin alfa administration.

Blood component replacement with fresh frozen plasma or cryoprecipitate.

Administration of vitamin K and folate.

❻ Nursing Diagnoses for DIC	Expected Outcomes
Tissue perfusion, alteration due to clotting in microcirculation	The patient will maintain all peripheral pulses
Increased fluid volume deficit due to bleeding	The patient's Hct, Hgb, and platelets will stabilize

Nursing Interventions

1. Assess vital signs frequently for signs of hemorrhagic shock (elevated HR, breathing, and decreased BP) *to identify and treat shock from DIC early.*

2. Administer oxygen *to decrease tissue hypoxia.*

3. Prepare to insert a pulmonary artery catheter *to measure volume replacement and ability of heart to handle fluids. Notify the physician if PAOP and CO readings drop, which can indicate shock.*

4. Prepare to administer blood products *to replace volume and clotting factors.*

5. Avoid the use of rectal temps and *suppositories, which can cause bleeding of intestinal mucosa.*

6. Monitor the skin under noninvasive sequential BP devices frequently.

7. Monitor all invasive sites for bleeding (nasogastric tubes, urinary catheters, ETT) *as they can be potential sites for increased blood loss/hemorrhage.*

8. Hold all invasive venous procedure sites for 15 minutes *to allow hemostasis to occur.*

9. Use gentle-tipped applicators for oral care. Do not include harsh alcohol-based mouth wash. *Prevents trauma and potential bleeding of the gingiva.*

10. Use electric razors for grooming *to prevent nicks, which can bleed excessively.*

11. Do not disturb clots that form such as in the oral cavity, *which can reactivate mucous membrane bleeding.*

12. Trend all hemodynamic and body system assessments *for signs of further tissue hypoxemia and bleeding.*

13. Observe for signs of MI, which include increasingly frequent chest pain, ST–T wave changes, and positive cardiac enzymes. *MI can occur if clots lodge in the coronary arteries.*

14. Observe for symptoms of PE, which include pleuritic chest pain.

15. Monitor the urinary output for signs of renal failure. Output should be greater than 30 cc/hr.

16. Keep the patient in a comfortable position, usually a semi-Fowler's position, *to minimize energy and help diaphragmatic drop by gravity.*

17. Provide emotional support to the patient and significant others.

CASE STUDY

Sixty-eight-year-old Patricia Cranton is admitted to the ICU through the ECU from a nursing home. Her admitting diagnosis is septic shock possibly from a long-term urinary catheter placed after a recent vulvectomy due to pelvic cancer. Her care includes chemotherapy several times a week at a local cancer center.

Vital signs: TPR = 103°F-126-36, BP 170/100, SaO_2 89%

ABGs: pH 7.30, pCO_2 55, pO_2 55, HCO_3 15

Labs: Na 150, K^+ 5.5, Cl 130, Phos 3, Ca^{++} 5, BUN 60, creatinine 2, Hct 25%, Hgb 8, RBCs 2,500, WBCs 2,500, neutrophils (segs) 25%, (bands) 9%

Urine culture: Pending

Chest x-ray: Patchy infiltrates in both lung fields suggestive of pneumonia

Body systems assessment reveals:

Neuro: A + O × 1 (disoriented to time and place; new onset)

    Lethargic with progressive difficulty to keep awake

    Only slight gag reflex

    Slow to follow commands; intermittent success in doing so

    Denies pain but states, "I'm having trouble catching my breath."

CV: Skin is warm and flushed

    S1 and S2 audible at apex without rubs/murmurs

    Peripheral pulses full and bounding with all +4/3

    Brisk capillary refill

Pul: Diminished breath sounds at the bases

    Unable to take a deep breath with coaxing

    Equal expansion of chest wall

Dull sounds percussed at the bases

On 100% nonrebreather

GU: Urine output via indwelling catheter foul-smelling, with shreds of white milky sediment

Output = 15 mL in the past 4 hours after ECU irrigated Foley

GI: Diminished bowel sounds throughout 4 quads

Stomach flat but soft protuberance

Spleen, liver unable to palpate; no tenderness in areas

QUESTIONS

1. From the above symptoms, describe what terminology related to sepsis this patient might be experiencing.
2. What do her ABGs indicate? What would cause you concern about them?
3. What assessment data confirms the probable location of Ms. Cranton's sepsis?
4. The resident asks you to confirm calculation of the patient's absolute neutrophil count (ANC). What value will you show her?
5. Prioritize collaborative care that the nurse would anticipate.

   It is decided to insert a pulmonary artery catheter to monitor fluid status.
6. What values in the PAP, PAOP, CO, and SVR would the nurse predict?

Despite aggressive therapy, Patricia spirals downward and the family decides Patricia has had enough. They know that she has expressed if she gets gravely sick she does not want to "go through anything more." She has left a living that includes mechanical ventilation and life support but not after a week. The medical and nursing staff, pastoral care, and the ethics committee confirm this decision. Patricia is started on a morphine drip, is extubated, and passes on a week after admission.

REVIEW QUESTIONS

1. An infectious disease physician and a medical resident are discussing the WBC count with a differential on a patient they suspect has sepsis. The nurse is aware that when they talk about a shift-to-the-left, they are referring to

   A. An increase in the band neutrophils
   B. A decrease in the basophils
   C. An increase in the eosinophils
   D. An increase in the lymphocytes

2. A patient is admitted with sepsis due to an indwelling suprapubic catheter that was poorly maintained at home. He is hypotensive and tachycardic with a low cardiac output and minimal renal perfusion. He will require intubation and mechanical ventilation, fluids, antibiotics, and other vasoactive medications to maintain his CO and BP. Which sequence of sepsis is this patient most likely in?

   A. Sepsis
   B. Severe sepsis
   C. SIRS (sudden inflammatory response syndrome)
   D. MODS

3. The nurse is looking at all laboratory and assessment data on a patient with MODS. Which of the following medications might be beneficial to this patient to reverse the inflammatory responses occurring in MODS?

   A. Dobutamine
   B. Heparin
   C. Antibiotics
   D. Xigris

4. The nurse is evaluating the results of a patient's CBC (complete blood cell count). Which of the following would indicate a severe bleeding problem?

   A. Red blood cell count of 5 million
   B. Platelets of 30,000
   C. White cell count of 15,000
   D. Band neutrophils of 5%

5. A nurse is evaluating an elderly patient who was admitted to the ICU with sepsis from an indwelling urinary catheter. Which of the following laboratory values might indicate the beginning of disseminated intravascular coagulation (DIC)?

   A. Increased urinary output
   B. Decreased prothrombin time (PT)
   C. Platelets less than 100,000/uL
   D. Decreased fibrin degradation products (FDP)

6. A nurse is scanning through the laboratory work and medication records to prepare a patient for a bone marrow biopsy. Which of the following medications should the nurse hold and notify the physician about before proceeding further with the preparation?

A. Clopidogrel (Plavix)

B. Cimetadine (Tagamet)

C. Vancomycin

D. Morphine sulfate

7. Preventing deep vein thrombosis and pulmonary emboli as possible complications of sepsis, the nurse would

A. Administer Xigris

B. Start warfarin (Coumadin)

C. Give vitamin K

D. Administer low molecular weight heparin

8. A patient is admitted to your ICU with severe respiratory distress. His secondary diagnosis is acute lymphocytic leukemia. You know this patient's profile indicates he is currently being treated with chemotherapy. You place this patient in neutropenic precautions but want to verify his absolute neutrophil count. You have a CBC that includes

Hemoglobin	8 g/dL
Hematocrit	25%
Total WBC	2,000
Neutrophils (segs)	50%
(bands)	7%
Eosinophils	5%
Basophils	0.5

Calculate the patient's ANC.

A. 70

B. 700

C. 1,140

D. 7,000

9. The nurse is teaching the family about entering the room of a patient on neutropenic precautions. The *priority* nursing measure the nurse needs to teach is

A. How to apply gloves before touching the patient

B. How to correctly form a mask to prevent exhaling on this patient

C. Wearing a gown when in direct contact with the patient

D. Hand washing

10. A patient is on neutropenic precautions for severe anemia from chronic renal failure (CRF). Which of the following would the nurse question in maintaining the plan of care?

   A Delivering flowers to the room.

   B. Including cooked foods delivered by dietary.

   C. Avoiding invasive procedures when possible.

   D. Removing and replacing peripheral IVs that are red or swollen.

ANSWERS

CASE STUDY

1. The elevated temperature, HR, breathing rate, and BP seem to indicate that Patricia is experiencing SIRS. The results of the urine cultures are pending; if they are positive she would have sepsis. Her urinary output is below that minimally accepted, and BUN and creatinine and her positive lung sounds and ABGs show there is lung involvement. This would indicate severe sepsis as two organs are involved. She does not have MODS at this time as no other organs show signs of failure.

2. ABGs: pH 7.30, pCO_2 55, pO_2 55, HCO_3 15
   The pH is below 7.35 indicating an acidosis. Next we need to find the primary target organ. Looking at the pCO_2 we find the patient is retaining CO_2, so she is in a respiratory acidosis. Next we look at HCO_3. Ms. Cranston is retaining acid because the HCO_3 is less than 22. She is also in a metabolic acidosis. Careful correction of these needs to occur as the combined acidosis and quick drops in the pH are not compatible with life. She is also severely hypoxemic with a pO_2 less than 80 mmHg.

3. Two things: She is currently undergoing chemotherapy and that can cause immunosuppression; we will look at the ANC to confirm this. Also, the presence of foul-smelling urine with white sediment suggests a urinary tract infection. The pending UTI will confirm this. The white cell count does not help out as it is below the normal level. This is due to neutropenia caused by chemotherapy. The crackles in lung fields and low SaO_2 may indicate lower lobe pneumonia.

4. ANC is calculated by taking the percentage of segmented and banded neutrophils and multiplying that percentage by the total WBCs.
   WBCs 2,500, neutrophils (segs) 25%, (bands) 9%
   25% + 9% = 39%, change to percentage = 0.39
   0.39 × 2,000 = 975
   This patient is neutropenic.

5. Prioritized collaborative care would include:
   Intubation and mechanical ventilation due to acidosis/hypoxemia.
   Be careful when administering fluids; she might go into fluid overload. She might need a pulmonary artery catheter along with urinary output and watching SaO_2/breath sounds to prevent pulmonary edema. Her Hct and Hgb indicate she may need blood transfusions.
   Confirming all cultures have been taken prior to starting antibiotics.
   Antipyretics like Tylenol.
   Neutropenic precautions.

6. The nurse might anticipate the following pulmonary artery pressures:
   CVP (low) due to vasodilatation
   PAP (high) due to pneumonia and possible left-sided failure
   PAOP (high) due to pneumonia and possible left-sided failure
   CO (high) due to compensation by catecholamine release confirmed by the hypertension
   SVR (low) due to liberation of endotoxins creating fluid translocating from the vasculature

CORRECT ANSWERS AND RATIONALES

1. A. A shift-to-the-left refers to an increase in the band neutrophils or immature neutrophils greater than 5%.
2. D. This patient shows cardiac (hypotensive, tachycardia, low CO) respiratory (need for mechanical ventilation) and renal involvement (minimal renal perfusion and need for fluids), so at least three systems are involved with failing to maintain homeostasis without intervention.
3. D. Xigris is the only medication that has properties to reverse inflammation and organ damage in MODS.
4. B. Since platelets control clotting of the blood, any platelet level below 150,000 can indicate bleeding potentials.
5. C. DIC is a syndrome of excessive clotting and then bleeding. It is indicated by decreased platelets, decreased urinary output, increased PT, and increased FDP.
6. A. Plavix is known to prevent platelets from aggregating and therefore increases the potential for bleeding in this patient.
7. D. The patient with sepsis is prone to develop DVT and PE, which can be life threatening. This is treated with turning, early ambulation, antiembolism stockings, sequential compression stockings, and low molecular weight heparin.
8. C. This value is calculated by adding the bands to the neutrophils then multiplying the sum by the total WBCs. This patient is neutropenic and you need to provide the correct care. Now institute neutropenic precautions.
9. D. Hand washing is the single most important measure for a patient who is immunocompromised.
10. A. Flowers can contain organisms that thrive in the water like *Pseudomonas*. All other actions are appropriate.

Final Exam Questions

Chapter 1

1. The critical care nurse is providing instruction to a patient with a tracheostomy. The patient and family will be caring for the tracheostomy at home. Which critical care competency BEST describes the role of the nurse in this situation?

   A. Systems thinking
   B. Advocacy
   C. Collaboration
   D. Facilitator of learning

2. A new critical care nurse is asking her mentor about the American Association of Critical Care Nurses Association. Which of the following statements by the mentor are characteristics of nursing organizations?

   A. Ensures pay per performance
   B. Ejects minimally competent nurses from service
   C. Protects the public
   D. Provides adequate staffing levels

3. A critical care nurse is developing a plan of care with the patient and significant other regarding use of a Hickman catheter implanted for dialysis. The standard that the nurse is addressing is

   A. Outcome identification
   B. Assessment
   C. Implementation
   D. Evaluation

4. In order to provide a culture free of errors, the nurse manager of the critical care area is encouraging her staff to report errors without undue penalty. Errors that cause potential harm to a patient are known as

    A. Advocacy
    B. Sentinel events
    C. Intensivist
    D. Competencies

5. While interviewing a prospective candidate for critical care nursing, the nurse manager mentions that the unit employs a critical care intensivist. Critical care intensivists are known to

    A. Increase critical care costs
    B. Increase mortality rates
    C. Decrease nursing staff to patient ratios
    D. Decrease mortality rates

6. The health care act that instituted increased penalties for breaches in confidentiality is known as

    A. HIPAA
    B. HRSA
    C. IHI
    D. IOM

Chapter 2

1. The nurse is assigned a newly intubated patient who becomes disoriented and combative. After least restrictive interventions, the health care provider is considering giving the patient a neuromuscular blocking agent (NMBA). Because these agents do not cross the blood-brain barrier, the nurse must

    A. Be sure to administer an antianxiety agent and/or pain medication with the NMBA.
    B. Make sure a chaplain and family visits the patient often for reality orientation.
    C. Administer the maximum allowable dose of antacid medication to relieve the patient's symptoms.
    D. Turn the patient at least once a shift as the patient will not be able to feel pain or pressure while undergoing therapy with NMBA.

2. A major cause of ventilator-acquired pneumonia (VAP) is aspiration of oral secretions. In order to prevent this complication of mechanical ventilation, the nurse should

    A. Keep the head of the bed flat and turn the patient less frequently.
    B. Ensure that no antiulcer medications are given and change the ventilator circuits every shift.

C. Provide frequent oral hygiene and meticulous suctioning procedures.

D. Survey the patient's vital signs but know that there is little we can do to prevent VAP in the patient who stays in the intensive care unit.

3. An experienced ICU nurse is teaching a new graduate about lung sounds in a patient with pneumonia. The new graduate states she is hearing soft, popping sounds on inspiration at both lung bases. These adventitious sounds are MOST LIKELY

A. Wheezes

B. Gurgles

C. Stridor

D. Crackles

4. The nurse is caring for a patient with chronic obstructive pulmonary disease (COPD). The nurse is observing the patient for signs of early respiratory failure. These symptoms/signs would include which of the following?

A. Bradycardia

B. Bradypnea

C. Hypotension

D. Tachycardia

5. A patient is post-operative for a pneumonectomy for metastatic squamous cell carcinoma. The nurse should anticipate all of the following with the exception of

A. Chest tube

B. Oxygen therapy

C. Frequent lung assessments

D. Chemotherapy

6. A nurse is palpating around a chest tube site and feels slight crackling around the site. This condition would be known as

A. Tactile fremitus

B. Stridor

C. Crepitus

D. Elastic turgor

7. A patient is admitted to the ICU in acute respiratory distress. The nurse should anticipate seeing which type of oxygen device in place?

A. Nasal cannula

B. Venturi mask

C. Aerosol mask

D. Nonrebreather

8. Analyze and determine what acid-base imbalance is indicated in the following example. A patient is admitted with acute respiratory distress, and after performing arterial blood gases the nurse sees the following results:

$$pH = 7.30, pCO_2 = 65, pO_2 = 45, HCO_3 = 22$$

A. Uncompensated respiratory acidosis
B. Partially compensated respiratory acidosis
C. Full compensated respiratory acidosis
D. Uncompensated respiratory alkalosis

9. A patient is placed on PEEP for acute respiratory distress syndrome (ARDS). The nurse notes a BP drop to 80/40 from 140/90 after being placed on PEEP. Which of the following might be a plausible reason for this drop?

A. The only reason for this is that the patient is going into shock.
B. This is a reaction to the anxiety and sympathetic stimulation before mechanical ventilation.
C. This might be due to PEEP decreasing venous return from increased intrathoracic pressure.
D. This is caused by the massive bleeding from ruptured alveoli from barotrauma.

10. A patient's ventilator alarms are going off. The nurse cannot find the cause of the alarms. The priority action of the nurse would be to

A. Call respiratory to troubleshoot the ventilator.
B. Manually resuscitate the patient until the problem can be found.
C. Turn the oxygen up on the ventilator and push the breathe button.
D. Tell the patient you have everyone paged stat and help will be there soon.

Chapter 3

1. A patient is admitted to your telemetry unit with Prinzmetal's angina (variant). The nurse is aware that this type of angina is usually treated with

A. Nitroglycerin
B. Sodium nitroprusside
C. Calcium channel blockers
D. Dobutrex

2. A nurse is assessing a patient's database for risk factors that could be modifiable to prevent coronary artery disease. Which of the following in the patient's database would be modifiable?

A. Hypertension
B. Family history
C. Increasing age
D. Race

3. A patient is experiencing signs and symptoms of left-sided heart failure. Which of the following would be consistent with this diagnosis?

   A. Ascites
   B. Elevated jugular venous distention
   C. Posterior tibial edema
   D. Crackles

4. Which of the following assessment findings in a patient with acute coronary syndrome would cause the nurse to withhold thrombolytic therapy?   **Select all that apply.**

   A. ST segment myocardial infarction
   B. Surgery within the past 2 months
   C. Need for frequent venipunctures
   D. Recent aspirin and heparin therapy
   E. Recent trauma
   F. Insertion of a central line
   G. Being 50 to 70 years old

5. A patient has just had a pulmonary artery catheter inserted to monitor severe heart failure. The nurse is reading the patient's pressures and notes a pressure of 28/0 mm Hg and a striking change from the previous pressures of 30/15. She also notes the patient is starting to have ventricular dysrhythmias. Which chamber has this catheter MOST LIKELY migrated to?

   A. The left ventricle
   B. The right atrium
   C. The right ventricle
   D. The left atrium

6. Your patient is to be discharged home after a heart transplant (orthotopic method). Which of the following would you include in his teaching plan?

   A. You will have to learn how to program a temporary pacemaker.
   B. You will have to stay on dobutamine as long as you have a transplanted heart.
   C. You will have to rise slowly in the morning as your BP may drop suddenly when you rise.
   D. You will always have two "Q" waves on your ECG.

7. A patient has been admitted to your medical unit with extreme hypertension. On physical examination you note a pulsating mass just to the left of midline in the upper abdominal area. Which of the following physical assessment procedures is **CONTRAINDICATED** based on the above information?

   A. Auscultation
   B. Deep palpation
   C. Light palpation
   D. Percussion

8. A patient has a pulmonary artery catheter inserted. When the nurse does the readings s/he sees a dampened pressure in the range of 7 mm Hg. The most likely cause for this is the catheter is

A. In the pulmonary capillary wedge position (PCWP or PAOP) and needs to be aspirated or the physician called to reposition it

B. In the right ventricle as dampened pressures are significant of the catheter migrating back to the right ventricle; the balloon needs to be inflated

C. In the central vein and needs to be inflated to pass through the tricuspid and pulmonic valves

D. In the right place and there is no cause for concern

9. A nurse is caring for a patient postoperatively after open-heart surgery. Which of the following interventions would be included in the care of this patient?

A. Systemic antirejection medications.

B. Annual angiography, echocardiography, and ultrasounds.

C. Temporary pacemaker.

D. Call the physician when two "P" waves are seen on a 12-lead ECG.

10. The patient has aortic stenosis. Which of the following would be an assessment finding in a patient with aortic stenosis?

A. A harsh blowing murmur over the 5th ICS, MCL

B. Right atrial hypertrophy and pulmonary low pressures

C. A soft radiating murmur over the 5th ICS, MCL

D. Left ventricular hypertrophy, lower systemic pressures

Chapter 4

1. A critical care nurse is analyzing a rhythm strip and finds that the atrial and ventricular rates are 120. The conduction times are normal. This rhythm is most likely

A. Normal sinus rhythm

B. First-degree AV block

C. Sinus tachycardia

D. Ventricular tachycardia

2. The nurse is measuring the waves and the intervals in a rhythm strip and notes the P-to-P interval is consistent. The characteristic this nurse is measuring is

A. Ventricular repolarization

B. Atrial regularity

C. Atrial rate

D. Ventricular conduction

3. The nurse is looking closely at ventricular contraction and is examining the first negative wave after the P wave. This is known as the

    A. ST segment
    B. R wave
    C. Q wave
    D. S wave

4. The nurse is assessing a patient's rhythm strip and notes multiple saw-toothed P waves for each QRS. This patient is most likely in a (an)

    A. Premature junctional contraction
    B. First-degree AV block
    C. Ventricular tachycardia
    D. Atrial flutter

5. A nurse notes that the PRI interval on a strip gets longer and longer with each heartbeat until there is a single P wave and no QRS. This rhythm is

    A. Complete heart block
    B. First-degree heart block
    C. Second-degree heart block; Mobitz II
    D. Second-degree heart block; Mobitz I or Wenckebach

6. The nurse is setting up quickly for emergency defibrillation in a patient with Ventricular Fibrillation (VF) without a pulse. Which of the following indicates successful setting up of this procedure?

    A. "I will depress the "synch" button on the defibrillator."
    B. "I will place the defibrillator pads in the anterior posterior position."
    C. "I will perform CPR until everything is ready to go."
    D. "I will run a strip to make sure I document a dot above each R wave."

7. A nurse is teaching a new critical care nurse about the settings for pacing. The nurse is talking about changing the strength applied to the pacemaker to override a patient's fast tachyarrhythmia. The mode she is talking about is

    A. The rate
    B. The mA
    C. The synchronous function
    D. The asynchronous function

8. A nurse is helping with a cardiac arrest victim. The patient is in asystole. Which of the following medications can she anticipate the physician ordering for a patient with asystole?

    A. Atropine
    B. Lidocaine
    C. Amiodarone
    D. Procainamide

9. A patient is placed on hypothermia therapy after a cardiac arrest. The nurse's role is to (select all that apply)

   A. Administer antipyretics if needed.

   B. Prevent sepsis.

   C. Insert an NGT to help with internal cooling.

   D. Keep the patient in profound hypothermia.

   E. Give antiarrythmics should they occur.

10. The patient is to have a cardioversion. Which of the following will the nurse perform to prepare the patient for this procedure?

   A. Set up for a chest tube.

   B. Ensure that a BVM is available at the bedside.

   C. Place the defibrillator without the synchronous mode depressed.

   D. Ensure the machine is set to fire on the T wave.

Chapter 5

1. A complication of receiving thrombolytic therapy in the vulnerable individual could be

   A. Extensive blood clotting

   B. An increase in CNS hemorrhaging

   C. Peripheral vasoconstriction

   D. Respiratory depression

2. To perform the patellar reflex examination, the nurse should position the patient

   A. Lying flat with the legs extended

   B. On the left side with the legs flexed

   C. Sitting with the legs hanging downward

   D. Standing with the knees slightly bent

3. Identify the muscle that is assessed to determine upper motor tract neuron disease when the Achilles tendon reflex test is performed.

   A. Biceps

   B. Brachioradial

   C. Triceps

   D. Gastrocnemius

4. **A nurse is assessing a patient's EOMs. Which cranial nerves would be involved in this assessment?**

   A. Optic/abducens/facial

   B. Olfactory/optic/oculomotor

   C. Oculomotor/trochlear/abducens

   D. Facial/vagus/trigeminal

5. **An individual who presents with a GCS (Glascow Coma Scale) of 6 is considered to be**

   A. In excellent health

   B. In a comatose state

   C. Oriented to person, place, and time

   D. Able to localize painful stimuli

6. **Change question to read: A nurse documents the patient's level of consciousness (LOC) as obtunded. The nurse is describing:**

   A. Responses require minimal external stimuli.

   B. The patient is drowsy and inactive, needing increased amounts of external stimuli.

   C. Vigorous and continuous external stimuli are needed to achieve a response.

   D. Reactions to increased external stimuli are rare and minimal.

7. **A comminuted skull fracture fits the description of**

   A. A broken eggshell.

   B. Occurring at the back of the skull.

   C. Outer skull is caved in.

   D. A hairline fracture.

8. **A nurse is examining the muscular strength of each extremity and is writing the response as 1/5. This means:**

   A. Absent muscle contraction.

   B. Normal muscle power and strength.

   C. A trace of muscle contraction is evident.

   D. Resistance against the examiner's muscle strength is weak.

9. **The nurse asks the patient to stick out his tongue. When the patient responds, his tongue deviates to the right. This response indicates possible damage to which cranial nerve.**

   A. VI – abducens

   B. VII – facial

   C. X – vagus

   D. XII – hypoglossal

10. A CAT scan reveals that an individual has sustained an SAH (subarachnoid hemorrhage). Which physical signs will best illustrate to the nurse a probable increase in ICP?

A. Absent verbal responses, decreased level of consciousness
B. Heightened awareness of the patient's environment
C. Spontaneous withdrawal from painful stimuli
D. Slurred speech, lateral eye deviation

Chapter 6

1. A nurse is performing an assessment of a trauma victim. In what phase of trauma care would the nurse examine each body region for additional injuries?

A. Definitive care
B. Secondary survey
C. Primary survey
D. Prehospital stabilization

2. A nurse is to administer massive transfusions to a patient who has been admitted to the ECU post industrial accident in profound hemorrhagic shock. After administering more than half his fluid volume in the first hour, the nurse should be observant for which of the following complications?

A. $K^+ = 2.5$ mEq/L
B. $Ca^{++} = 12$ mEq/L
C. Platelet count of 250,000 cm^3
D. pH 7.20, pCO_2 45, HCO_3 10

3. A patient is admitted to the hospital in Class III hemorrhage. The nurse is aware that the patient will exhibit which of the following signs/symptoms in this stage of hemorrhagic shock?

A. Heart rate of 100
B. Bradypnea
C. Drop in MAP of less than 60
D. 30% to 40% blood loss

4. A patient is admitted to the ICU post surgical wiring of a Le Fort III facial fracture. Which of the following would be contraindicated in this patient's nursing care?

A. Insertion of a nasogastric tube for nausea
B. Administration of a simple mask
C. Monitoring the site for redness, irritation, and exudate
D. Assessing the surgical site for symmetry

5. A nurse is monitoring the chest tube output of a patient who has been diagnosed with a left massive hemothorax. The nurse has recorded over 500 mL output in the last 2 hours. Which is the next step the nurse should take?

A. Continue to monitor the output; this is normal in a massive hemothorax.

B. Clamp the chest tube, call the physician, and prepare the patient for surgery.

C. Prepare for blood and IV fluid to stabilize the patient and notify the trauma surgeon.

D. Monitor the patient's vital signs and SaO_2. Prepare the patient for surgery after notifying the physician.

6. A patient is admitted with a right tension pneumothorax after a ski pole s/he fell on created a sucking chest wound. Which of the following signs/symptoms would confirm the presence of a tension pneumothorax?

A. Tracheal deviation to the right; diminished breath sounds on the left

B. Trachea midline; hypertension and tachycardia

C. Tracheal deviation to the left; diminished breath sounds on the left

D. Tracheal deviation to the right; absent breath sounds on the right

7. A new nurse is being orientated to the emergency room. A call comes from the local EMS that they are bringing in six family members from a household fire. This nurse would anticipate the type of burns she will be caring for to be

A. Radiation burns

B. Thermal burns

C. Chemical burns

D. Electrical burns

8. A patient is admitted to the ECU with thermal burns that involve the anterior and posterior surfaces of the legs. The nurse would estimate the body surface area (BSA) burned to be

A. 4.5%

B. 9%

C. 18%

D. 36%

9. A patient is admitted to the burn unit after stabilization in the ECU. During report, the nurse caring for this patient learns the patient weighs 165 lb, has a body surface area burn of 70%, and is ordered 4 mL of LR per kilogram. The nurse is checking the amount of fluid this patient should have during the first 12 hours of the burn injury. How many milliliters should this patient receive in the first 12 hours?

A. 2,100 mL

B. 5,000 mL

C. 10,500 mL

D. 22,000 mL

10. **A patient is admitted with a spinal cord injury (SCI) from an axial loading injury from diving into a swimming pool head first. The nurse's FIRST priority nursing diagnosis for this patient would be**

A. Risk for decreased cardiac output due to lack of innervation of the spinal column

B. Impaired gas exchange due to inhalation of pool water

C. Risk for altered tissue perfusion (spinal) due to lack of spinal cord innervation to the extremities

D. Risk for ineffective breathing pattern due to swelling of the cord and lack of innervation to respiratory centers

Chapter 7

1. **A patient is scheduled for discharge after having been treated for an adrenal crisis. Which comments by the patient indicate that she understood the nurse's discharge teaching instructions?   Select all that apply.**

A. "I must take my steroids for 10 days."

B. "I must weigh myself every day to make sure I do not eat too many calories."

C. "I must notify my physician prior to any dental work."

D. "If I feel weak or dizzy, I must call my doctor."

E. "I will not be concerned if I feel like I have the flu."

F. "I need to obtain and wear a Medic Alert bracelet."

2. **The nurse understands that the anatomic feature controlling pituitary function in the patient is (are) the**

A. Midbrain

B. Pons

C. Adrenal glands

D. Hypothalamus

3. **A nurse's first-line treatment measures administered to a patient during an Addison's crisis include all EXCEPT**

A. Blood glucose management

B. Intravenous hydrocortisone

C. Antihypertensive medications

D. Intravenous fluid replacement

4. **The positive results of Trousseau's and Chvostek's signs in a patient indicate to the nurse a state of**

   A. Hypercalcemia
   B. Hyperparathyroidism
   C. Decreased phosphate levels
   D. Hypocalcemia

5. **Characteristics of Cushing's syndrome in a patient could be improved by all of the following except**

   A. Administration of steroids every other day
   B. A diet high in protein and calcium
   C. A diet low in calories, sodium, and carbohydrates
   D. An increase in steroid therapy

6. **The nurse can expect a patient with diabetic ketoacidosis to reveal which type of respirations?**

   A. Cheyne-Stokes
   B. Kussmaul's
   C. Agonal gasps
   D. Dyspneic

7. **The nurse knows that the patient should receive the following medication as thyroid replacement therapy:**

   A. Tapazole
   B. PTU
   C. Decadron
   D. Synthroid

8. **The only insulin most suitable for intravenous use is**

   A. Ultralente
   B. Regular
   C. Lispro
   D. NPH

9. **An example of a first-generation sulfonylurea used to treat a patient with diabetes mellitus is**

   A. Avandia
   B. Glucophage
   C. Tolinase
   D. Prandin

10. CAT scan results indicate to the nurse that the patient has a normal-functioning thyroid gland, which can be described as

    A. Thyroiditis
    B. Thyromegaly
    C. Euthyroid
    D. Myxedema

Chapter 8

1. Proper pharmacologic management is important in the care of the patient on hemodialysis (HD). When caring for the HD patient, which of the following medications would the nurse question and hold in a patient with chronic renal failure until after HD?   **Select all that apply.**

    A. Digoxin
    B. Folic acid
    C. Vitamin B6
    D. Os-cal
    E. Renagel capsules
    F. Procrit

2. A nurse is reviewing the laboratory values in a patient with chronic renal failure. Which of the following are consistent with a patient before dialysis?

    A. Serum creatinine 1 mg/dL
    B. Serum potassium 5.8 mEq/L
    C. Hemoglobin 13 g/dL
    D. Urine creatinine clearance 125 mL/min

3. A patient has been treated with hemodialysis for chronic renal failure (CRF). You are told in report that the patient has a right upper arm arteriovenous (AV) fistula. Upon assessing this patient it is critical to determine the patency of this AV fistula by the presence of

    A. A murmur and a pulse deficit
    B. Silence when auscultating the fistula
    C. A bruit and thrill
    D. Steal syndrome located in the left upper arm

4. When administering Kayexalate to a patient in ARF, the nurse should be sure to

    A. Monitor for Steal syndrome.
    B. Observe for a drop in sodium levels.
    C. Watch for the return of normal T and P waves.
    D. Administer sorbitol and/or cleaning enemas after the medication.

5. Which of the following types of dialysis requires a temporary externally inserted access site?

A. All types of dialysis
B. Only hemodialysis (HD)
C. Hemodialysis (HD) and continuous renal replacement therapy (CRRT)
D. Peritoneal dialysis

6. The nurse is assessing a patient for peritonitis before performing peritoneal dialysis (PD). Which of the following assessment findings would confirm the presence of peritonitis?   **Select all that apply.**

A. Clotting of the PD catheter
B. WBCs 20,000 mm^3
C. Cloudy dialysate output
D. Tenderness at the insertion site
E. Temperature 97.2°F
F. Slightly blood-tinged exudate after PD catheter insertion

7. A patient with transient hypertension related to heart failure is admitted to your unit. The nephrologist has ordered slow continuous ultrafiltration (SCUF) continuous renal replacement. As a nurse with experience performing this type of dialysis, you know it is the treatment of choice for which of the following?

A. Fluid volume overload
B. Cardiogenic shock
C. Disequilibrium imbalance
D. Severe azotemia

8. A patient on hemodialysis suddenly becomes hemodynamically unstable with a mean arterial BP of 60. The best form of dialysis for this patient is

A. To continue with HD
B. Peritoneal dialysis
C. Intermittent HD
D. CRRT

9. A patient has been requiring chronic treatments of hemodialysis through a right forearm arteriovenous (AV) graft. The nurse knows that planning this patient's care requires

A. Frequent BP monitoring in the right arm
B. IV sticks and laboratory work to be taken from the graft site
C. Notifying all members of the health care team to avoid BPs on the right arm
D. Starting IVs in the right arm

10. A patient is starting on spironolactone (Aldactone) for high blood pressure unresponsive to hydrochlorothiazide (HCTZ). During the morning assessment the nurse notes the patient is disoriented to time and place. The patient also states he has had cramps in his legs all night. Although the cardiac rhythm is unchanged from the previous shift, the next course of action the nurse should perform is to

A. Perform a more thorough neurological assessment and continue to monitor the patient.

B. Check the patient's last potassium level; the symptoms might indicate hyper-kalemia.

C. Administer both medications and call the physician to report these new symp-toms.

D. Hold both drugs until the physician is notified; this could be a rebound effect of the diuretics.

Chapter 9

1. Upon examining the extremities of a patient suspected of having a hematologic problem the nurse notes pinpoint red tiny dots around both ankles of the patient. The nurse would chart these findings as

A. Hematoma

B. Petechiae

C. Hematopoiesis

D. Jaundice

2. The nurse suspects that a patient might be in septic shock. Which of the follow-ing laboratory values points in this direction?

A. Increased serum ferritin and increased basophils

B. Decreased iron-binding capacity and increased eosinophils

C. Increased D-dimer and increased FDP

D. Increased fibrinogen levels and decreased INR

3. A nurse is monitoring a patient's status after a bone marrow biopsy. Which of the following would follow the standard of nursing care?

A. Check vital signs once a shift immediately after the procedure.

B. Feed the patient ASAP to ensure adequate nutrition.

C. Monitor the site for bleeding.

D. Institute neutropenic precautions until test results return.

4. It is decided to institute drotrecogin (Xigris) in a patient with severe DIC. Which of the following would the nurse perform to safely administer this medication? Xigris can cause

   A. Severe clotting; monitor for edema and redness in extremities.

   B. Hemorrhage if the patient has had recent surgery or stroke within 3 months. Notify the physician.

   C. Monitor the aPTT for severe elevation, which can indicate pending hemorrhage. Continuously monitor this test.

   D. Pain at the insertion site while being administered through an epidural catheter. Give the patient morphine sulfate if this occurs.

5. The nurse is interviewing the son of an unconscious patient admitted to the ICU with severe sepsis secondary to acute myelogenous leukemia. The son tells you the patient self-administers an "injection to prevent blood transfusions." The son is most likely describing

   A. Epoetin alfa (Epogen)

   B. Aminocaproic acid (Amicar)

   C. Dobutamine (Dobutrex)

   D. Intropin (dopamine)

6. You are the mentor for a new graduate who started 2 weeks ago in the ICU. Jointly you are caring for a patient post septic shock who has recently been extubated off the ventilator. Which statement by this new nurse would the mentor question?

   A. "I will encourage the family to bring in this patient's favorite foods. I believe he likes fresh baked apples."

   B. "I will take his temperature rectally."

   C. "I need to talk to the family about flowers. We can keep them in his/her room."

   D. "I should stop his friend with a cold from visiting him."

7. The nurse is monitoring a patient admitted to the ICU with chronic lung disease in acute respiratory distress. Systemic inflammatory response syndrome (SIRS) is suspected. Which of the following would add to this suspicion?

   A. Temperature 99.8°F

   B. Bradycardia

   C. Tachycardia

   D. Bradypnea

8. In order to be most effective and efficient when obtaining cultures for sensitivity in patients with hematological problems, the nurse should

   A. Give antibiotics after all cultures have been obtained.

   B. Start antibiotics as soon as they are available.

    C. Obtain urine and sputum cultures first, then give antibiotics. Get other cultures when time permits.

    D. The timing of these events is not critical. The nurse should do them when he or she has the time.

9. A nurse is assessing a patient for risk factors in determining the susceptibility to disseminated intravascular coagulopathy (DIC). Which of the following can lead to an increased risk?   **Select all that apply.**

    A. Burns

    B. Chronic obstructive lung disease

    C. Hyperkalemia

    D. Pericarditis

    E. Abruptio placenta

    F. Acute hemolytic reaction

    G. Bacterial infection

10. **The nurse must monitor a patient with DIC for complications. Complications of DIC include**

    A. Myocardial infarction

    B. Leukemia

    C. Fetal demise

    D. Crushing traumatic injury

Correct Answers and Rationales

Chapter 1

1. D. Although the nurse could use others to help, such as respiratory therapy (collaboration), use systems thinking to provide additional resources in the critical care unit/home. The role of the nurse here is facilitator of learning as he or she is teaching.

2. C. Nursing organizations protect the public by ensuring that safe standards of practice are adhered to by their members. Pay per performance and staffing levels are generally thought of as institutionally driven, and the State Boards of Nursing deal with minimally competent nurses if they commit professional standard infractions.

3. A. Outcome identification can only be done after assessing the patient and significant other's educational needs. Implementation is done after identification of outcomes and includes steps to reach those outcomes. Evaluation is done of the outcomes after interventions have been implemented.

4. B. Sentinel events are unplanned events that occur that can result in potential harm to the patient. Advocacy involves acting on the behalf of a patient. Synergy means increasing energy and maintaining competencies to help protect the nurse from sentinel events.

5. D. A critical care intensivist is a physician specifically trained in the needs of critical care patients.

6. A. HIPAA is the Health Insurance Portability and Accountability Act and provides patient confidentiality. HRSA is the Health Resources Administration, IHI is the Institute for Health Care Improvement, and IOM is the Institute of Medicine.

Chapter 2

1. A. Although reality orientation with spiritual care as well as turning the client and preventing ulcers are important, the patient can still feel pain/anxiety, so administering medications to reduce those is critical.

2. C. There is much the critical care nurse can do to prevent VAP. Keeping the HOB elevated can prevent vomiting and aspiration. Antiulcer medications are important, although hydrochloric acid blockers can increase alkaline vomitus and promote VAP. It is well documented in the literature that poor oral hygiene and unsterile suctioning procedures can increase VAP.

3. D. Crackles are soft popping sounds heard in the lung periphery during auscultation. Gurgles are heard in the larger airways and indicate mucus in the larger airways. Stridor is a harsh, snoring sound that indicates imminent airway closure.

4. D. In early respiratory failure, all vital signs are elevated except the patient's temperature. The other choices are seen in late failure.

5. A. Chest tubes are usually placed in a partial lung removal such as a lobectormy or segmental resection. In a pneumonectomy, the place where the lung was needs to fill in with exudate so a chest tube is usually not placed.

6. C. Crepitus is the popping felt when a nurse is palpating around a chest tube that has leaked air into the subcutaneous tissues. Tactile fremitus is the vibration a nurse feels when palpating a chest wall. Stridor is a harsh, loud sound that indicates impending airway closure, and elastic turgor is when the skin stays elevated when you pinch it.

7. D. The nonrebreather supplies almost 100% oxygen as it has a reservoir that traps oxygen and when the patient exhales, his or her CO_2 flows out of two valves on either side of the mask.

8. A. The pH is below 7.35, which indicates an acidosis. The CO_2 is above 45, so the patient is retaining CO_2, indicating the acidosis is respiratory. The HCO_3 is 22, which indicates a normal value, so the kidneys are not compensating for this problem. Therefore, the patient is in an uncompensated respiratory acidosis with hypoxemia.

9. C. PEEP causes an increase in intrathoracic pressure and therefore decreases the amount of blood from entering the heart. This can cause a drop in BP. Shock is not a complication of PEEP. This drop is too significant to be a patient's anxiety or sympathetic stimulation. Barotrauma can be caused by PEEP, but it usually is in the form of a pneumothorax.

10. B. Always support the patient first by manually ventilating him with a BVM device with the oxygen up to the highest setting. No other answer is acceptable as the first priority.

Chapter 3

1. C. Variant angina is caused by coronary artery spasm. To make the arteries less responsive to spasm a calcium channel blocker is generally used.
2. A. Hypertension is modifiable with diet, exercise, weight loss, and medications. The others are what one is born with (family history, race) or inevitable (aging).
3. D. Crackles indicate left-sided failure as they are caused by increased pressure in the left ventricle backing up into the pulmonary circuit. All other signs are from peripheral venous congestion.
4. B and E. Any recent surgery or trauma is a contraindication because of increased incidence of bleeding in patients. An ST segment MI is an indication for thrombolytic therapy. Venipunctures should be decreased in frequency, and central lines must be monitored for bleeding but are not a contraindication. Pressure must be held longer and the site observed for further bleeding. Age is not a deterrent to administering thrombolytics.
5. C. Since the diastolic pressure goes down to zero in this reading and the patient is having ventricular dysrhythmias, the catheter is probably in the right ventricle. The nurse could try to wedge the catheter to float it back into the PA. It is impossible for a PAC to go into the left side of the heart; therefore, A and D are incorrect. A right atrial pressure would be a mean value and much lower than the RV **or** PA pressures. It also would not go down to a zero reading.
6. C. Since patients with an orthotopic transplant have denervated hearts, they have to rely on circulating catecholamines to increase their heart rates and this takes several minutes. A temporary pacemaker and dobutamine are usually only used immediately postoperative and patients do not go home on these devices as the norm. They also have two P waves: one from the donor and their own native P wave.
7. B. Deep palpation is contraindicated in this instance as the pulsating mass could be an AAA. Deep palpation could cause it to rupture.
8. A. A dampened pressure is either from the central vein or the PCWP (PAOP). This pressure is too high to be CVP, which is around 2–6 mm Hg, so it is a PCWP (PAOP). If the nurse leaves it in this position, it blocks off distal blood flow to the lungs creating a pulmonary infarction. If the catheter migrates to the RV, the pressures would not be dampened but would have large fluctuations from 30 to 0 and can have premature ventricular contractions (PVCs) to boot. There is most definitely cause for concern in this instance as a pulmonary infarct can be caused by a wedged catheter.
9. C. All OHS patients have temporary pacemakers as a quick access to heart rate if edema causes heart blocks and bradycardias. The other choices are most common in heart transplantation.
10. D. Fluid from aortic stenosis would back up into the left ventricle creating left ventricular hypertrophy for a period of time. The ventricle would have to work hard to maintain BP. A murmur would be heard over the right 2nd ICS.

Chapter 4

1. C. Sinus tachycardia is normal except for the rate, which is over 100. First-degree AV block has a prolonged PRI and everything else is normal. In ventricular tachycardia, the ventricular rate is fast, but there are no P waves and the QRS is wide and bizarre.

2. B. The P-to-P interval shows us that the P waves are regular and marching on time. The atrial rate refers to counting the P waves and multiplying them by 10. Ventricular conduction is the QRS measurement, and ventricular repolarization is looking at the T wave to see that it is upright, rounded, and symmetrical.

3. C. Q wave is the first negative wave after the P wave. The ST segment is after the QRS and indicates the pause between ventricular depolarization and repolarization. The R wave is the first positive wave after the P wave, and the S wave is the first negative wave after the R wave. Deep Q waves are indicative of an MI if they are consistent in certain leads that look at the heart.

4. D. Atrial flutter is known by its regular, multiple P waves that all march out on time and are known as flutter waves.

5. D. Second-degree heart block, Mobitz type I or Wenckebach, is known for its characteristic prolongation of the PRI until there is a blocked or nonconducted P wave. In complete heart block the atrial and ventricular rhythms are regular because the atria and ventricles beat independently. First-degree heart block is prolongation of the PRI. Mobitz II has a consistent PRI and some QRS are not conducted.

6. B. Because this situation is an emergency and early defibrillation is critical, the nurse uses the anterior posterior pad position. Time wasted on CPR will delay defibrillation time, so getting the defibrillator ready is a priority. CPR can be performed later. A strip is only needed in a cardioversion as the machine is synched to avoid the T wave and fire on the R.

7. B. The mA is the amount of electricity applied to the heart. It needs to be turned up to capture the heart when the heart is brady or tachy. The rate refers to how fast the pacemaker is set. The synchronous function is when the pacer fires only when the heartbeat slows down too much or speeds up too fast. The asynchronous function is set so that the pacer is firing all the time.

8. A. Atropine is used to help increase the heart rate. The other medications are used in VT or VF.

9. B, C, and E. The nurse's role is to prevent sepsis by suctioning, turning, and providing infection control. An NGT is inserted to induce mild hypothermia until a cooling blanket can be obtained. Antiarrhythmics can be common as the heart may still be cranky. Antipyretics are not needed as patients do not have fevers with mild hypothermia.

10. B. A patient may not breathe well after a cardioversion, so a BVM is important to have on hand. A chest tube is not needed as pneumothorax is not a complication of this procedure. The defibrillator is placed on the synchronous mode to avoid the T wave and to fire on the R wave.

Chapter 5

1. B. Thrombolytic therapy breaks down fibrin that is present in blood to cause blood clotting. With the absence or decrease of fibrin, hemorrhaging and internal bleeding is a strong possibility.
2. C. In order to cause contraction of the quadriceps muscle, the patient should be sitting with the legs dangling downward as the test is performed.
3. D. The gastrocnemius muscle should contract, causing plantar flexion of the foot when this test is performed.
4. C. These nerves are specific to eye movement, pupillary constriction, and accommodation.
5. B. A GCS of 7 or less generally describes a comatose state in the patient with a neurologic deficit. A: Requires a GCS of 15 to be considered normal and in good health. C: The patient who is oriented to person, place, and time would earn a 5 on the GCS. D: The patient would earn a 5 on the GCS for the best motor response giving the patient a total of 10 points for C and D. In actuality, this patient was only assigned 6 points, describing a patient in a comatose state.
6. D. Responses do occur, but not very well and not very often. A: The patient would be alert. B: The patient would be lethargic. C: The patient would be considered stuporous.
7. A. B describes a basilar skull fracture. C describes a depressed skull fracture. D describes a linear skull fracture.
8. C. According to the muscle strength grading scale, a trace of muscle strength exists at the 1/5 level.
9. D. The hypoglossal (12th cranial nerve) is responsible for tongue movement. A: Abducens (6th cranial nerve) controls the lateral deviation of the eye. B: Facial (7th cranial nerve) controls tears, salivation, facial expressions, and eyes closing. C: Vagus (10th cranial nerve) controls the voluntary acts of swallowing and phonation and the involuntary acts of the heart, lungs, and digestive tract.
10. A. Bleeding that is extending into the subarachnoid space will compromise the patient's ability to appropriately respond to verbal commands or questions. Pressure on the brain from bleeding will create cerebral edema, causing a deterioration in the patient's level of consciousness. B, C, and D are responses that can be attributed to neurological deficits created by other factors such as traumatic brain injury, seizure activity, or side effects of medications.

Chapter 6

1. C. This describes the primary survey; E – exposure, where the patient is undressed and examined for additional injuries; A – definitive care—the time when specific injuries are addressed such as surgery or suturing; B – secondary survey where a more detailed approach is conducted in a head-to-toe examination of the patient; D – the ABCs of trauma care are initiated at the trauma scene.

2. D. The patient with massive transfusion is prone to lactic acidosis, which is a form of metabolic acidosis indicated with a pH that is low (acidosis) and an HCO_3 that is low (metabolic acidosis). Hyperkalemia, hypocalcemia, and low platelets can occur as well. These values indicate hypokalemia, hypercalcemia, and normal platelets.

3. D. Class III hemorrhage consists of 30%–40% of blood loss, a heart rate greater than 120, tachypnea, mental status changes, and a drop of 20 mm Hg in the MAP.

4. A. Insertion of a nasogastric tube could possibly perforate the sinuses and wind up in the brain in a patient with severe facial fractures.

5. B. This patient is hemorrhaging and the left lung can fill up with blood from an unexpected bleed in the chest. Clamp the chest tube to prevent massive hemorrhage, notify the physician, and prepare the patient for an exploratory thoracostomy.

6. C. The pressure from a tension pneumothorax pushes the trachea away from the affected side. Since this is a right tension pneumothorax, the trachea is deviated to the left and the left side has diminished or absent breath sounds.

7. B. Thermal burns are caused most frequently by residential fires and involve tissue destruction from heat applied to the skin layers. Radiation and chemical burns are most frequent in commercial or industrial accidents. Electrical burns involve lightning or exposure to electricity in household incidents.

8. C. According to the Rule of Nines, each leg is 9% of the BSA, so both anterior/posterior portions would be 9% + 9% or 18%.

9. C. The fluid to give according to the Rule of Nines would be calculated as 165 divided by 2.2 = 75 kg.

$$75 \text{ kg} \times 70 \text{ (BSA burned)} \times 4 \text{ (mL ordered)} = 10{,}500 \text{ mL}$$

10. D. In an SCI, the level of injury, especially with an axial loading injury, can compromise the innervation of the cord to the diaphragm, which controls breathing patterns. The patient may die from hypoventilation, so keen observation and early intubation may be necessary to support this patient.

Chapter 7

1. C, D, and F. Dental work can cause additional physical stressors, so the patient's physician needs to know about the dental work so that steroid therapy dosages can be adjusted as needed. Fatigue, weakness, and dizziness are signs of inadequate steroid therapy and the physician should be notified. A Medic Alert bracelet is essential to communicate the patient's history of Addison's disease. A 10-day treatment of steroids is not adequate for people with Addison's disease. Instead, steroid treatment is done over a lifetime, because someone with Addison's does not produce enough steroids. Daily weights should be assessed to monitor changes in fluid balance, not caloric intake. The flu is another physical stressor that may require steroid adjustment and the physician should be notified if the patient has the flu.

2. D. Pituitary hormone functions of secretion and inhibition are regulated by the hypothalamus.

3. C. Patients with an Addison's crisis present with symptoms of hypotension. Giving anti-hypertensive medications is an unacceptable treatment measure.

4. D. Positive Trousseau's and Chvostek's signs indicate tetany as a result of low calcium levels and hypoparathyroidism.

5. D. Cushing's syndrome is associated with excessive production of corticosteroids. Dosages of steroid therapy could be re-evaluated and either tapered down or given every other day, but not increased.

6. B. The patient will have deep, rapid Kussmaul's respirations in an effort to remove excessive carbon dioxide buildup from the body.

7. D. Synthroid is used to treat hypothyroidism.

8. B. Regular insulin is the only type of insulin that can be used intravenously and still be effective.

9. C. Tolinase is a first-generation sulfonylurea. Glucophage is a biguanide. Prandin is a meglitinide, and Avandia is a thiazolidinedione.

10. C. Euthyroid is the descriptive term used for a normal thyroid gland.

Chapter 8

1. B, C, and F. Folic acid and vitamin B6 are water-soluble and HD can remove them. Procrit is removed by dialysis. The other medications are commonly given to a patient in CRF.

2. B. In chronic renal failure, the kidneys retain potassium leading to a hyperkalemia. All other values are normal. In CRF the serum creatinine is usually elevated. The hemoglobin and urine creatinine clearance are lower than normal.

3. C. When an artery and vein are anastomosed as with an AV fistula, turbulence of increased arterial flow through this area creates a swishing sound (bruit) that can be heard on auscultation and a pulsatile vibration under the site during palpation (thrill).

4. D. Kayexalate is a phosphate and potassium-binding resin and works in the intestines to remove those substances. One of the side effects is constipation, which can be relieved by sorbitol and/or enemas.

5. C. Both CRRT and HD require that a patient have a temporary central venous access site. PD requires an internally inserted catheter.

6. B, C, and D are indicative of peritonitis. Elevated WBCs greater than 10,000 mm^3 indicate an infection, cloudy dialysate output shows organisms growing in the peritoneum, and tenderness is a symptom of infection. Clotting of the site is usually due to fibrin deposits or kinking of the PD catheter. A temperature of less than 100°F is considered normal as with bloody dialysate after the initial catheter insertion.

7. A. SCUF therapy requires that a patient has enough systolic BP to drive the dialysis. Therefore, its best use is for fluid removal. A patient in cardiogenic shock would not have a systolic BP high enough for this type of therapy and might need CVVHDF. It acts slowly, and therefore problems with disequilibrium do not occur as with HD. Solutes are not removed in this therapy, so it would not filter out particles needed for azotemia.

8. D. CRRT is used with hemodynamically unstable BP as it is a slower and gentler process. To continue with any form of HD would compromise the patient's BP with extracorporeal circulation without fluid replacement. PD is contraindicated in hypotension.

9. C. The right arm in this patient is his or her lifeline for dialysis and every effort should be made to prevent trauma to this graft. Therefore, BPs, IV sticks, and laboratory work should be drawn on the left arm.

10. B. Muscular cramping and changes in the level of consciousness might indicate that hyperkalemia is resulting from this potassium-sparing diuretic.

Chapter 9

1. B. Hematomas are large bruises. Hematopoiesis is the formation of the blood cell line. Jaundice is yellow discoloration of the mucous membranes, sclera, and skin from excreted bilirubin.

2. C. The increased D-dimer and FDP levels show that clots are being lysed. This is indicative of sepsis, as it causes massive inflammation and activates the clotting cascade.

3. C. Bone marrow biopsies are done on patients with suspected abnormal blood cell lines. The platelets, which cause clotting, are part of this line. If levels are low, the patient can bleed. VS should be done q 15 minutes for the first hour, then according to protocols. Patients are given sedation prior to this procedure; check the gag reflex before liquid/solid food. Neutropenic precautions are not necessary unless the patient is immunocompromised.

4. B. Hemorrhage is the most common side effect; so recent bleeding by surgery or hemorrhagic stroke would preclude using this medication. It is given for severe clotting. The aPTT is an invalid test for this medication and it is contraindicated for introduction through an epidural catheter.

5. A. Epoetin alfa is used to prevent exposing the patient to complications from blood transfusions. All of the other medications are given intravenously.

6. C. Fresh flowers harbor dangerous pathogens. Fresh fruits can carry fungi and molds. Rectal temps can cause exposure to *Escherichia coli* and possible bleeding. Visitors and staff with cold can enter the room but PPE must be applied. Staff can ask for reassignment as they have more frequent exposure.

7. C. The diagnosis of SIRS is made on the basis of temperature higher than 100.4°F or lower than 96.8°F, tachycardia, tachypnea, and elevated white cell counts.

8. A. All cultures should be obtained before starting on antibiotics or the drugs can interfere with the results.

9. A, E, F, and G can leave the patient prone to DIC.

10. A. If coronary arteries are blocked due to clotting, the patient can have chest pain, ST elevation, and positive enzymes. The other medical problems are causes of DIC.

Index

Note: Page numbers followed by *f* denote figures; page numbers followed by *t* denote tables.